Operative Techniques in Epilepsy

John P. Girvin

Operative Techniques in Epilepsy

Springer

John P. Girvin
Department of Clinical
Neurological Sciences
Western University
London, ON
Canada

ISBN 978-3-319-10920-6 ISBN 978-3-319-10921-3 (eBook)
DOI 10.1007/978-3-319-10921-3
Springer Cham Heidelberg New York Dordrecht London

Library of Congress Control Number: 2014957641

Printed on acid-free paper

Springer is part of Springer Science+Business Media (www.springer.com)

Preface

The impetus leading to the authorship of this book was derived from the many young resident and fellow neurosurgical trainees who lamented the fact that there were limited comprehensive resources that covered purely *technical* aspects of neurosurgery, especially those of epilepsy surgery. This is not to say that there are not good articles and books in the literature dealing with epilepsy surgery, but rather that there is a paucity of literature primarily devoted to considerations of functional cortical localization and the surgery of the majority of the epilepsies. The usual complaint that I hear from the trainees is that most articles dealing with epilepsy surgery are in large part confined primarily to the results of the surgery, rather than any significant details of the techniques and surgical anatomy employed in the surgery. This monograph is entirely limited to what I believe are the most important operative aspects of neurosurgery in general, but particularly those associated with so-called epilepsy surgery and, again, more particularly resective surgery.

Some of the comments and discussions will be too elementary for many readers. I make no apologies for this, as the primary objective of the monograph is to be of use to all young surgeons, from first-year residents (PGY1) to more experienced and sophisticated epilepsy surgery fellows and recently graduated consultants. The amount of writing lent to the use of appropriate coagulation, electrocortical mapping, and the technique of subpial dissection reflects the importance I attach to these principles in the surgery of the central nervous system.

I have not included an exhaustive bibliography, but I have included many original articles that are less likely to have appeared in the lists of current everyday literatures of residents' programs. Some of these older articles are just as important and in some cases perhaps more important as resource references than many of the more recent references. However, the last decade has witnessed a remarkable increase in the numbers of medical journal articles that can be retrieved easily from the Internet and particularly from universities' medical libraries. Many of them have made it easy to retrieve the majority of articles from the twentieth-century literature and now even many of those of the nineteenth century. Thus, now the reader should be able to find from them a broad, comprehensive insight into the literature pertaining to whatever category of interest she/he might wish to pursue.

At the end of some of the chapters dealing with the common cortical sites of epilepsy surgery, I have made reference to the "Safe Limits of Resection." The observations in these sections have been derived from the combination of the uses of local anesthesia and intraoperative cortical stimulation, which have been the primary historical tools for defining the functional localization of the human cerebral cortex. The operations of nearly all my patients were conducted under these circumstances, and thus individual chapters have been devoted to local anesthesia and electrocortical stimulation in this book. Indeed the use of local anesthesia is not anywhere near as important now with the sophistication of imaging and instrumentation as many decades ago, but there is no doubt that its use is mandatory in many neurosurgical operations, and my personal view is that every neurosurgeon should feel comfortable using it. The provision of these safe limits of resection is simply noted, as I believe they are helpful guides in the conduct of many resections of the cortex in the immediate vicinity of what I will refer to as eloquent cortex. These are, in essence, reviews of functional cortical localization for which I have drawn heavily on the comments of the Montreal School of Epilepsy Surgery, especially those of Drs. Penfield and Rasmussen, in addition to my own.

Springer's publishing mandate requires bibliographic references to be at the end of each chapter, and thus is the case with this monograph. Springer has also allowed me to still place the whole bibliography at the end of the book, which I requested, so that it may help the reader to easily locate where each bibliographic reference has been cited in the book. Within the Bibliography, each reference, per se, has a number in bold, within square brackets (**[...]**), which identifies the chapter, section, and subsection (by their numbers) in which that particular reference has been cited.

The Index is similar to that of many other books in that there is a cross-reference to where some of the various subjects of the Index can be found in the text of the book. The places where the indices are cited are identified, as in the preceding paragraph, by a combination of the chapter, section, and subsection numbers; boldface for the numbers suggests a greater significance of the cross-reference and even more by an associated asterisk (*).

I have already indicated that this monograph is not confined to clinical results, and thus it is not helpful with regard to statistically significant outcome assessments. Having said that, infrequent clinical examples are used wherever I felt the text description requires them.

There are many that I would like to acknowledge who have contributed through the years to the content of this manuscript. However, my fear of leaving some out who deserve to be so acknowledged leads me to follow the path of not becoming involved in trying to accurately determine when and where names, which I can remember, should be recorded. However, putting this aside, I do believe that my major acknowledgment would be attributed to the patients upon whom I have operated. I feel a responsibility to thank them for how much they have contributed to our neurosurgical understanding of the functional localization within the human cerebral neocortex. This has been and continues to be achieved from their tolerance and acceptance of being operated upon awake – often with a dreaded feeling of the unknown, of what such an operation might bring, and often with a sense of volunteerism in their willingness to accept extension of the times required to conduct electrocortical stimulation purely for academic purposes. As surgeons, we are forever indebted to all of them. Witnessing the acceptance and the behavior of patients undergoing these types of operation, particularly the young teenagers and adolescents, is always an inspiration and cannot help but make one feel that this is the "stuff" that makes one proud to be a member of the human race!

I thank the young residents and fellows who continually question our methods and who have led to a number of improvements in surgical techniques, either directly by their independent suggestions or indirectly through discussions associated with the surgical aspects that are described in the following chapters. I would be remiss in not thanking my neurosurgical colleagues from all of whom I have learned and who became part of the staff of the UWO (University of Western Ontario; now, as of three years ago, known as "Western University") Department of Clinical Neurological Sciences and its Epilepsy Surgical Program; these included Drs. Howard Reichman, Andrew Parrent, Ram Sahjpaul, and David Steven.

I particularly would like to acknowledge and thank very much Ms. Caren Erlichman and Mr. Tom Adam for their so freely provided unending expenditure of time on my behalf, as without their help I would have very unlikely been able to obtain the necessary Permissions for publication of this book. And, finally, I thank my wife, Bettye, for the many hours without conversation to which she has been committed during the preparation of this monograph.

Finally, it is my responsibility to indicate that within the monograph any errors in interpretation, failure to provide the reader with a text easy to understand, failure to have acknowledged pertinent articles, or errors in presenting the accuracy of reports to which I have referred are entirely attributable to me, for which I apologize in advance.

London, ON, Canada John P. Girvin

Contents

History of Epilepsy Surgery 1

1.1 Pre-twentieth Century

The poor understanding of epileptic disorders in the nineteenth century gave rise to what now would be considered a somewhat remarkable list of surgical and nonsurgical management schemes; these included remedies such as a variety of peculiar diets, bloodletting, magic, religious prayer, ligation of cerebral arteries, etc. In each epoch of time, the treatment of diseases or disorders was most often related to what was considered to be the causes of them at the time. Thus, witchcraft, herbs and plants of all kinds, fetishism, and amulets, often inscribed with sacred incantations, were all used at one time or another, particularly prior to the Renaissance.

At about the time of the Renaissance, epileptic seizures, also increasingly known as a *falling sickness* (see particularly Temkin 1971), began to be recognized as a physical ailment, rather than magical or occult abnormalities, evil spirits, demons, or irreligious disorders. Metals of various types became a popular treatment. There were many operations by a number of surgeons in the early half of the nineteenth century whose patients had epilepsy. Perhaps Dudley in 1828 might be considered as one whose primary operations could indeed be considered *epilepsy operations* (see Cutter 1930), but it was really towards the end of the century when epilepsy surgery took its place as a specialized surgery.

An example of a rather remarkable, but not necessarily isolated, report exhibiting the lack of understanding of the basic tenants of epilepsy was that of Alexander in 1883. He reported on his management of epilepsy in the 1870s and early 1880s through the ligature of the vertebral arteries. The report concerned 21 patients, the majority of whom had bilateral vertebral artery ligations. Three were doing *quite well* for nearly a year, nine others were *free from fits* sufficiently long "that it may be said a cure has resulted, or is likely to result," and eight were "improved in so many respects, or are improving so steadily, that the operation would be justifiable were no better results ever obtained!" His conclusion was "I now think that ligature of the vertebral arteries ought to take its place as a recognized operation for the cure

J.P. Girvin, *Operative Techniques in Epilepsy*,
DOI 10.1007/978-3-319-10921-3_1

of epilepsy …." It is difficult to know what type of person Alexander was and what might have been his knowledge of epilepsy as he stated, regarding a patient who had a retroflexed uterus, "It may be said, that had the retroflexed uterus been brought into place, the ligature of the vertebrals might have been unnecessary." The detail of this paper is not to condemn Alexander, but rather to exhibit the ignorance of the understanding of the substrate of epileptic seizures in parts of the nineteenth century. This is particularly so, given that the publication was not only just 3 years prior to the publication by Horsley (vide infra) but that it was in the prestigious journal, *Brain*.

It was really towards the end of the nineteenth century when there became an increasingly widespread understandable awareness of epilepsy. It was also in this period when the first effective drug against epilepsy was discovered, e.g., bromine.

Sir Victor Horsley, at the age of 29, carried out a surgical operation with the specific objective of removing a cerebral cortical posttraumatic epileptic focus and thereby abolishing seizures on May 25, 1886. This is usually characterized as the *first* of such specific operative interventions, which is not completely accurate. However, it was really this particular operation that has led to Horsley being acknowledged as the father of epilepsy surgery. Certainly, it was a *first* from the point of view of the use of the developing neuroscientific evidence, which was burgeoning at the time. However, similar types of such operations are attributed to Duretus in the sixteenth century (noted by Penfield and Jasper 1954). Other early attempts in the USA included those of Dudley (1828) of the Transylvania University Medical School in Lexington, Kentucky (see also Patchell et al. 1987), Billings (1861), and Lloyd and Deaver (1888). Smith provided a survey of the cases in the USA up to 1852 (Smith 1852). In 1888, similar *Horsley operations* were carried out by Keen and by Nancrede (1896). By the end of 1886, Horsley had carried out nine operations similar to that of the one in May of the same year (1887). O'Leary and Goldring provide a very good nineteenth-century review of the initiation of surgical attempts at dealing with epileptic patients and the consequent advances during the latter part of the century (1976), and for those who enjoy history, Fox's first chapter in his *Dandy of Johns Hopkins*, although brief, provides a very interesting history of the beginning of surgery in 10,000 BCE (1984).

In the undertaking of his initial operation, Horsley was both influenced and encouraged to operate on this patient of Hughlings Jackson by Jackson himself. The latter, in turn, had been influenced by the studies of the localization of function within the motor cortex, occurring about the same time, by Hitzig (1900).

It is rather interesting that after epilepsy became recognized as a bona fide disease entity, rather than a psychiatric disability, its acknowledged appearance in many historically important figures began to emerge more often, e.g., Socrates, Greek philosopher (469–399 BCE); Julius Caesar (100–44 BCE); Saint Paul, the Apostle (5–15 CE); Joan of Arc, French saint (1412–1431); Napoléon Bonaparte (1769–1821); Lord Byron, English poet (1788–1824); Fyodor Mikhailovich Dostoyevsky (1823–1881); Alfred Nobel (1833–1896); and Vincent van Gogh (1853–1890).

1.2 Twentieth Century

In the early twentieth century, a stream of prominent German neurosurgeons who operated under local anesthesia provided a significant boost to the quality, experiential background, and frequency of the epilepsy operations (Krause 1909, 1924; Krause and Schum 1931; Foerster 1925, 1926, 1929a, b, 1934, 1936a, b; Foerster and Penfield 1930; Foerster and Altenburger 1935). The success of this led to further operations typical of those that Horsley had conducted on the nine patients by the end of 1886.

In the early part of the twentieth century in North America, when epilepsy surgery was in its infancy, there was a general view among neurologists, especially in the USA, that surgery was of little value in the management of epilepsy. Dr. Wilder Penfield, after studying neurophysiology with Sherrington in Oxford and cerebral morphology with Pío del Río Hortega in Madrid, trained with Foerster in Breslau and then went on to Montreal in 1928 where he developed the Montreal School of Epilepsy Surgery that was so prominent in the training of epileptic surgeons who eventually chaired most of the epilepsy centers throughout the world in the middle of the twentieth century. The review of the influence of the Montreal school has been well documented by others (O'Leary and Goldring 1976; Feindel 1986; Meador et al. 1989; Feindel et al. 2009; Olivier 2010). Parallel to Penfield in Montreal were similar initiatives in the USA by Sachs (1935) and particularly Bailey and Gibbs (Bailey et al. 1935; Bailey and Gibbs 1951). Interestingly, Cushing conducted two operations on patients, under local anesthesia, in 1908 (1909). Documentation of the very significantly important Chicago school has undergone a similar review by Hermann and Stone (1989).

The Chicago (Bailey and Gibbs 1935; Bailey et al. 1951) and Montreal (Penfield and Steelman 1947) schools devoted to epilepsy surgery began in the second quarter of the twentieth century and gained momentum over the middle part of the century, especially the school in Montreal, championed by Drs. Herbert Jasper and Theodore Rasmussen, in addition to Dr. Penfield. Over this era, trainees, the majority of whom had had all or at least some of their formal training at the Montreal Neurological Institute, led epilepsy units worldwide. A plethora of publications over the last half of the century outlined the contributions of the surgical management of intractable epilepsy, which gave impetus to the appreciation of the contributions of neurosurgery in the management of intractable epilepsy (Penfield 1939, 1947, 1950, 1954a, b; Penfield and Evans 1935; Penfield and Steelman 1947; Penfield and Flanigin 1950; Penfield and Welch 1949, 1951; Penfield and Baldwin 1952; Penfield and Paine 1953, 1955; Penfield and Jasper 1954; Rasmussen 1963, 1975a, b, 1977, 1983a, b, c; Rasmussen and Jasper 1958; Rasmussen and Branch 1962).

This heralded the onset of the modern era of epileptology, electroencephalography, and epilepsy surgery in North America. Penfield, using the techniques of cortical stimulation in conscious patients that he learned from the German school, undertook comprehensive stimulation of the cortex, arriving at his now famous *homunculus*—the cortical localization of human motor and sensory function in the pre- and postcentral gyri.

In the Western medical community, there were many physicians, around the time of the introduction of, and in the early history of, the use of epilepsy surgery, who seemed certain that surgery was not destined to be of significant value in the treatment of epilepsy. Comments such as that of Professor J.A.V. Bates typified this view at the time; he indicated that "…the role of surgery in the treatment of epilepsy is uncertain," except for that of hemispherectomy in the case of hemispheric porencephalic cysts (1962). He indicated that "It may be suggested that the surgeon is merely replacing one scar by a second and larger one" (e.g., the surgical scar arising from the operative intervention). There is some truth to this, in that there is always some surgical scar left behind by any surgery of the central nervous system and such a scar is indeed a potential etiology of an epileptic focus. However, as will be emphasized later, the basis of epileptic surgery is that a very large (epileptogenic) scar is removed while at the same time only a very small, usually insignificant, scar is left behind. The latter part of the twentieth century witnessed a wealth of observations that led to a striking increased recognition that surgery was the preferable management in patients in whom medically intractable epilepsy was demonstrated. There were a number of reasons for this eventuality, but perhaps one of the more important was the failure of the introduction of the ideal predictable pharmaceutical anticonvulsant silver bullet.

While the foregoing was devoted to the improved understanding of all components associated with epilepsy, I would be remiss in failing to very briefly note that there were similarly many, many advances that have to do with medicine in general and surgery in particular in the twentieth century. The early part of the century witnessed many changes to the improvement of neurological surgery. These included the introduction of blood transfusion, antibiotics, safer general anesthesia, and better sterile technique in the operating rooms.

The middle of the century saw the development of the beginning of imaging with the advent of cerebral angiography, pneumoencephalography, ventriculography, and the use of radioactive tracers for scanning the brain. The understanding of electroencephalography (EEG) and the increased sophistication of its use, including ECoG (electrocorticography), was an exciting advancement in this era. Included within this latter group are the expansions of the safety limits of the use of low cerebral blood flow, hypotension, and hypothermia.

The latter part of the century witnessed even more significant improvements, which included those in (1) EEG technology, (2) medical imaging, (3) the technology associated with general anesthesia, (4) the use of longer lasting and more effective local anesthesia and its use with neuroleptanalgesia, and (5) the remarkable improvements in lighting, miniaturization of ocular lenses, and instrumentation associated with the so-called minimally invasive surgery.

References

Alexander W. The treatment of epilepsy by ligature of the vertebral arteries. Brain. 1883;5:170–87.

Bailey P, Gibbs FA. The surgical treatment of psychomotor epilepsy. JAMA. 1951;145:365–70.

Bailey P, Green JR, Amador L, Gibbs FA. Treatment of psychomotor states by anterior temporal lobectomy. A report of progress. Res Publ Ass Nerv Ment Dis. 1935;31:341–6.

Bates JAV. The surgery of epilepsy. In: Williams D, editor. Modern trends in neurology, vol. 3. Washington: Butterworths; 1962. p. 125–37.
Billings JS. The surgical treatment of epilepsy. Cincinnati Lancet Obs. 1861;4:334–41.
Cushing H. A note upon the faradic stimulation of the postcentral gyrus in conscious patients. Brain. 1909;32:44–53.
Cutter IS. Benjamin W. Dudley and the surgical relief of traumatic epilepsy. Int Abstr Surg. 1930;50:189–94.
Dudley BW. Observations on injuries of the head. Transylvania J Med. 1828;1:9–40.
Feindel W. Electrical stimulation of the brain during surgery for epilepsy—historical highlights. Int Anesthesiol Clin. 1986;24:75–87.
Feindel W, Leblanc R, Nogueira DE, Almeida A. Epilepsy surgery: historical highlights 1909–2009. Epilepsia. 2009;50(S3):131–51.
Foerster O. Zur Pathogenese und Chirurgischen Behandlung der Epilepsia. Zentralbl Chir. 1925;52:531–49.
Foerster O. Zur operativen Behandlung der Epilspsie. Dtsch Z Nervenh. 1926;89:137–47.
Foerster O. Sur Pathogenese und chirurgischen Behandlung der Epilepsie. Zentralbl Chir. 1929a;52:531–49.
Foerster O. Beiträge zur Pathophysiologie der Sehbahn und der Schsphäre. J Psychol Neurol Lpz. 1929b;39:463–85.
Foerster O. Uber die bedeutung und reichweite des lokalisation-sprinzips im nervensystem. Verh Dtsch Ges Inn Med. 1934;46:117–211.
Foerster O. Sensible corticale Felder. In: Bumke O, Foerster O, editors. Handbuch der Neurologie, vol. 6. Berlin: Springer; 1936a. p. 1–448.
Foerster O. The motor cortex in man in the light of Hughlings Jackson's doctrines. Brain. 1936b;59:135–59.
Foerster O, Altenburger H. Elektrobiologische vorgänge an der menschlichen hirnrinde. Dtsch Z Nervenheilkd. 1935;135:277–88.
Foerster O, Penfield W. The structural basis of traumatic epilepsy and results of radical operation. Brain. 1930;53:99–120.
Fox WL. Chapter 1. Neurological surgery before Walter E. Dandy: a brief introduction. In: Dandy of Johns Hopkins. Baltimore: Williams & Wilkins; 1984. p. 1–7.
Hermann BP, Stone JL. A historical review of the epilepsy surgery program at the University of Illinois medical center: the contributions of Bailey, Gibbs, and collaborators to the refinement of anterior temporal lobectomy. J Epilepsy. 1989;2:155–63.
Hitzig E. Hughlings Jackson and the cortical motor centres in the light of physiological research. Brain. 1900;23:544–81.
Horsley V. Brain-surgery. Br Med J. 1886;2:670–5.
Horsley V. Ten consecutive cases of operation upon the brain and cranial cavity to illustrate the details and safety of the method employed. Br Med J. 1887;1:863–5.
Krause F. Die operative behandlung der epilepsie. Med Klin Berlin. 1909;5:1418–22.
Krause F. Die Sehbahnen in chirurgischer Beziehung und die faradische Reizung des Sehzentrums. Klin Wschr. 1924;3:1260–5.
Krause F, Schum H. Die spezielle Chirugie der Gehirnkrankheiten. In: Kuttner H, editor. Neue Deutsche Chirugie, 3 Bände. II. Band. Die epileptischen Erkrankungen. Enke, Stuttgart; 1931;49a:482–6.
Lloyd JH, Deaver JB. A case of focal epilepsy successfully treated by trephining and excision of the motor centres. Am J Med Sci. 1888;96:477–87.
Meador KJ, Loring DW, Flanigin HF. History of epilepsy surgery. J Epilepsy. 1989;2:21–5.
Nancrede NB. The operative treatment of Jacksonian and focal epilepsy. Ann Surg. 1896;24:122–30.
O'Leary JL, Goldring S. Chapter 16. Role of neurological surgery in the treatment of epilepsy. In: Science and epilepsy: neuroscience gains in epilepsy research. New York: Raven; 1976. p. 227–50.
Olivier A. Epilepsy surgery at the MNI: from Archibald to the creation of the Shirley and Mark Rayport fellowship in surgery of epilepsy. Epilepsia. 2010;51 Suppl 1:97–100.

Patchell RA, Young AB, Tibbs PA. Benjamin Winslow Dudley and the surgical treatment of epilepsy. Neurology. 1987;37:290–1.
Penfield W. The epilepsies: with a note on radical therapy. N Engl J Med. 1939;221:209–18.
Penfield W. The supplementary motor area in the cerebral cortex of man. Arch Psych Zeit Neurol. 1950;185:670–4.
Penfield W. Combined regional and general anesthesia for craniotomy and cortical exploration. Part I. Neurosurgical considerations. Curr Res Anesth Analg. 1954a;33:145–55.
Penfield W. Temporal lobe epilepsy. Br J Surg. 1954b;41:337–43.
Penfield W. Bilateral frontal gyrectomy and postoperative intelligence. Chapter XXIII – symposium on gyrectomy, part 1. Res Publ Ass Nerv Ment Dis. 1947;27:519–34.
Penfield W, Baldwin M. Temporal lobe seizures and the technique of subtotal temporal lobectomy. Ann Surg. 1952;136:625–34.
Penfield W, Evans J. The frontal lobe in man: a clinical study of maximum removals. Brain. 1935;58:115–33.
Penfield W, Flanigin H. Surgical therapy of temporal lobe seizures. Arch Neurol Psychiatry. 1950;64:491–500.
Penfield W, Jasper H. Epilepsy and the functional anatomy of the human brain. Boston: Little, Brown and Co; 1954. p. 896.
Penfield W, Paine K. Results of surgical therapy for focal epileptic seizures. CMAJ. 1955;73: 515–31.
Penfield W, Steelman H. The treatment of focal epilepsy by cortical excision. Ann Surg. 1947;126:740–62.
Penfield W, Welch K. Instability of response to stimulation of the sensorimotor cortex of man. J Physiol. 1949;109:358–65 [1.2, 7.5].
Penfield W, Welch K. The supplementary motor area of the cerebral cortex: a clinical and experimental study. AMA Arch Neurol Psychiatry. 1951;66:289–317.
Penfield W, Paine K. The results of surgical therapy for focal epileptic seizures. Proceedings of the fifth international neurological congress, Lisbon; 1953. [1.2]
Rasmussen T. Surgical therapy of frontal lobe epilepsy. Epilepsia. 1963;4:181–98.
Rasmussen T. Cortical resection in the treatment of focal epilepsy. In: Purpura DP, Penry JK, Walter RD, editors. Advances in neurology, vol. 8. New York: Raven; 1975a. p. 139–54.
Rasmussen T. Surgery for epilepsy arising in regions other than the temporal and frontal lobes. In: Purpura DP, Penry JK, Walter RD, editors. Advances in neurology, vol. 8. New York: Raven; 1975b. p. 206–26.
Rasmussen T. Surgical treatment of epilepsy. CMAJ. 1977;116:1369–70.
Rasmussen T. Hemispherectomy for seizures revisited. Can J Neurol Sci. 1983a;10:71–8.
Rasmussen T. Characteristics of a pure culture of frontal lobe epilepsy. Epilepsia. 1983b;24: 482–93.
Rasmussen T. Surgical treatment of complex partial seizures: results, lessons and problems. Epilepsia. 1983c;24 Suppl 1:S65–76.
Rasmussen T, Branch C. Temporal lobe epilepsy: indications for the results of surgical therapy. Postgrad Med. 1962;31:9–14.
Rasmussen T, Jasper H. Temporal lobe epilepsy: indications for operations and surgical technique. In: Baldwin M, Bailey P, editors. Temporal lobe epilepsy. Springfield: Charles C. Thomas; 1958. p. 440–60.
Sachs E. The subpial resection of the cortex in the treatment of Jacksonian Epilepsy (Horsley operation) with observations on areas 4 and 6. Brain. 1935;58:492–503.
Smith S. The surgical treatment of epilepsy, with statistical tables, comprising all recorded cases of ligature of the carotid artery; and also of trephining the cranium by American surgeons. NY J Med. 1852;220–42.
Temkin O. The falling sickness. 2nd ed. Baltimore: The Johns Hopkins Press; 1971.

2 Techniques in Epilepsy Surgery

2.1 The Use of Bipolar Coagulation

2.1.1 The Physical Principles of Bipolar Coagulation

There are *general* characteristics of epilepsy surgical technique that facilitate the accomplishment of satisfactory cortical resection. These are all aimed at increasing the gentleness of the surgery and thereby reducing potential injury from the surgery while particularly providing protection of the juxtaposed cortex at the same time. They include the appropriate use of bipolar coagulation, irrigation, suction, and cottonoid patties. The importance of these characteristics with respect to the quality of all branches of neurosurgery cannot be overemphasized!

One of the most important components in neurosurgical technique is the appreciation of the benefits of good coagulation. Perhaps even more important is the understanding of what *good coagulation* is and how to achieve it. Physically, the use of bipolar coagulation is characterized by the passage of electrical current between the two poles of the coagulator, e.g., the two blades of the bipolar coagulation forceps. The route, or routes, of current passage will involve whatever conducting material exists between the blades of the forceps. That is to say, *any* conductive electrical pathway(s), which exist(s) between the blades of the forceps, irrespective of how far they may be from the shortest route between the blades, will conduct some fraction of the current when the coagulator is activated. These pathways consist of any biological fluids or tissue, e.g., cerebrospinal or extracellular fluid, parenchyma, cells, blood, saline, etc. If there are a number of such pathways, then they are said to be *in parallel*. That is to say, they are parallel to one another, and, as such, they will all conduct some part of any electrolytic current passing through the area from one blade of the coagulating forceps to the other. In other words, they will share the available current to varying degrees. There are a number of variations, but the primary one consists of the resistances of the various segments of the current pathway. The larger the resistance (i.e., the lower the conductance) of a given segment, the smaller will be the share of current traversing that segment. Conversely,

J.P. Girvin, *Operative Techniques in Epilepsy*,
DOI 10.1007/978-3-319-10921-3_2

the greater the conductance of a particular pathway, the greater will be the share of current traversing that pathway. Thus, the reader will appreciate that the ideal preparatory achievement when using coagulation is to isolate the tissue that is to be coagulated, to as great an extent as possible, such that as much as possible the current will in fact travel through that targeted tissue, e.g., a blood vessel in most situations. There are a number of aids that can be utilized to achieve this isolation, which can be continually emphasized further on in this section.

If the conducting surfaces of the bipolar forceps are large, then the amount of current flowing between any two points of the pair of forceps, at a given strength of current, is small. This is illustrated in Fig. 2.1a. In this illustration, the current is equally distributed through the entire conducting medium that is in contact with the metal surfaces of the two bipolar forceps. Thus, if a small blood vessel was placed anywhere in the pathway under the circumstances outlined in the figure, only a very small amount of current would travel through the blood vessel, per se. The remainder of the current would travel through the other segments of the conducting medium, providing no help in coagulating the targeted tissue for the coagulation. This wasteful conduction of current is often referred to as the *shunting* of current, i.e., shunting it away from the primary pathway through which the proposed coagulation is aimed.

Figure 2.1b depicts the situation in which the illustrated elements are the same as in Fig. 2.1a except that the blades of the bipolar forceps are insulated except at the tips of the blades. Thus, all the segments of the current pathway travel between the blades and hence are concentrated between the two blade tips, the only parts of the forceps lacking insulation. With large areas of the forceps blades insulated, there is a significant reduction in the large amount of current (as in Fig. 2.1a) that is simply shunted away from the vicinity of the opposing tips, where the coagulation is to take place. Figure 2.1b also exhibits what was noted earlier that *any* potential bona fide segment of the pathway that is capable of carrying current would do so. In Fig. 2.1a, the current segments traveled the same distances between the non-insulated forceps and hence had equal shares, or fractions, of the current. Figure 2.1b illustrates that the farther away a segmental path is from the conducting metal points, the smaller is the fraction, or share, of the current it accommodates, depicted by thinner lines of the farther away (from the points of the forceps) segments of the pathway. In this situation, all of the current travels between the two small, non-insulated tips of the coagulating forceps, and thus nearly all of the current will follow a pathway through the tissue on either side of which the forceps tips are placed. Further, it can be appreciated that the *shunting* of current noted in the immediate foregoing can be largely abolished by removing the excess conducting medium around the targeted tissue. This will be addressed further on (*vide infra*).

Not only might the number of pathways be of importance in coagulation, but the composition of the conducting pathway will also influence the amount of current carried by the potential segments of the pathway. If the composition in a single pathway, for example, is a simple electrolyte solution such as saline, then the current will simply travel through the solution as a homogeneous electrolytic current, which is the same at any point or segment within the pathway, because the

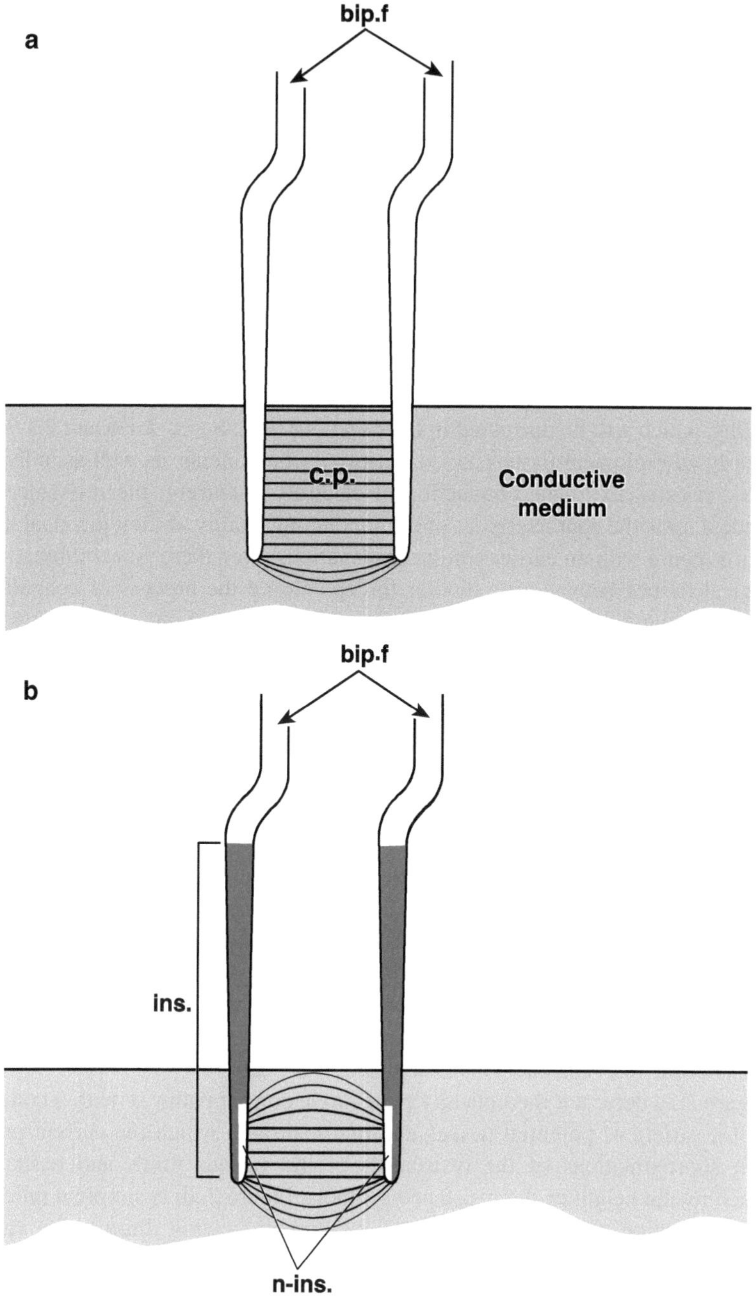

Fig. 2.1 Current pathways involving insulated and non-insulated bipolar coagulation forceps. Potential current pathways in the use of bipolar forceps, at a given strength of coagulation, without insulation (**a**) and (**b**) those with insulated forceps blades (except for the internal opposing surfaces of the tips). In the latter, the current pathways are more compact and more concentrated in the vicinity of the small non-insulated areas at the tips of the forceps. The amount of the current is proportional to the illustrated thickness of the theoretically depicted pathways. *bip.f* bipolar forceps, *c.p.* conducting pathway, *ins* insulation on forceps, *n-ins* non-insulated internal tips of the forceps

resistance is uniform throughout the saline solution. [An example of this is the function of a kitchen toaster, i.e., all of the heating coils are the same thin, equally resistant wires. Thus, the heat generated by the total matrix of wires is homogeneous throughout.] In such a circumstance, if the current is gradually raised, then a level will be reached where the current is sufficiently strong to create enough thermal energy to bring to the boiling point the immediate environs between the tips of the forceps, i.e., this is reflected in bubbles at the tips of the forceps. In a given current pathway, the amount of current required for this phenomenon to occur is related, in a positive correlation, to the resistance of the pathway. The generation of the bubbles may produce sufficient amplitudes of mechanical perturbations (vibrations) in that the experienced surgeon can physically appreciate the mechanical, vibratory transmissions up through the handles of the forceps! (This is usually not appreciated until a few seconds after the onset of the current, especially in using lower current strengths, which will be discussed in later sections, e.g., Sects. 2.1.6 and 2.1.7.)

Nearly all biological tissues have electrolytic components, as well as individual intrinsic resistances to the conduction of electrolytic current; the resistances are dependent upon the characteristics of the conducting quality of their physical makeups. In keeping with an earlier similar explanation, when there is a combination of biological tissues between the bipolar forceps during the process of coagulation, then each tissue will conduct a share of the coagulating current; each share will be inversely related to its intrinsic resistance. If within a given single current pathway there are components with varying resistances, then these components are said to be *in series* along this pathway. If the components have different resistances, then the heat generated within a given segment will vary depending upon the resistance of the component; the greater the resistance of a given component, the greater will be the heat generated by a given current traveling through it. For example, components containing protein, e.g., tissue such as blood, blood vessels, meninges, and brain parenchyma, have a much greater resistance to current flow than do solutions that are primarily electrolytic, such as saline and pure extracellular fluid (including cerebrospinal fluid). Because of their increased resistances, the flow of current through these protein-containing components will result in the generation of greater quantities of heat than in those components consisting primarily of a simple electrolyte. Contrariwise, the pathways, which have smaller resistances, will conduct greater amounts of the total current. This is depicted in Fig. 2.2.

Figure 2.2a depicts a theoretically pure single current pathway with a composition of a variety of potential tissues and fluids through which the current passes. Rough approximations of the resistances of the various fluids and tissues are depicted by the height of the resistance symbols. Figure 2.2b is simply a reflection of the generation of heat as a result of the current flowing through the various resistances.

Given the foregoing discussions, the ideal situation for the achievement of satisfactory coagulation is when the pathway through which the electrolytic current passes contains primarily the tissue targeted for the coagulation. Taken a step further, the absolute ideal environment of a current pathway, then, would consist of targeted tissue being the *only* significant coagulable component in the pathway;

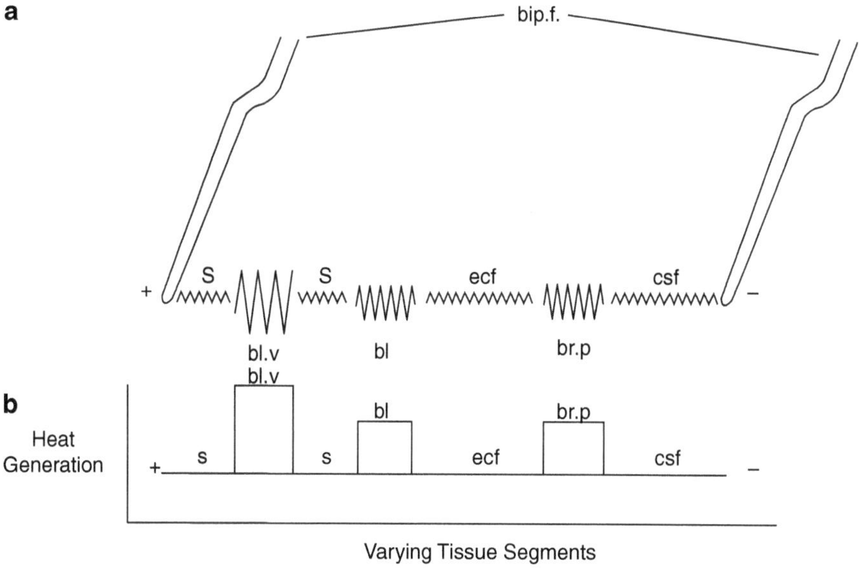

Fig. 2.2 Differential resistances of tissues within a theoretically single segmental current pathway between the bipolar coagulation forceps. (**a**) Exaggerated separation of the forceps blades, exhibiting a theoretic single pathway, through which current is flowing, which consists of varying components, with different resistances, within the pathway. (**b**) The inferior part of the diagram depicts the heat generation in the different components of the current pathway. *bip.f.* bipolar forceps blades, *bl* blood, *bl.v* (*blv*) blood vessel, *br.p.* (*brp*) brain parenchyma, *csf*, cerebrospinal fluid, *ecf.* extracellular fluid, *R* resistance, *S* saline, R^{blv}, R^{bl}, R^{brp}, R^{ecf}, R^{s}, and R^{csf} represent the resistances of blood vessel, blood, brain parenchyma, extracellular fluid, saline, and cerebrospinal fluid, respectively, where $R^{blv} > R^{bl} \approx R^{brp} >> R^{ecf} \approx R^{s} \approx R^{csf}$ (see text)

more often than not, this would consist of a bleeding point. Thus, in this situation there would be no excess blood or excess saline or other electrolytic fluid irrigation in the current pathway, under which circumstances the proteinaceous blood vessel can be broken down and destroyed, leaving behind the residual *coagulum* of that tissue. To again reiterate an earlier notation, if saline irrigation can be utilized to dilute, or clear, the pathway of potentially coagulable substances, except that which is to be coagulated, then the quality of the coagulation event is optimized!

2.1.2 The Separation of the Blades of the Bipolar Coagulating Forceps

Section 2.1.1 was directed purely at the consideration of the environment between bipolar blades during the use of coagulation. This section is simply a brief consideration regarding the distance between the blades of the forceps during coagulation, and as such it is somewhat redundant. I have chosen to accept the redundancy as a number of overlapping features lead to satisfactory coagulation. No surgeon is unaware that if the blades of the forceps touch one another, then there is no resistance to the flow of current between the blades. Thus, quite irrespective of what other pathways might exist, all of the current will flow directly from one blade to the other, leaving none to traverse the tissue targeted for coagulation, which, of course, has resistance. In this case, the current is purely an electrical current between the two forceps blades, i.e., there is no, or insignificantly little, intervening electrolytic current passing through tissue.

The ideal separation will be the smallest that can be maintained without the blades actually contacting one another on the one hand but yet on the other hand as close together as possible in order to include primarily the bulk of the tissue to be coagulated. This ideal separation will provide a pathway through which the majority of the current traverses this tissue, thereby minimizing the amount of current necessary to achieve the coagulation. The minimization occurs through optimally reducing the amount of current that is shunted through pathways, which does not contribute to the coagulation of the tissue in question. This is depicted diagrammatically in Fig. 2.3. Figure 2.3a demonstrates forceps blades that are too far apart and, additionally, an excess of (conducting) fluid between them. In Fig. 2.3b, the excess fluid has been largely removed, but the blades remain too far apart. As a result, there will still be some wasteful *shunting* of current on either side and around the blood vessel. Figure 2.3c illustrates the ideal—the removal of all the excess fluid and the marked increased reduction of the separation of the forceps blades. Both of these alterations reduce the amount of current required for the achievement of a simple satisfactory coagulation.

Blood flowing within a blood vessel will carry away varying amounts of heat surrounding it. If it is a bleeding vessel that is being coagulated, then the separation of the blades of the bipolar forceps should be small enough to obliterate the flow, thereby providing static blood inside the vessel, which is much more easily coagulated than flowing blood (*vide infra*).

2.1.3 Saline Irrigation

In keeping with the tenets of the foregoing, the ideal coagulating pathway consists of pure electrolytic components with the only exception being that of the component to be coagulated. As noted in the foregoing, saline irrigation, or irrigation with some other equivalent electrolyte, aids in achieving this by primarily washing out other components, whose coagulation would be simply unnecessarily shunting current away from the tissue being coagulated. The primary *other* component in most instances is blood. If there is blood along the pathway, then it will absorb current and heat and will elevate the requirement for the necessary current to coagulate that at which the coagulation is being aimed. Thus, adequate saline irrigation will keep the pathway an electrolytic current pathway, except for what is being coagulated. Its use, of course, is only helpful if an excessive amount of the saline (electrolytic) solution is *not* left in the environment of the current pathway.

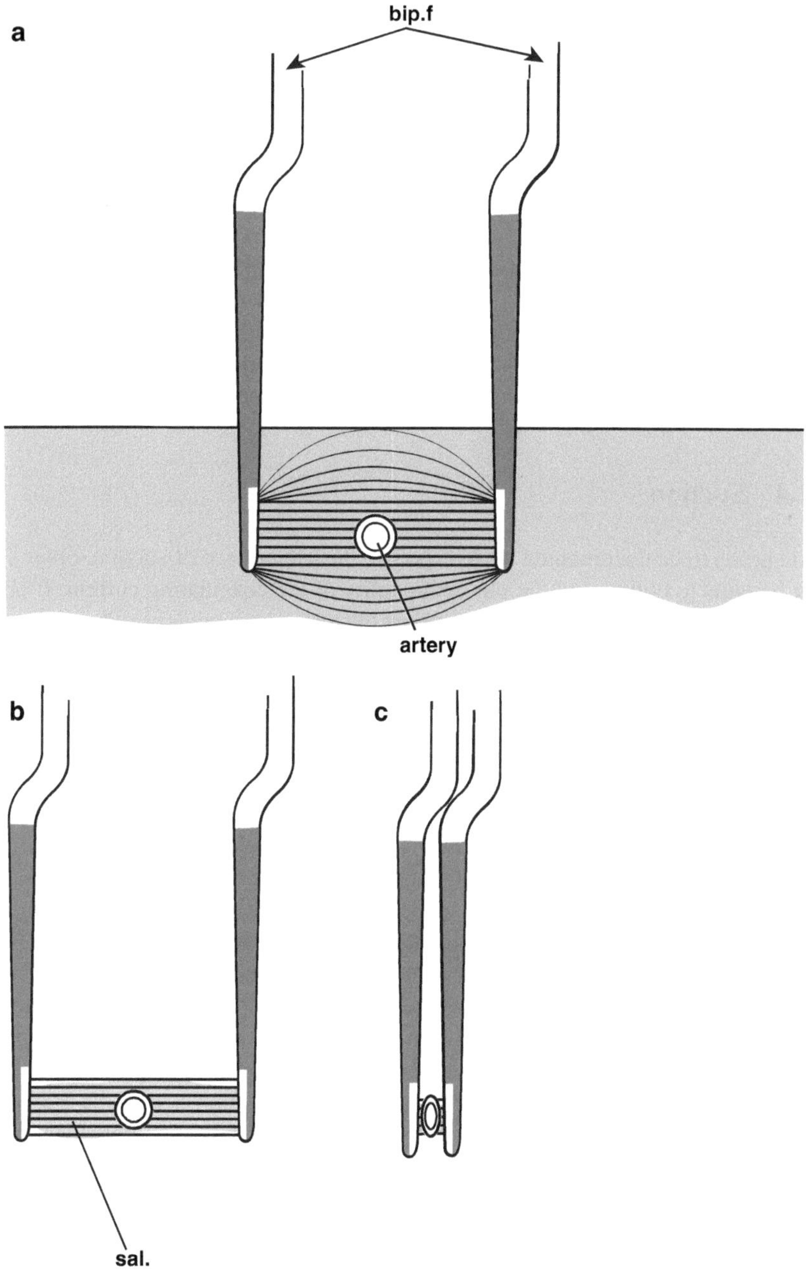

Fig. 2.3 The effects of separation of forceps in bipolar coagulation. Diagrams demonstrating the advantages of reducing the separation of bipolar coagulating forceps blades to a minimum; (**a**) illustrates forceps blades that are too far apart and with an excess of fluid between the blades and around the blood vessel; (**b**) is the same diagram as (**a**), but with the excess fluid having been removed (thus a reduction of unnecessary *shunting* current); (**c**) shows the blade separation reduced to a minimum thus reducing the distance of the current pathway between the blades and insuring that within the pathway the primary composition is the targeted tissue (e.g., blood vessel, parenchyma, etc.). *bip.f.* bipolar forceps, *sal* saline (see text)

In summary, gentle saline irrigation of the site of coagulation facilitates the removal of proteinaceous-containing substances that may unnecessarily raise the required strength of current to achieve the satisfactory coagulation of the tissue to be coagulated; its effect is by virtue of providing a better quality environment for the conduction of electrolytic current. This abolishes the case of high current and increased amounts of blood that leads to a coagulum on the forceps, which is associated with all the aggravations well known to the neurosurgeon!

I would be remiss in not acknowledging the *irrigating* bipolar forceps. For the surgeon working alone or without an experienced assistant, there is no adequate substitute for a good pair of irrigating bipolar forceps with the irrigation regulated to just provide the appropriate saline moisture at the end of the forceps during the course of significant requirements of ongoing coagulation.

2.1.4 Suction

Little needs to be documented with respect to the importance of suction, other than as it pertains to optimizing the physical quality of the coagulating current. It obviously must be gentle enough not to damage the tissue immediately surrounding the point of suction, e.g., also one of the strategies to reduce postoperative lesions arising from the surgery. However, from the physical aspect, the suction is important in reducing any excess electrolyte solution, which has been utilized to cleanse and to keep moisturized the area to be coagulated. As noted in the foregoing, this applies also to other tissue, the coagulation of which is not germane to the desired tissue to be coagulated. Leaving excess saline fluid around this area, if it contacts both blades of the forceps, will electrically provide *in parallel* pathways (see Figs. 2.1 and 2.3a), which will *shunt* current through it without making any contribution to the desired coagulation. Since the electrolytic (saline) pathways have less resistance than that which involves the point to be coagulated (which will be protein in content), the former may conduct the majority of the current, and the latter will receive insufficient current to effect the appropriate coagulation in much the same way as noted in the foregoing section which dealt with the separation of the blades of the coagulating forceps. The removal of this excess saline has the same effect as narrowing the separation of widely separated forceps blades, i.e., it minimizes the loss of current through noncontributory pathways (illustrated in Fig. 2.3a, c). Once again, the importance of the gentleness of the application of the suction cannot be overemphasized.

In summary, during normal epilepsy surgical resection, the pressure of the suction should be lowered such that it will not damage tissue to which it might be applied, when the outlet hole on the handle of the suction cannula is uncovered. Given this as the starting point, then the regulation of the force of suction may be controlled by gently rolling the thumb over the outlet hole. At the same time, *any* unwanted potentially injurious event from too much suction can be prevented instantly by rolling the thumb off the hole.

2.1.5 Cottonoid Patties

The use of cotton patties in any neurosurgical procedure has many attributes. One of these is its protective effect during the use of higher levels of suction without traumatizing the underlying brain parenchyma. For example, there are unusual cases when the suction must be raised to high levels, e.g., high enough to damage brain tissue if applied directly to it. A typical such case involves the bleeding that may occur during the removal of an arteriovenous malformation and which can be sufficient to preclude satisfactory vision of the underlying operative field. The safety to underlying brain parenchyma can be achieved through the use of cottonoid patties. The use of a cottonoid greatly increases the efficiency of removing only the blood, of providing easier visual access to the bleeding point(s), and of significantly reducing the potential of damaging brain parenchyma or small fragile vascular vessels.

In addition to the foregoing, the use of suction applied to cotton patties allows the safe application of pressure for the occlusion of the flow of blood from bleeding vessels. The object is to achieve a bloodless field in which to conduct optimal coagulation. Bleeding arteries, if sufficiently large, may be impossible to coagulate without significantly reducing or abolishing its flow at the point from which it is escaping. In such a situation, if the flow is not stopped or at least significantly reduced, it may simply carry away enough or *all* of the localized heat generated by the coagulation current, thus precluding a heat-generating coagulum from forming in the vessel's lumen and halting the flow of blood. As noted earlier, once the blood is static, it can be easily coagulated with the result of a significantly sized coagulum.

Under this circumstance, I have witnessed surgeons attempting to control the situation by either increasing the force of suction, in order to remove the blood, or the strength of the coagulation current, in order to provide enough heat to effect coagulation, or both. Both of these require a change in at least one of the technical essentials at this point in the surgery. Both of these potential changes may eventually aid in achieving coagulation of the bleeding vessel. However, I believe very strongly (!) that both of these are not only completely unnecessary but require more time (adjusting the required alterations at the time and then readjusting them back again when the bleeding is controlled) and are also much less likely to achieve a satisfactory coagulation. This can usually be rectified by either significantly reducing or obliterating the blood flow through the very safe use of pressure, applied by the suction cannula on a cottonoid patty over the bleeding arterial vessel. This is demonstrated in Fig. 2.4. In Fig. 2.4a, an appropriately sized cottonoid patty is placed over the end of the bleeding vessel, and Fig. 2.4b simply demonstrates the suction cannula being pressed down with sufficient force to collapse the lumen of the vessel, thus stopping any flow of blood. In response to the occasional neurosurgical resident or fellow saying "but won't your way of dealing with the bleeding vessel take more time?" (i.e., the very few seconds longer!), I have no concern about saying *Yes*. The reason for this lack of concern will become clear when seeing the section on current strength (*vide infra*, Sect. 2.1.6).

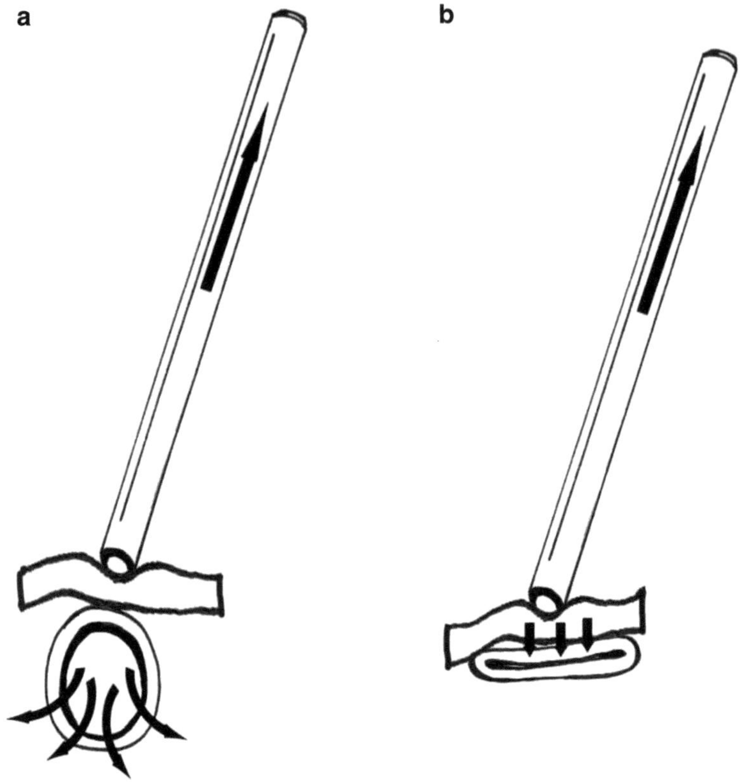

Fig. 2.4 The effect of flowing blood on the quality of coagulation. This illustrates the obliteration of the flow of blood through a bleeding vessel by the application of sufficient pressure applied to the vessel through the use of a suction cannula on a cottonoid patty. (**a**) The application of an appropriately sized patty over the bleeding point. (**b**) The application of sufficient force of the suction cannula on the patty to occlude the bleeding foramen

Perhaps the most useful information that I was privileged to have learned about the use of a cottonoid patty from Dr. Rasmussen (personal communication) was that the quality of its use is dependent upon it being kept the appropriate size, moist, and used on bleeding surfaces only for short periods of time, e.g., a matter of a few minutes. It was Dr. Rasmussen's practice, in the face of continual need of patties in a given area, to change them every few minutes. He always was concerned about leaving the patties long enough to reduce capillary bleeding but not long enough to become physically attached to the parenchyma; in the case of the latter, the removal often removed the very small blood clots, which would then simply rejuvenate the bleeding problem for which the patties had been placed in order to stop. This is a small point but with a very large importance! Dr. Rasmussen also *always* placed patties for a few minutes on the inside of leptomeningeal barrier(s), immediately following its exposure by subpial resection of its parenchyma. Practice quickly leads to an intuitive appreciation of how long to leave the patties before removing or exchanging them without physically altering the tissue from which the bleeding is occurring.

When I returned to London, Ontario, to practice, I encountered the then current practice of using cottonoid patties only when they were attached to long strings, the view being that this was the only certain way to determine, through the mandatory counts at the end of the operation, that none had been left intracranially. Operating with Dr. Drake (personal communication), we not infrequently used small pieces of gauze and cottonoid patties to stop aneurysmal bleeding and often to actually leave them in place around aneurysmal clips in order to increase the long-term bond around peculiarly shaped aneurysmal necks. There was *never* any evidence in these patients of *any* concerns with respect to the cotton left behind around aneurysms. The result was that I gave rise to changing the traditional practice, as stated at the beginning of this paragraph, i.e., that only the use of large stringed cottonoids could be used. The change consisted of the scrub nurses' preparations for operations that included taking a large sheet of cottonoid and cutting it into pieces, the sizes of which varied from some as small as 2×2 mm to some as large as 2×5 cm! These were used throughout the operation, as required. The large commercial patties with attached strings were used only infrequently, primarily in operations when their placement inside the ventricle was required. I have been asked "how do you know that you haven't left some of the cottonoids in the brain?" My answer is: "I really don't know for certain ..." and "further, I have little doubt but that some have been left from time to time," but "there has never been a concern, to my knowledge," i.e., just as there was never a concern when leaving them around aneurysms!

2.1.6 The Strength of Coagulating Current

One of the most difficult aspects of coagulation to appreciate is that the optimal current is the *least* current required to carry out the coagulation. High currents often bring about increased tissue damage, which is to be avoided at all cost. One of the most important aspects of neurosurgery in general and epilepsy surgery in particular is to make certain that any parenchyma left behind is as healthy as possible! The reason for this with respect to epilepsy surgery is that there is a significant concern that the cortex of epileptic patients has a greater inherent potential epileptogenicity than that of non-epileptic patients. Quite irrespective of whether this is true or not, one of the principles of neurosurgery is that any surgical procedure should be associated with the least possible amount of damage arising from the surgery, per se.

Potential tissue damage from mild increases in the strength of coagulation is perhaps of less concern than other concerns about raised strengths of current, especially relatively large increases. One of the most annoying aspects to utilizing higher than required strengths of current is that these strengths often lead to the coagulum, the solidified mass resulting from the coagulation, adhering to the bipolar forceps. Every neurosurgeon has had colleagues who talk about *sticky* forceps or who continually complain about the forceps being clogged with coagulated blood, necessitating their nearly continual cleaning by the operating nurse or technician. This can lead to an unnecessarily tremendously increased time of operation. One can often see that the use of bipolar coagulation in the hands of these same colleagues may be associated with actual sparking when the forceps blades are close together! The *sticky* forceps is not the fault of the forceps, nor necessarily the fault of the technique. Rather, it is nearly always the result of the use of unnecessarily high levels of coagulating current. It may be avoided by lowering the current of coagulation or aided by the application of sufficient saline irrigation.

The drawbacks of the use of excessively high levels of coagulation current cannot be overemphasized. Yes, the initial coagulation, at high levels, may occur earlier when applied, but in addition to the foregoing noted concerns, its use often coagulates only short segments of what is to be coagulated, and these segments are very akin to burnt toast in which the brittle burnt portions are much more fragile and likely to crumble when divided or incised in some manner or when moved around with retraction or the ongoing surgery. Under these circumstances, the current, itself, may result in a spontaneous incision in the area of the forceps blades, often associated with incomplete obliteration of the flowing blood. For those who understand the injurious aspects of electrical stimulation of the cortex will recognize that such high currents lead to what is called an *electrolytic* injury. In coagulation, this injury leads to a small, fragile, unstable coagulated area, which at its worst may incise the area to be coagulated. Compare this to low coagulation current, which utilizes heat rather than electrolytic current and hence coagulates a longer segment, with an intrinsic stronger coagulum, and which is not only much less likely to crack, crumble, or snap when it is incised but will *never* spontaneously cut the bleeding vessel at the point of coagulation before the coagulation is satisfactorily completed.

2.1.7 The Ideal Components of Optimal Coagulation

There is no more important surgical strategy than that relating to high-quality coagulation as part of all subdisciplines of neurosurgery but particularly in cerebrovascular and epilepsy surgery.

As already discussed, *saline irrigation* to maintain the electrolytic component of the current pathway, *suction*, and *cottonoid patties* for assistance to reduce unnecessary excess conductive material and parenchyma in the current pathway, a small *separation of the blades* of the bipolar coagulating forceps, and most important of all the use of the *lowest satisfactory coagulating current* for the best quality coagulation. Table 2.1 outlines these components.

The ideal in training residents in this practice is the achievement of a coagulation *field* which is bloodless, which is moist from irrigation, and which involves obvious occlusion of the vessel being coagulated, often in which the saline around the tips of the forceps is *boiling*, i.e., small bubbles from the heat can be seen, as well as being felt by the surgeon in her/his hand and not associated with continual clotting of blood on the forceps. I have been made fun of by many trainees about using the expression *make it boil*. Sometimes it is only an extra second or two of application of coagulating current that is required to achieve the boiling point! The evidence of the optimal

Table 2.1 The components of ideal optimal coagulation

Cottonoid patties
Low coagulating current
Narrow separation of the blades of the forceps
Moisture from saline irrigation
Suction

use of all the foregoing principles associated with bipolar coagulation can be found in the cases when the operating surgeon can complete an operative procedure without requiring *any* cleaning of the forceps! (Yes, that *is* possible!) That is to say, he/she requires no, or very few, requests of the scrub nurse to *please clean the bipolars*!

Coagulation is easier, more efficient, more localized, safer, and more effective when the current is used at as low levels as possible. It is also the quality of this type of coagulation in which recurrent bleeding is less likely and that gives rise to the smallest potential *lesion* arising from the coagulation, per se. I have never been involved with a trainee, who has not become enamored with these advantages associated with the use of very low levels of coagulating current in subpial dissection. (In general neurosurgery, the closest equivalent to the strength of coagulating current suggested here would be that used over the surface of the spinal cord.)

2.2 Subpial Dissection

2.2.1 Introduction

The time-honored technical surgical procedure by which cortical epileptogenic foci are removed is the so-called subpial dissection or subpial resection. It is a technique which has at its basis the removal of the cortex as non-injuriously as possible and has now been in use since the latter part of the nineteenth century. It would seem that it was introduced by Horsley (1886, 1887) and was often referred to in the literature as the *Horsley operation*. Indeed, Sachs, in 1935, discussed the technique and called it the *Horsley operation*. It was, however, Penfield's Montreal (Neurological Institute) school that drew most attention to the technique (Penfield and Evans 1935; Penfield 1939; Penfield and Baldwin 1952). Penfield noted the importance in carrying out resections "along fissure lines whenever possible" in that "this method seems to decrease the likelihood of postoperative epilepsy" (1947). Steelman showed in experimental animals the smaller scar left behind using this technique, in comparison with the then existing general neurosurgical method of cortical removal (1949).

The rationale of the technique of subpial resection is threefold: (1) the selective removal of the epileptogenic tissue, (2) the minimization of the post-resection scar, and (3) the preservation of the anatomical and physiological health of the remaining cortex (the cortex left behind). Before addressing these objectives, the anatomy will be briefly reviewed.

2.2.2 Anatomy of the Cerebral Cortex and Leptomeninges

A discussion of the technique of subpial dissection is best initiated with a simple review of the anatomy of the cerebral gyri and the membranes (meninges), as it is an understanding of this anatomy that is necessary to understand the strategy and technology of resecting tissue subpially. Figure 2.5 discloses a diagrammatic representation of cortical gyri and their covering meninges. The external meningeal covering (membrane) of the whole of the central nervous system is the dura mater. That part of the dura mater covering the brain is strongly adherent to the inner surface of the cranial vault. Lying under the dura mater is the arachnoid membrane—a somewhat fragile membrane that is directly applied to the undersurface of the dura mater. However, it is not adherent to the dura mater, and thus between them is a potential space, which is referred to as the subdural space. A pial membrane, also somewhat fragile, covers the parenchyma of the nervous system. Between these two membranes lies the subarachnoid space (e.g., *below* the arachnoid membrane). These two membranes are collectively known as the leptomeninges.

There are further aspects in Fig. 2.5 that are worth emphasizing as a prelude to a discussion of subpial dissection. Note that the arachnoid membrane follows the same course as the dura mater in that it covers primarily the most extrinsic anatomy of the brain. Thus, in that course, it covers primarily the externally exposed (*surface*) cortex and does not cover the cortical surfaces, which reside within the sulci. Occasionally, the cortex that is not visibly exposed when the dura mater is removed is referred to as the *hidden* or *buried* cortex; the cortex within the sulci falls into this category. The entire cerebral cortex, including not only the exposable surface but also that within the sulci, is covered with the thin, delicate pia mater membrane. Thus, while all cortices have a pial investment, all cortices do not have the somewhat stronger investment of the arachnoid membrane. The combination of these two membranes, as noted earlier, constitutes the *leptomeninges* or the *leptomeningeal membrane*. This combination of membranes is of primary importance in the discussion of subpial dissection. While there is no such membrane covering the sulcal cortex, there is this dual combination over the surface of the gyri and within the *fissures*. This is of significance with respect to any surgery in and about the Sylvian fissure.

The subarachnoid space contains the cerebrospinal fluid (CSF) and the vasculature irrigating the underlying cortex. The arterial vessels, which are responsible for the irrigation of this cortex, must penetrate the pia mater to gain access to the cortical parenchyma to which it supplies the nutrients responsible for its health. Similarly, the veins penetrate the pial membrane, in the opposite direction, to carry away the unwanted by-products of metabolism, also responsible for the health of the cortex.

It is worth emphasizing the significant importance in understanding the difference between the strengths of the meningeal investments in the two situations. The leptomeningeal investment is much stronger, and thus more potentially protective of the underlying structures, than the very thin pial membrane alone. As a result, subpial resection of the cortex within sulci is associated with a greater risk of injury to the pia mater, the vasculature traveling through it, and even possibly the cortex on the other side of the sulcus.

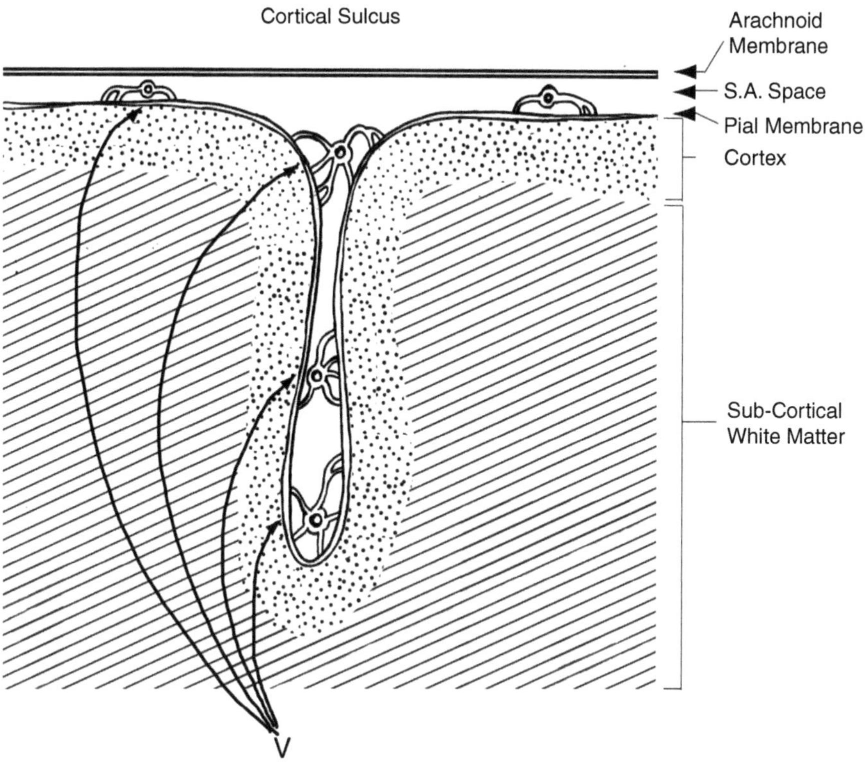

Fig. 2.5 The anatomy of cerebral gyri. Diagrammatic representation of a cerebral sulcus and part of the associated cortical gyri. Overlying the cortical surfaces of the gyri is the pial membrane, which is adherent to the cortex. Outside of this is the so-called subarachnoid space, which contains cerebrospinal fluid. It is *so called* because there is a thin membrane lying over (external to) the space known as the arachnoid membrane; the fluid rests between the arachnoid and pial membranes, e.g., the subarachnoid space. Outside of the arachnoid membrane is the very solid, thick, and strong membrane known as the dura mater (not shown in the diagram), which is intimately adherent to the inner surface of the cranial vault. Note that the arachnoid membrane covers only the exposed (exterior) surfaces of the gyri. The *buried* cortex, within the sulci, is covered only with the somewhat delicate pial membrane. *v* vasculature, with branches, which penetrate the pia to irrigate the underlying cortex (arteries) or to remove its metabolic products (veins)

2.2.3 The Technique of Subpial Dissection

The technique of subpial removal of the cortex, as noted earlier, forms the basis of epilepsy surgical technique. Nearly all surgeons, who have been introduced to the technique during training, will utilize the technique in *all* surgery, irrespective of whether the surgery involves the removal of epileptic foci or the normal run of neurosurgical procedures involving the entrance and removal of brain parenchyma.

The technique involves the separation of the unwanted cortex from its pial or leptomeningeal investment and adjacent parenchyma, leaving completely healthy the juxtaposed cortex that is left behind. This can be achieved through the gentle use of a blunt instrument, e.g., the bipolar coagulation forceps, and/or with the use of suction. When a blunt instrument is used, such as a Penfield #1 or #4 dissector, it is wedged between the cortical surface and meningeal investment. Through a series of manipulations of the tip of the dissector, the latter is gradually advanced between the cortex and leptomeningeal investment. Often this requires facilitation with the use of a small cottonoid patty, upon which the suction cannula can be applied, and with added pressure the underlying area of the cortex may be *held* in place, as it were, from moving with the manipulation of the dissector. This is really simply a form of counter-traction (see Fig. 2.6a). Frequently, the applied pressure of the cottonoid patty in this way may provide the majority of the force bringing about separation of the cortex from the pia by stepwise *pulling* the cannula/patty/cortex in the opposite direction (Fig. 2.6b). Finally, the separation may be achieved by simply removing the underlying parenchyma (primarily the cortex) with suction, as shown in Fig. 2.6c, e.g., *subpial resection*. All three of these methods of achieving subpial separation of the membrane and the underlying parenchyma may be used alone, but in general they are nearly all utilized intermittently throughout a cortical resection. The one advantage of using primarily the blunt dissector in the separation (Fig. 2.6a) is that the cortex usually will be sufficiently preserved to provide the neuropathologist with an intact specimen of the cortex. When conducted with care, the separation can nearly always be achieved easily, safely, and satisfactorily. This is especially the case when the periphery of the resection is somewhat removed from the actual epileptic focus. Under these circumstances, the cortex is closer to being normal or indeed definitely normal. Under normal circumstances, it has very little adherence to its overlying pial membrane in addition to its soft intrinsic structure, both of which provide a more easily removed tissue.

To reiterate the foregoing, the next three subsections will cover the objectives of subpial dissection/resection: (1) the selective removal of the epileptic focus, (2) the minimization of the postoperative scar, and (3) the insurance in the health of the parenchyma left behind.

2.2.3.1 The Selective Removal of the Cortical Scar

The foregoing has centered on the instances, which represent the majority, i.e., where the subpial resection is through more *normal* tissue than the tough, gliotic tissue that may be encountered in some cases. In the case of dense gliotic scars, the intrinsic strength of adherence between the cortex and its meningeal investment may be such that it simply cannot be separated in the initial attempt. This can be dealt with in two ways. Attempts always allow some measure of removed tissue. Dr. Rasmussen (personal communication) taught that if this is left for a few minutes while working elsewhere, the second, third, or later attempts often allow the achievement of its complete satisfactory removal. There is no doubt that this is a very beneficial and historically proven typical Rasmussen teaching! The other alternative is to isolate these very adherent sections of the cortex and simply leave them intact. So long as the *isolation* is complete, there will be no deleterious effects postoperatively.

In the foregoing, the use of counter-traction was mentioned, particularly that relating to Fig. 2.6b, c. The importance of the use of counter-traction will rise throughout

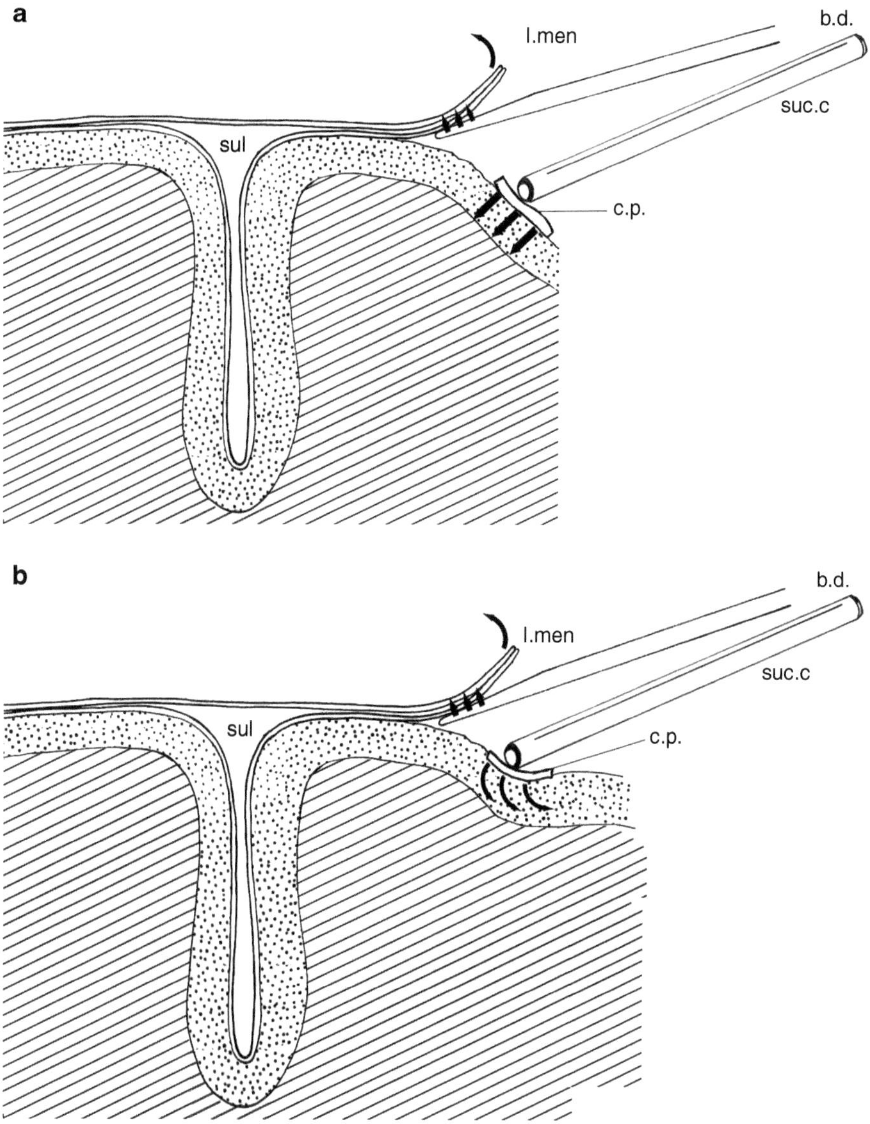

Fig. 2.6 Aids in assisting the conduct of subpial dissection. Subpial dissection, with separation of the cortical epileptogenic surface from its overlying meningeal investment: (**a**) through the use of a blunt instrument, with or without the facilitation of *holding* the cortex stable with the use of a cottonoid patty and suction cannula; (**b**) same as figure (**a**), but using the applied pressure of the cottonoid patty and cannula to *pull* the cortex from the blunt instrument; (**c**) through the removal of the cortex, by simply using suction. *b.d.* blunt dissector, *c.p.* cottonoid patty, *l.men.* leptomeninges, *suc.c.* suction cannula, *sul.* sulcus

c

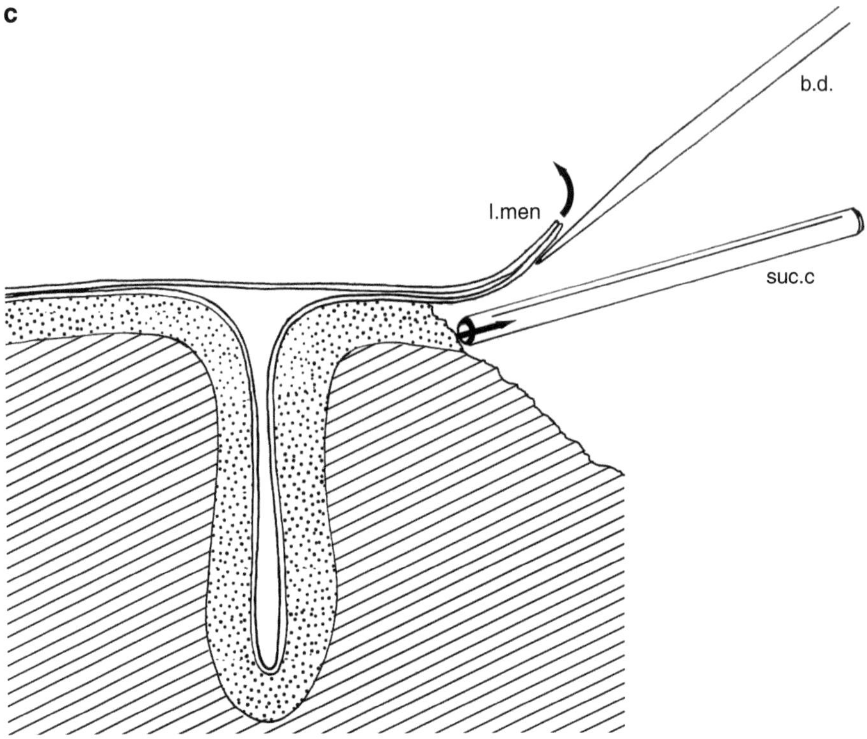

Fig. 2.6 (continued)

a consideration of the techniques associated with subpial resection. In Fig. 2.6a, it was used to provide stability of an area of the cortex such that it would not move in the direction of the applied force of the blunt dissector separating it from its overlying membrane. Without this stability, the movement of the cortex commonly may significantly reduce the achievement of the separation, especially in the cases where there is significant adherence between abnormal cortices and their overlying pial or leptomeningeal membranes. Figure 2.6b depicts the reverse of Fig. 2.6a in that the overlying membrane is being held stable by the blunt dissector, while the combined cottonoid patty and suction cannula traction force achieves separation by *pulling* the cortex away from its overlying membrane. Both of these represent cases of traction and counter-traction—the traction being the blunt dissector in Fig. 2.6a and the patty/cannula in Fig. 2.6b. The more delicate the tissue is in the dissection, the greater is the necessity of using traction and counter-traction to minimize the risk of injury to tissue that is being removed. A good example of this is when one side of a sulcus is normal and should be preserved and the other side is considered to be part of the epileptic focus and is to be removed. In cases where the so-called *eloquent* cortex happens to reside on one side, then it *must* be preserved as a residuum of the dissection.

Figure 2.7 illustrates the traction and counter-traction balance through the use of a blunt dissector, in this case the tips of a bipolar coagulation forceps (or a cottonoid patty under its tips), and the combination of the cottonoid patty/suction cannula during the subpial removal of the cortex from the right side of a sulcus while preserving that on the left side. In Fig. 2.7a, the force of the applied suction is counterbalanced by the forceps, which are used to hold the delicate pial membrane from moving towards the suction and being removed or injured. The counter-traction (applied by the forceps tips) may be unnecessary if the cortex is soft and nonadherent. However, often the force of the suction requires being raised to

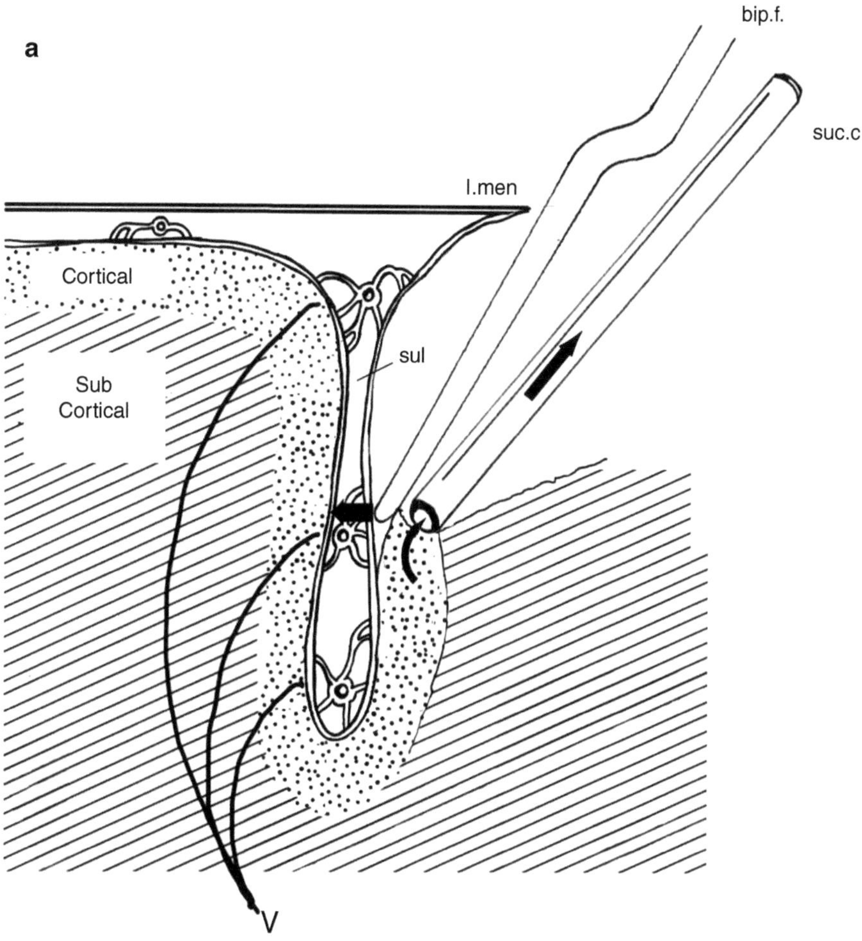

Fig. 2.7 The importance of counter-traction in subpial resection. The application of counter-traction has a number of clear-cut advantages in carrying out subpial dissection (see text). The counter-traction can be achieved simply with the use of (**a**) the bipolar forceps or (**b**) probably the safest, and preferred, way of using a cottonoid patty under the blades of the forceps or the suction cannula. *bip.f.* blades of coagulation forceps, *c.p.* cottonoid patty, *l.men.* leptomeninges, *suc.c.* suction cannula, *sul* sulcus, *tr.* traction, *v* blood vessels within the sulcus; ⬅ (*thick arrow*) counter-traction

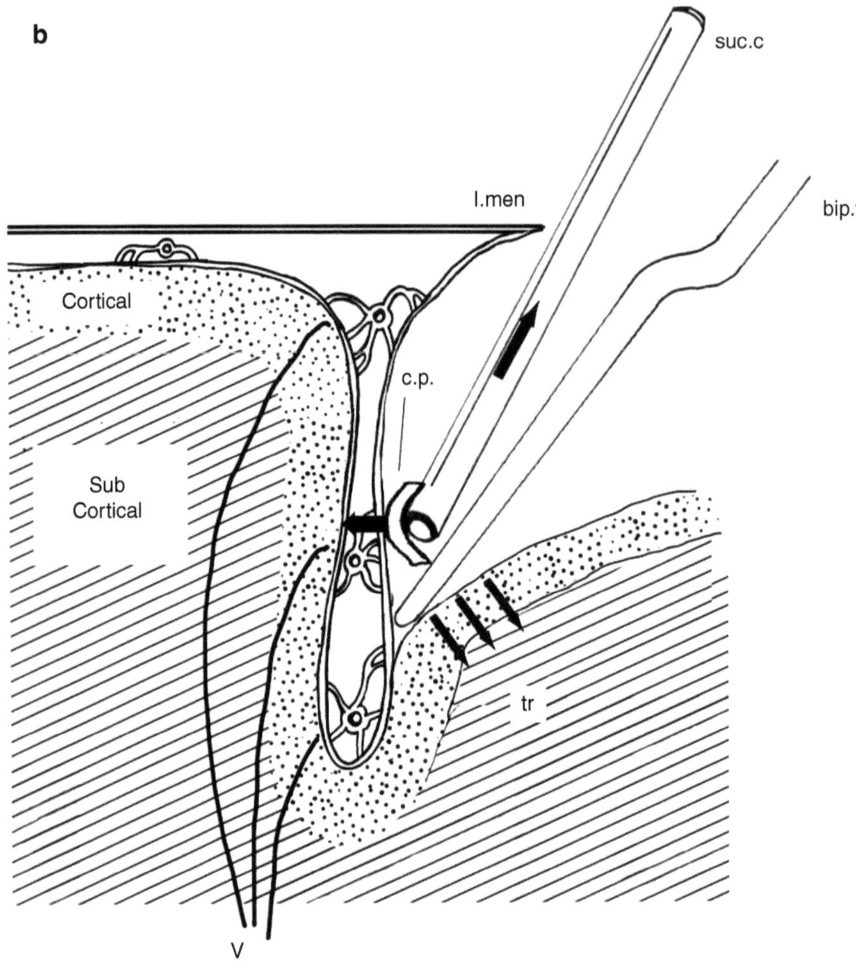

Fig. 2.7 (continued)

a point where it cannot safely be applied directly onto the pial membrane. Figure 2.7b is the reverse of Fig. 2.7a in that the cottonoid patty combination is used for counter-traction, opposing the traction of the forceps. Perhaps the greatest concern about not providing reliable traction and counter-traction in the sulci is that not only is the pial membrane delicate and fragile, but also there is fragile vasculature in the subarachnoid space between the two pial membranes within the sulcus supplying the cortex on either side of the sulcus, which can also be compromised (see Sects. 2.2.3.2 and 2.2.3.3).

Although never mentioned in textbooks, there is frequently a minor amount of venous bleeding from very tiny veins at the very bottom of sulci. There is no reason for coagulation in these instances. A small cottonoid patty can be placed on the point of bleeding and the saline moisture suctioned from it. This, left in place for a very few minutes (*à la Rasmussen*), is usually all that is required for abolishing the bleeding from these very small venous vessels.

Continuing on from the last section (Sect. 2.2.3), Fig. 2.8 illustrates the side of an epileptogenic focus, which is to be removed. Figure 2.8a shows two adjacent gyri, separated by a sulcus. On one side of the sulcus (the right side), there is the epileptogenic cortex, while on the other (left) side there is the normal cortex. The objectives of the subpial resection are to remove the epileptogenic cortex, e.g., the epileptic focus, while at the same time leaving the remaining surrounding cortex completely intact. The resection of the epileptogenic cortex may amount to the removal of only a few gyri, a large area of the cortex, or a lobe of the brain. Irrespective of the size of the resection, it is the *margin* between the cortex to be resected and the cortex to be left behind that is the area of most importance in the removal of the cortex subpially.

Figure 2.8b, using the same Fig. 2.8a, illustrates that the postoperative resection line, e.g., a margin between healthy and epileptogenic cortices, discloses the very small postoperative scar following the uneventful subpial removal of the abnormal cortex. Note the normality of the pial membranes on either side of the sulcus, e.g., one side being that which had been a part of the epileptogenic cortex (right side) and that on the other side which remains as a normal-appearing investment of the healthy cortex.

2.2.3.2 The Minimization of the Post-resection Scar

Any surgery involving the cerebral cortex that requires incisions in, and removal of, the cerebral parenchyma will leave postoperatively, in the vicinity of that tissue removal, a scar. The scar is simply the result of the surgical *trauma*! This is not new. Penfield noted in 1947 "...no cerebral incision or removal is quite free of the threat of subsequent epilepsy." Recognizing this, any surgery of the brain requires that the *trauma* of the surgery leaves as little evidence of traumatic residuum as possible. This is important in all the sub-disciplines of neurosurgery, but it is certainly most important in the surgery of epilepsy, particularly if the theory of those who believe that the cortex of individuals with chronic epilepsy have a propensity for epileptic foci throughout their cerebral cortex are correct.

As noted in the foregoing, Fig. 2.8b demonstrates the very small scar, at the bottom of the sulcus, which remains following a satisfactory resection. This scar is not part of the previously depicted epileptogenic focus but rather that arising as a result of the surgical resection, per se. It is this scar that the epilepsy surgeon wishes to minimize in order to reduce the theoretical potential of producing a scar that might give rise to postoperative seizures. All of the aspects discussed to this point, e.g., gentleness in the surgical technique, low current for coagulation, the use of cottonoid patties, saline irrigation, etc., help to achieve this end, i.e., the minimization of this scar.

Figure 2.8c, like Fig. 2.8b, is a postoperative view of a very unsatisfactory surgical resection. The very small postoperative scar that is so common at the margin of the resection, as seen in Fig. 2.8b, is in this case unnecessarily large. In addition to the latter, the pial membrane having covered the abnormal cortex has been

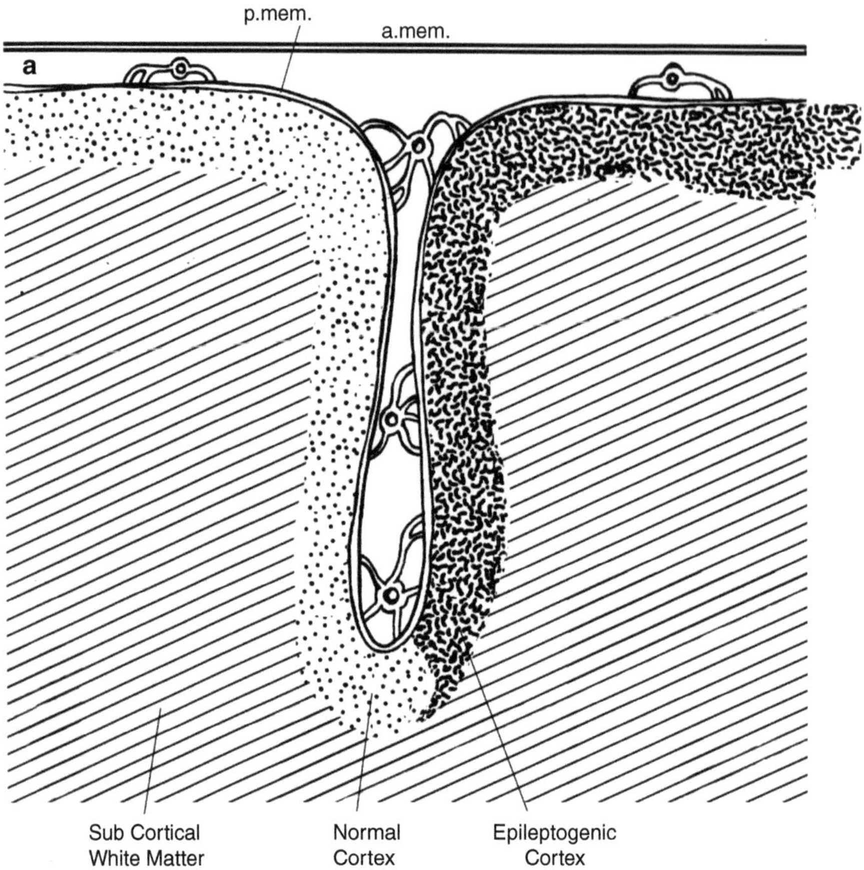

Fig. 2.8 The selective removal of the epileptogenic cortex and postoperative anatomy. (**a**) A diagram of a cortical sulcus, which represents a small segment of the periphery of an epileptic focus, which is to be removed surgically; the cortex on the left side of the sulcus is normal, while that on the right is part of the epileptogenic cortical focus. (**b**) Illustrates the same gyri and sulcus after the satisfactory removal of the segment of the epileptogenic cortex; the remaining cerebral parenchyma is normal, except for the very small postoperative scar left in the depth of the sulcus, which initially had been the margin between the epileptogenic scar and normal cortex; other than the small scar, the parenchyma left behind is normal and healthy. (**c**) Using the same illustration of the anatomy of the sulcus shown in (**a**, **b**), this figure depicts the opposite to the very satisfactory resection of the epileptogenic tissue of figure (**b**); that is, there is a large scar in the depth of the sulcus and a significant scar in the other side of the sulcus as a result of a rent in the pia matter during the resection that resulted in destruction of a sulcal artery, which in turn has resulted in an infarct in the normal cortex across the sulcus. This is a very unsatisfactory resection! *a.mem.* arachnoid membrane, *art.* small artery/arteriole, *l.men.* leptomeninges, *p.mem.* pial membrane, *sas* subarachnoid space (Redrawn, with permission, from Girvin (1992))

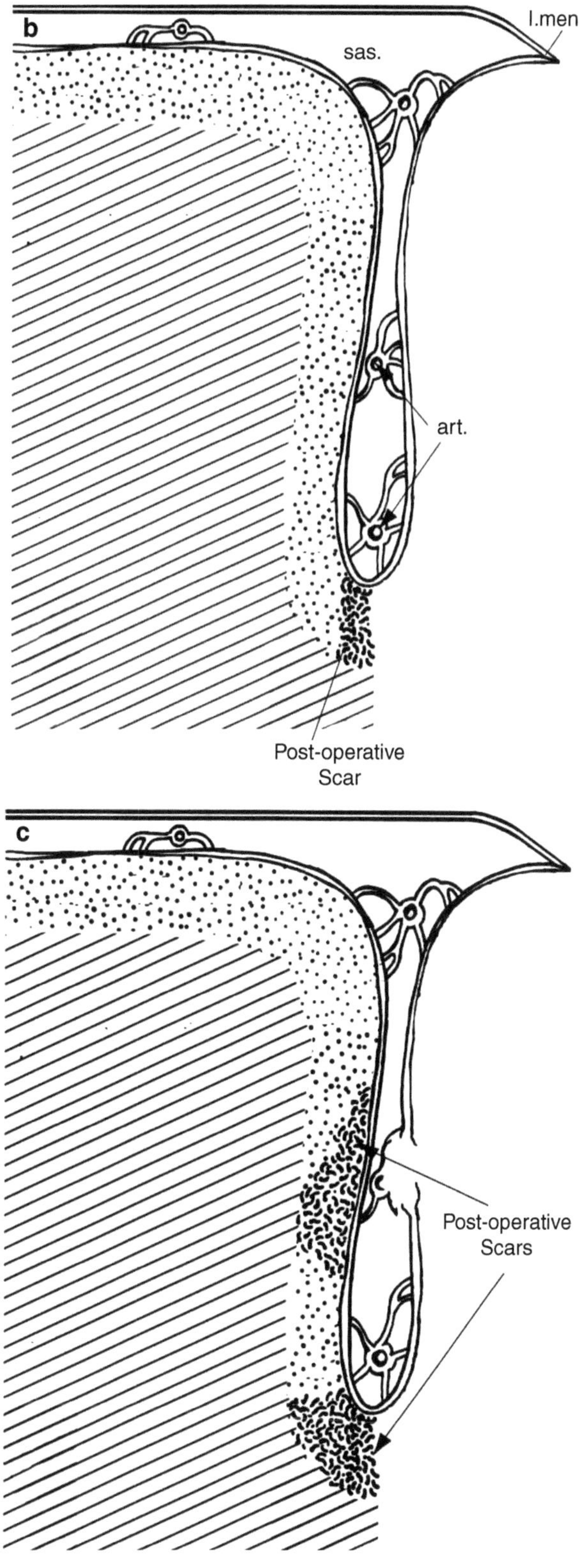

Fig. 2.8 (continued)

violated, and a small vessel in the underlying subarachnoid space has been occluded, resulting in an infarct in the normal cortex across from the violated pia. There may be no clinical risk from this small infarct other than the birth of another epileptogenic focus, but if the cortex happened to be the *eloquent* cortex, then there may well be some associated neurological impairment. It is worth noting that this damage can be produced mechanically through the use of perfectly normal surgical instrumentation but which has been used without sufficient care. Among the most likely causes would be excessive retraction, coagulation, or suction. As noted in the foregoing, such a lesion may be of absolutely no future significance, but a surgically marred technique such as this, if it is accepted as normal practice, will become associated at some point with postoperative neurological deficits and/or the appearance of a new seizure disorder! The take-home message from a discussion such as this is that any school of epilepsy surgery must be obsessively devoted to the knowledge and the abolition of practices that might give rise to postoperative surgical scars.

2.2.3.3 The Preservation of the Health of the Remaining Cortex

As has been emphasized repeatedly in the forgoing comments, it is most important to maintain the health of the cortex that is remaining behind, adjacent to the removed epileptogenic cortex. This is probably the most important part of the subpial resective technique. Certainly, it is the most difficult part of the technique to achieve with purity. In addition to the importance of avoiding mechanical injury to this cortex during the resection, the health of the remaining marginal cortex is dependent upon both the preservation of normal blood supply and the preservation of its neuronal connectivity. These are considered in the following narrative relating to the corticectomy (see Sects. 5.2, 5.3, and 5.4).

2.2.4 Retraction with Normal-Sized Retractors

This has been relegated to a separate section, not because of any complexity, but because of its importance in protecting the health of cerebral parenchyma being left behind following any surgical procedure involving retraction of that parenchyma. When retraction of large segments of cerebral parenchyma is required in order to achieve satisfactory vision of the operative field, the retraction should *always* be applied to the tissue that is being removed, not to that which is to remain. Very often the conditions suggest that perhaps the easier retraction would be that of the healthy cortex that would remain behind at the termination of the surgery. This situation of what tissue to which the traction should be directed during the course of surgery is commonly encountered in epileptic operations. This is especially the case when completing the isolation of the neocortex of the temporal lobe in an anterior temporal lobectomy (aTLY) and even more so in the case of a radical frontal lobectomy and in corticectomies of all sizes. Other than perhaps mildly altering the morphological specimens, there is no concern about using the retractor on the parenchyma being removed. However, it is evidence of carelessness and unsatisfactory retraction when bruising of parenchyma, which is being left behind, is seen following the removal of the retractor at the termination of an operation!

Interestingly, the choice of the wrong tissue to retract has most often, in my experience, had to do with the handedness of the surgeon. I maintain that part of resident training is mandatory inclusion of bimanual use of *all* the instrumentation. This is briefly dealt with in one of the following sections (Sect. 2.4).

2.3 Anatomical Measurements of Functional Areas of the Cortex

In most chapters, there will be a notation of various measurements, which help to identify functional areas of the cortex, without the benefit of direct cortical stimulation. Thus, these may provide some helpful hints to the surgeon in cases where the patient is not awake and thus cannot be stimulated satisfactorily and communicated with directly. Such examples include the use of general anesthesia, a very prolonged postictal coma/confusion following a seizure in an awake patient, etc. Although some of these measurements are reasonably accurate with respect to identifying functional cortical areas, they can only be taken as reasonable guides. That is to say, these measurements lack the *absolute certainty* of the identification of various locales of cortical functional localization when dealing with patients under general anesthesia. The reader, no doubt, will be aware that this author's bias leans towards the use of local anesthesia, whenever possible, and always in cases where an accurate knowledge of the location of the so-called functional cortex is mandatory in order to achieve optimal surgical outcomes.

How are such areas identified? The time-honored way of measuring the amount of temporal cortex removed as part of an anterior temporal lobectomy (aTLY) was introduced by Dr. Penfield. He used his own dissector, now called a Penfield #1, by placing it concave side down over the middle temporal gyrus of the cortical surface. The dissector is then gently pushed forwards on the cortex until it stops against a bony part of the anterior middle fossa. The distance between the tip of the #1 dissector and the chosen posterior resection boundary of an anterior temporal lobectomy (aTLY), or where the speech center has been localized, or where a particular anatomical structure is located is able to be determined. Making these types of measurements many times leads to a reasonably accurate assessment of where various anatomical structures and/or physiological functional areas of the temporal lobe cortex are located, even though the tip of the dissector does not reach the most anterior aspect of the lobe. Thus, this is like any surgical instrument in that once the surgeon is ensconced and comfortable in the continual use of a given instrument, her or his experiential background often adopts its use, irrespective of perhaps other better similar instruments. This has been the case in my experience. I do not believe that the Penfield #1 dissector is necessarily the best instrument with which to measure the various distances of functional areas from the poles of the frontal, temporal, and occipital lobes, but that is the measuring instrument to which I was initially introduced, and as is so often it is the one I became accustomed to using when I started in practice. For the most part, it was satisfactory in my experience. The standard criteria for gaining the best repetitive accuracy in measurements with this dissector are to place it (1) with the concave side down (against the cortex), (2) anteroposteriorly along the middle temporal gyrus (MTG), and (3) *parallel* to the MTG, e.g., the whole of the dissector. The latter is probably the most difficult to achieve comfortably.

Figure 2.9a demonstrates the side and flat views of the Penfield dissector (P.d.). Figure 2.9b, c illustrates views of the placement of the dissector from both the lateral and the inferior surfaces of a right temporal lobe, respectively. They both demonstrate the fact that the tip of dissector fails to reach the actual anterior tip of the temporal lobe, e.g., the anterior extent of the middle fossa. Because of this fact, it was always important to place the dissector more than once, until the best accuracy was obtained. It is also this feature that lessens the precision of this particular method of measuring more posteriorly situated structures or cortical areas of the temporal lobe, as all such measurements are the distances posterior to the tip of the dissector as opposed to being able to clearly indicate that they were posterior to the tip of the temporal lobe. The drawback of using the dissector is the stiffness of the instrument, which precludes being able to extend it to the anterior extent of the middle fossa while following the surface of the lobe.

Having used the Penfield #1 dissector for these measurements for over 30 years, I came to the conclusion that there was a better, more repetitively accurate manner of making such measurements, especially with respect to the frontal lobe. One day, while attempting to accurately measure the distance from the tip of a left frontal lobe back to the speech center and the Rolandic fissure, I chose to use a simple #8 pediatric urinary red rubber catheter. Each repetitive measurement was nearly exactly the same! I really cannot say that that was also the case with the Penfield dissector! I have used this method since that time in Jeddah in 2003. This is simply illustrated in Fig. 2.10 through a and b figures, which are similar to Fig. 2.9c, b respectively, in which the Penfield dissector was utilized for the same measurements.

In measuring the distances behind the tip of the temporal pole, there is a discrepancy of ~5 mm between the smaller measurement using the Penfield dissector and the larger measurement using the pediatric red rubber catheter. In any of the measurements, the catheter should be placed a sufficient number of times—an exercise that takes only a few seconds—such that a satisfactory reliable repeatability of measurement can be achieved. Once familiarity with the use of whatever method of measuring is used is sufficient, then it may be applied to any measurements from the poles of the temporal, frontal, or occipital lobes with relative confidence in its reliability. [I now accept that the use of the red rubber catheter is much more easily conducted physically and requires fewer attempts to obtain a repeatable accurate measurement. Thus, from here-on-in the measurements in this book will be the result of the use of the pediatric red rubber catheter.]

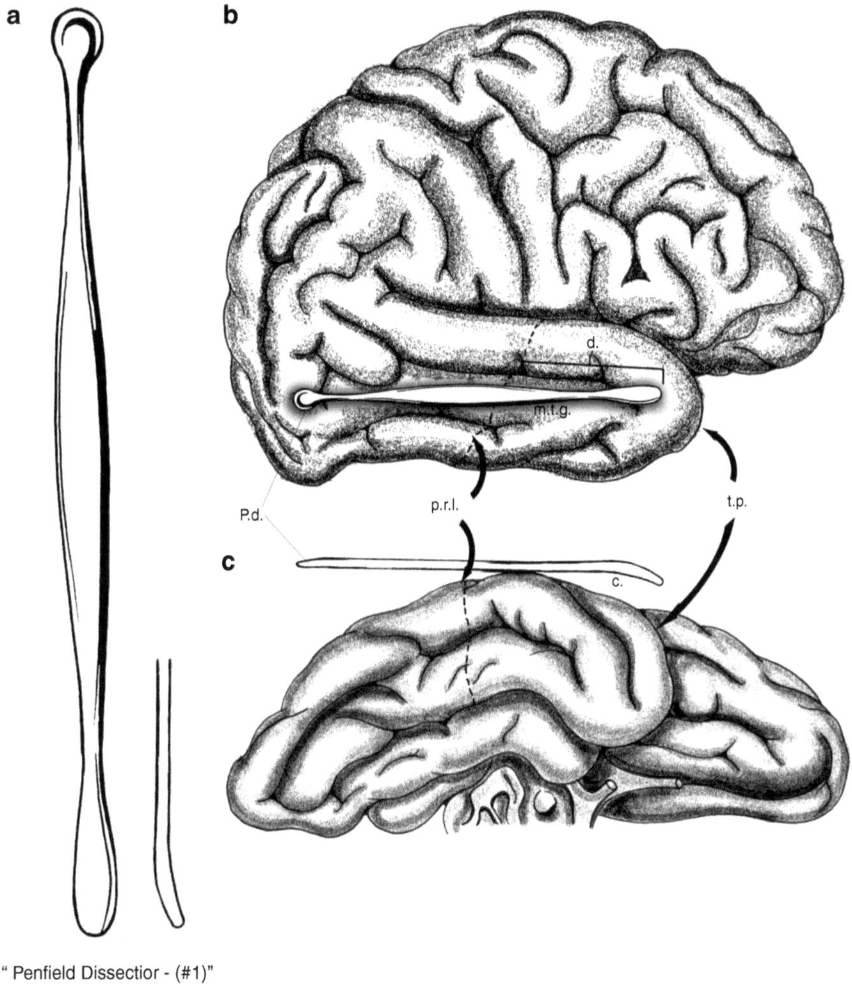

Fig. 2.9 The use of the Penfield #1 dissector to make measurements. The Penfield #1 dissector may be used to measure back (posteriorly) from the end of the dissector against a lateral part of the bony anterior wall of the middle cranial fossa to a given distance. The latter may include a number of functions (i.e., see text). (**a**) An illustration of the Penfield #1 dissector. (**b**) An illustration of the lateral aspect of the right temporal lobe and the dissector lying anteroposteriorly along the middle temporal gyrus. (**c**) An illustration of the inferior surface of the right temporal lobe, demonstrating the dissector laying across the lateral surface of the lobe. Note that the concave end of the dissector is facedown against the cortex, that the axis of the stem of the dissector is as parallel as possible to the surface of the temporal cortex, and that the dissector does not actually reach the tip of the temporal (lobe) pole, i.e., the most anterior aspect of the middle fossa. *P.d.* Penfield #1 dissector, *c.* concavity of the dissector, *m.t.g.* middle temporal gyrus, *d* distance between a given location (in this case the p.r.l.) and the tip of the dissector, *p.r.l.* posterior resection line, *t.p.* tip of the temporal lobe

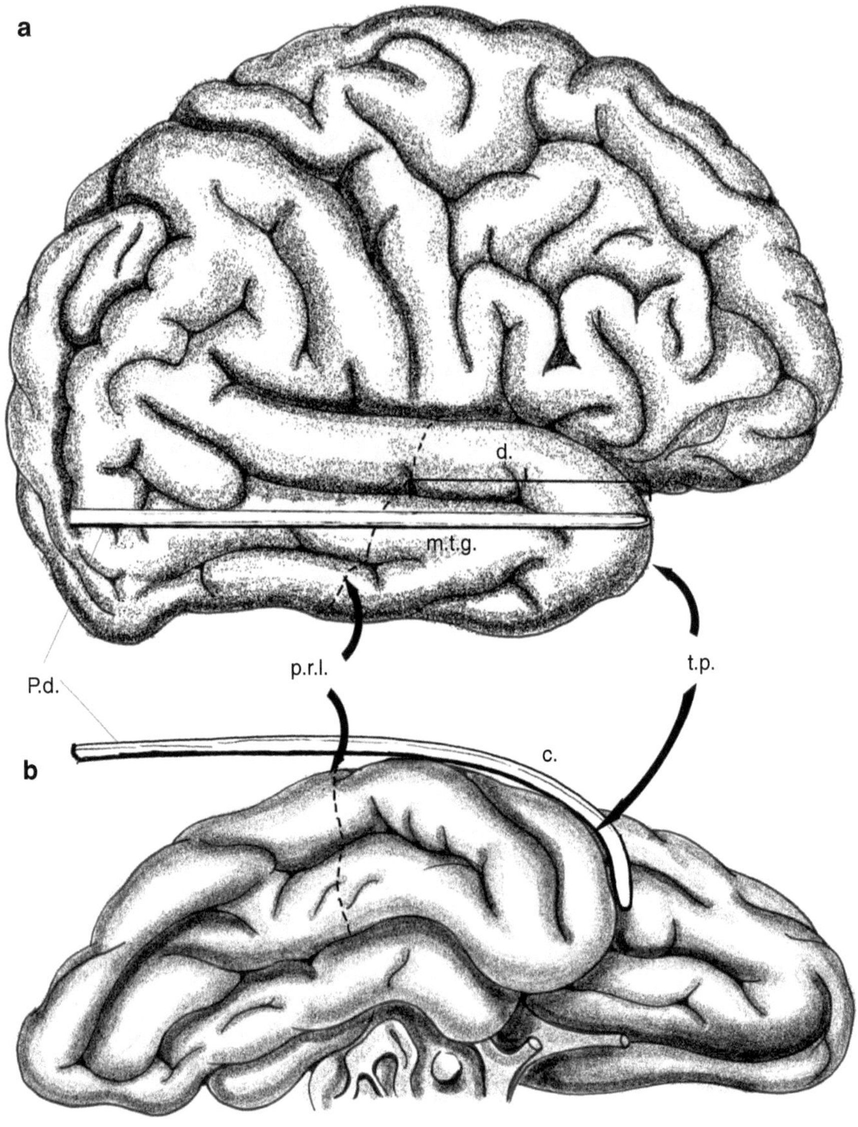

Fig. 2.10 Measurements of functional cortical localization with a red rubber catheter. The use of a pediatric urinary (#8) catheter for identifying the various distances from the poles of the cerebral lobes to the locations of functional cortical areas or to determine the location of the placement of the appropriate distances of the *safe* surgical resection lines from the tips of the poles of the lobes. In this particular case, the diagrams of the lateral (**a**) and inferior (**b**) surfaces of the right temporal lobe are depicted, much as had been shown in Fig. 2.9b, c, using the Penfield #1 dissector. *m.t.g.* middle temporal gyrus, *d* distance between a given location (in this case the p.r.l.) and the tip of the dissector, *p.r.l.* posterior resection line, *r.r.c.* red rubber catheter, *t.p.* tip of the temporal pole (e.g., anterior extent of the middle cranial fossa)

2.4 The Mandatory Bimanual Instrumental Use!

"You can't be a basketball player unless you can use both hands!" That expletive is the one that I have used monotonously during the training of many residents. In my own experience, the majority of fellows who came to London (usually to spend time with Dr. Drake and hence had been trained elsewhere, i.e., those who had not been subject to my harassment during the course of their residency training!) became intent on using one hand or another for handling particular instruments. The instruments that often fell into this category were coagulation forceps, the suction cannula, or micro-dissectors.

I believe that during subpial dissection the instrument used for retracting cerebral parenchyma should *always* be directed against that parenchyma that is being removed, not that which is to be left behind at the termination (as outlined in Subsect 2.2.4). In carrying out a linear subpial dissection of significant length, there will usually be a reversal, or reversals, in direction during the completion of the dissection. In this situation, if the instruments are not changed from one hand to the other, then the functions of the instruments, remaining the same, will be reversed in which case the instrument which is most likely to injure the parenchyma will end up, in one direction or another, being in contact with the parenchyma which is to be left behind—healthy. The instrument with which I have the most concern being in contact with the parenchyma to be left is the suction cannula, which will not have a cottonoid patty at its end when sucking away parenchyma. I realize that this may seem somewhat anal (!), but it is sad to see the cannula taking significant bites of tissue from what is to be left as healthy functioning parenchyma; it is even worse if the suction force has been elevated to an unnecessary level.

References

Girvin JP. Chapter 11. Temporal lobectomy. In: Apuzzo MLJ, editor. Neurosurgical aspects of epilepsy. American Association of Neurological Surgeons; 1992. p. 157–70.

Horsley V. Brain-surgery. Br Med J. 1886;2:670–5.

Horsley V. Ten consecutive cases of operation upon the brain and cranial cavity to illustrate the details and safety of the method employed. Br Med J. 1887;1:863–5.

Penfield W. The epilepsies: with a note on radical therapy. N Engl J Med. 1939;221:209–18.

Penfield W. Bilateral frontal gyrectomy and postoperative intelligence. Chapter XXIII – symposium on gyrectomy, part 1. Res Publ Ass Nerv Ment Dis. 1947;27:519–34.

Penfield W, Baldwin M. Temporal lobe seizures and the technique of subtotal temporal lobectomy. Ann Surg. 1952;136:625–34.

Penfield W, Evans J. The frontal lobe in man: a clinical study of maximum removals. Brain. 1935;58:115–33.

Sachs E. The subpial resection of the cortex in the treatment of Jacksonian Epilepsy (Horsley operation) with observations on areas 4 and 6. Brain. 1935;58:492–503.

Steelman HF. Technique of cortical excision: an experimental study of postoperative cicatrization. Arch Neurol Psychiatr. 1949;62:479–92.

Surgery Under Local Anesthesia 3

3.1 Philosophy of the "Traditional" Use of Local Anesthesia

The beginning of epilepsy surgery in the English-speaking world was largely the result of the simultaneous establishments of abiding interests in the surgical treatment of epilepsy in Chicago and Montreal in the middle third of the twentieth century. The Montreal school (Montreal Neurological Institute, McGill University) initiated the use of local anesthesia in operations associated with the removal of epileptogenic foci. The rationale underlying the abiding interest that the Montreal school developed for the use of local anesthesia is exemplified in an observation of Penfield, who noted that when he and Foerster (Foerster and Penfield 1930) began conducting radical excisions for the treatment of focal epilepsy, large parts of the dominant hemisphere were considered "forbidden territory," because of the concern of producing dysphasia (Penfield and Roberts 1959, p.103). He noted that "a method of *mapping the speech cortex* by using electrical interference on the surface at the time of operation" was developed at this time. He went on to indicate that experience with the mapping was responsible in part for "the growing ability to predict speech area limits …" (p. 104). It is a combination of experiences such as this that has given rise to the knowledge of the localization of function in the human cerebral cortex.

Quite irrespective of the location of the epileptic focus, the use of local anesthesia became the standard in Montreal. The Montreal school was so prolific in the training of epileptologists and epilepsy surgeons during the middle of the twentieth century that the use of local anesthesia became a standard at the institutions to which their trainees became attached. Its use was not only a standard at the MNI, but as a result it also became the standard at the majority of surgical institutions worldwide. Because of this and the worldwide influence of the Montreal school, the use of local anesthesia became synonymous with epilepsy surgery, over the early and middle parts of the twentieth century. This synonymy was not seriously challenged until the latter part of the last (twentieth) century.

J.P. Girvin, *Operative Techniques in Epilepsy*,
DOI 10.1007/978-3-319-10921-3_3

The challenge to the practice of carrying out epilepsy surgery under local anesthesia became more understandable in the face of a number of rather important advances, which have evolved over the course of some 50 years. These included (1) the increasing experience of surgery, which led to a reasonably standard operative technique, especially in the case of anterior temporal lobectomy (aTLY); (2) the increased knowledge of the pathology and the location of epileptic foci, underlying the seizures of temporal lobe origin, residing in the antero-infero-mesial structures; (3) the increasing lack of dependence upon the intraoperative electrocorticography (ECoG) for the determination of the epileptic focus; (4) the remarkable improvement in identifying small morphological abnormalities through the continually improving medical imaging and the associated correlations between these and the electrographically identified epileptic foci; (5) the rather striking improvements in general anesthesia and neuroleptanalgesia, which, even when intraoperative ECoG is necessary, fail to adversely affect the ECoG, as it did in the early and middle part of the twentieth century; and (6) the use of preoperatively implanted ECoG electrodes, which not only provide evidence of localized epileptogenic discharges but also allow the preoperative electrocortical stimulation, which may provide the necessary functional localization to carry out the eventual operation satisfactorily under general anesthesia.

Why did the use of local anesthesia become such an integral part of epilepsy surgery in Montreal? Probably the primary reason was the dependence of the intraoperative ECoG for the localization of epileptic foci, in the early part of the twentieth century, and the concern of the effect of general anesthesia on the ECoG. The authenticity of this view was derived from a number of observations. Without going into a detailed bibliography in this regard, a single example will suffice. Burns, in 1951, showed the reduction of excitability of electrographic activity in isolated slabs of feline cortex with *any* general anesthetic. Pasquet noted the deleterious effects of general anesthesia on the ECoGs of patients undergoing operations for epilepsy (1954). In the latter part of the century, there was a strong advocacy against this notion. However, as noted in the foregoing, apparently the improvements in general anesthetic agents have considerably reduced the deleterious effects of general anesthesia on the quality of the ECoG, and, as also noted, this has provided a more justified current challenge to the use of local anesthesia than many years ago.

While the use of local anesthesia is considered by some to be unnecessary, there is also a notion by some individuals that it leads to less satisfactorily achievable qualities of outcome. The reason given for this view is that when patients are awake there are possible restraints placed upon the surgeon as a result of potential discomfort of the patient (Wyler and Hermann 1988). Nevertheless, there is much to be said about the importance of the observations that have been made possible from its use in human patients. There is no doubt that its use in all patients undergoing surgery for the management of epilepsy cannot be justified by simple reference to its historical importance. On the other hand, there is similarly no doubt that in a small portion of operations, at least, it is mandatory (see below) in order to take advantage of the best surgical license. Whereas it is not necessary in most temporal lobectomies and

Table 3.1 Patients in whom satisfactory operative procedures under local anesthesia are difficult to achieve

Mentally retarded
Insufficient behavioral maturity (e.g., <9–11 years of age)
Pathological anxiety and/or claustrophobia

certainly not in the nondominant lobectomies, it is necessary in operations close to, or within, those areas of the cortex, which might be inadvertently injured without the certain knowledge of the location and the function of the juxtaposed cortex involved in the surgery.

The proponents of the use of local anesthesia point out that the many, many observations made from stimulation of the human brain under conditions of awake patients have been of inestimable importance to our understanding of the functional localization within the human neocortex. One of the legacies of these observations is the markedly enhanced appreciation of the safe limits of surgical resection of the cortex. The proponents will also point out that the ease of conducting operations under local anesthesia, when they become necessary, is markedly enhanced when the operating room team has carried out such operations relatively routinely. Finally, a further by-product of the use of local anesthesia is the training of operating room nurses, technicians, young anesthetists, and young surgeons in its characteristics, which then allows them to return to their institutions with comfortable roles in the practice. The latter has certainly been the case at our institution (the University of Western Ontario), where many such individuals in all these disciplines have been so trained over many years. The proper training of operating room teams in the use of local anesthesia in neurosurgical operations also usually results in the likely *preclusion* of the procedure developing into a miniature three-ring circus on the occasions when the use of local anesthesia is required in their home institutions!

Let us return to the question of whether the use of local anesthesia is necessary. When is it necessary? If all of the above-noted advancements to the conduct of surgery under general anesthesia have been used, then perhaps it might be argued that it is nearly never necessary. However, the argument on the other side pertains to the confidence that the managing team has in these preoperative advances in safely conducting resective operations in the immediate vicinity of the important functional, i.e., *eloquent*, cortex. If this confidence is lacking in *any* way, then local anesthesia should be utilized, as surely there can be argument that the safety of the patient and the confidence in the surgical license of the operating surgeon are both significantly enhanced with the patient awake. In most such cases, the resections will involve those areas of the cortex associated with sensorimotor or speech function or the immediately adjacent cortex. This author would *always* use local anesthesia in these cases.

A discussion of the indications for the use of local anesthesia must be combined with references to those cases in which local anesthesia cannot commonly be utilized (see Table 3.1). There is an age below which local anesthesia simply cannot be employed, even in the face of what is determined to be a patient with optimal behavioral development. This age is usually in the early adolescence period, e.g., 10–12 years of age (see Girvin 1986a). I have had young children in the 9–10 year age group that I felt absolutely certain would be able to undergo satisfactory operations under local anesthesia, but most of the time I was disappointed with these attempts in this age group. Pasquet noted the difficulties with the satisfactory conduct of craniotomies under local anesthesia in this specific age group as early as 1954. The so-called wake-up procedures or the use of deep neuroleptanalgesia has been advocated as appropriate alternatives, but in my hands these have never been entirely satisfactory and certainly never as satisfactory as the crisply carried out, routine awake operations in the appropriately chosen cases. However, in making that statement, it is probably very important to consider the fact that nearly all such procedures many years ago were carried out with barbiturate drugs, especially sodium pentothal, as opposed to the current, much more advantageous, use of intravenous propofol, a short-acting, nonbarbiturate sedative agent (Diprivan™: *di*iso*pr*opyl *IV an*esthetic).

Other potential patients in whom the use of local anesthesia may be difficult are those in the category of the mentally retarded. In the case of a mentally retarded patient, the judgment of the operating team, on an individual basis, is an important opinion with respect to whether the use of local anesthesia is likely to be satisfactorily achieved. It is worth mentioning that this can be a very, very difficult consultative opinion by which to reach certainty, as it is remarkably surprising how well some such patients do under local anesthesia, when the initial view is that a satisfactory operation almost certainly could not be achieved without general anesthesia. However, this is the exception, not the rule. Finally, there is a small group of patients who, because of the inability to deal with the envisioned anxiety and/or claustrophobia surrounding the operation, simply cannot reach an appropriate level of preparedness. In order to minimize the possibility of the latter, the draping of the patient is of major significant consequence (see Sect. 3.4).

Finally, reference will be made to other alternative strategies to this more *traditional* method of achieving the advantages of an awake patient under local anesthesia (*vide infra*, Sect. 3.9).

3.2 Preparation of the Patient

The most important preparatory undertaking in advance of a neurosurgical operation to be undertaken with the patient awake is indeed the *preparation of the patient*, per se. The appropriate preparation of the patient facilitates the surgeon's conduct of the surgery, facilitates the anesthetist's and nurses' responsibilities in the operating room, and facilitates the reduction of the normal apprehension and stress of the patient during the procedure. All of these contribute significantly to the ease of obtaining a good-quality operation. Penfield taught that hesitation on the part of the patient to undergo such an operation is probably sufficient to defer the operation (1954).

What is the *appropriate preparation*? This has been discussed in detail elsewhere (Girvin 1986a) and will be briefly reviewed in the following. In general terms, it is the achievement of a somewhat intangible cognitive and psychological preparedness. It is most important to provide the necessary communication and reassurance that guarantees that the patient understands *fully* the sequential steps of the procedure, particularly with respect to when he/she may or may not be uncomfortable, and that the whole team is there for one reason—the combination of both the comfort of the patient and the discharge of the individual responsibilities of the team that guarantee the best possible final outcome of the surgery. My own practice is to tell the patient that no matter how important he/she might have perceived to be in other situations, he/she is the most important individual in the operating room on that day. It is easily worth the time that it takes to educate the patients with respect to the anatomy and the pain sensitivity of the structures associated with the operation, e.g., scalp, cranium, periosteum, and meninges, and to advise them as to when these structures are likely to be involved in the operative sequence. In this education, it is important to let them know that the brain tissue, per se, is *not* associated with pain. (Although the manipulation and cauterization of brain tissue can very occasionally cause discomfort, this is so very, very rare that it does not demand the necessity of a discussion of its possibility!)

The patients should be told that the injections of local anesthetic will be done with a very fine needle such that they may not feel the penetration of the skin from the needle, that they will feel the injection of the local anesthetic per se, that all the injections will take no more than a very few minutes (usually no more than two or three), and that the majority of any discomfort they might feel will be over once the injections have been made. [This is certainly not always true of the operations in the middle fossa, e.g., anterior temporal lobectomy (aTLY), but I have nevertheless indicated such!] This is particularly true with pure central craniotomies when it is uncommon to feel any further discomfort after the scalp injections.

This practice of communication continues throughout the operation. The biggest reason for failure to achieve satisfactory operations under local anesthesia is the failure to continually warn the patient about *every* possible procedural event that may be associated with discomfort, physical movements of the head, or potentially mechanically disturbing auditory signals. The latter may be no more than the painless use of a curette or rongeurs to trim bone or an air drill producing holes in the bone. The risk of the absence of this constant communication in a patient who is tense, waiting with fear for the next perception of unannounced sudden pain or the sudden crunching of bone, can be catastrophic. Thus, *every* time bone is to be rongeured, the patient should be told "you are going to hear some crunching of bone, but it will not hurt you … coming … now!" Once patients become aware that everything is announced beforehand, regarding what they might hear or feel, they will relax and be much less anxious participants.

The importance of compassionate anesthetists and nurses, rounding out the operating room team, can similarly not be overemphasized. The fundamentals of compassion and full communication remain the important behavioral characteristics of *all* members of the team. This will be continually reemphasized throughout this monograph. It is a feeling of accomplishment when the day arrives when the surgeon is aware and appreciative that the combination of the anesthetist and the operating room nurses/technologists has, as a matter of course, simply taken over the prime role of making certain that the patient, in turn, is comfortable and engaged as part of the team.

3.3 The Preoperative Use of Local Anesthesia

3.3.1 The Local Anesthetic Agent

Historically, local anesthesia was carried out through the use of what is now considered to be short-acting anesthetics, e.g., Xylocaine. These anesthetics lasted for varying times, ranging from 90 min to 3 or 4 h. Thus, most operations required at least a further injection of the scalp in the event of any prolonged operations and nearly always during the closure. This was time consuming, labor intensive, and emotionally difficult for both patient and surgeon. The introduction of bupivacaine hydrochloride (Marcaine™) in the 1960s changed this considerably and, together with the increasing number of good neuroleptanalgesic agents, utilized by experienced anesthetists, should be given the credit for the current much more satisfactory surgery under local anesthesia than any other factor. It also makes one look back with admiration upon the original surgeons and their patients who labored with what might be considered now as seemingly rather inhumane practices in the early part of the twentieth century.

3.3.2 The Initial (Preoperative) Regional Anesthetic Blockade

The author's methodology in the use of local anesthesia has been reported elsewhere for epileptic operations (Girvin 1986a) and for operations not necessarily associated with epilepsy (Girvin 1986b) but will be reviewed here. The use of a 0.5 % solution of bupivacaine hydrochloride with 1:200,000 epinephrine for regional blockade will normally last for something of the order of 8–10 h. The recommendation is to conduct regional scalp blocks a couple of hours prior to the scheduled time of the operation. Injecting the local anesthesia well before the operation provides the ability to carry this out in a private setting, rather than in the operating theater, per se, where many of the operating room teams are streaming around in carrying out their preparations. When it is conducted in a more private environs, the patient is much more at ease, is in a more comfortable position for the injections (e.g., on a bed or stretcher, rather than the operating table in the OR), and is past the time of the majority of the discomfort when arriving in the OR, and there is far less reason to hurry in any way! Further, this early preoperative injection, using a fine #25 gauge needle, given 2 or more hours beforehand, minimizes the already very minimal risk of bupivacaine toxicity. (For an 8 a.m. start, I injected the scalp at 6–6:30 a.m.)

Figure 3.1a, b discloses, respectively, the courses of the five nerves that innervate the scalp and the sites of injections which bring about satisfactory anesthetic blockades of the areas of innervation. For the normal adult, 20 ml of the anesthetic agent (0.5 % bupivacaine) is utilized, which allows 3–5 ml to be used for each of the scalp nerves to be blocked. The five nerves responsible for the innervation of the scalp are as follows:

The *greater occipital n.* is often farther lateral than is usually thought to be the case. It is approximately half way between the mastoid process and the inion. It can often be easily localized by the appreciation of a palpatory depression just below the nuchal line, which is the site of emergence of the nerve through the deep fascia. Localization is further enhanced by the application of pressure to this point, which usually results in unusual discomfort, often with a burning component to the sensation, when compared with pressure applied to adjacent tissues.

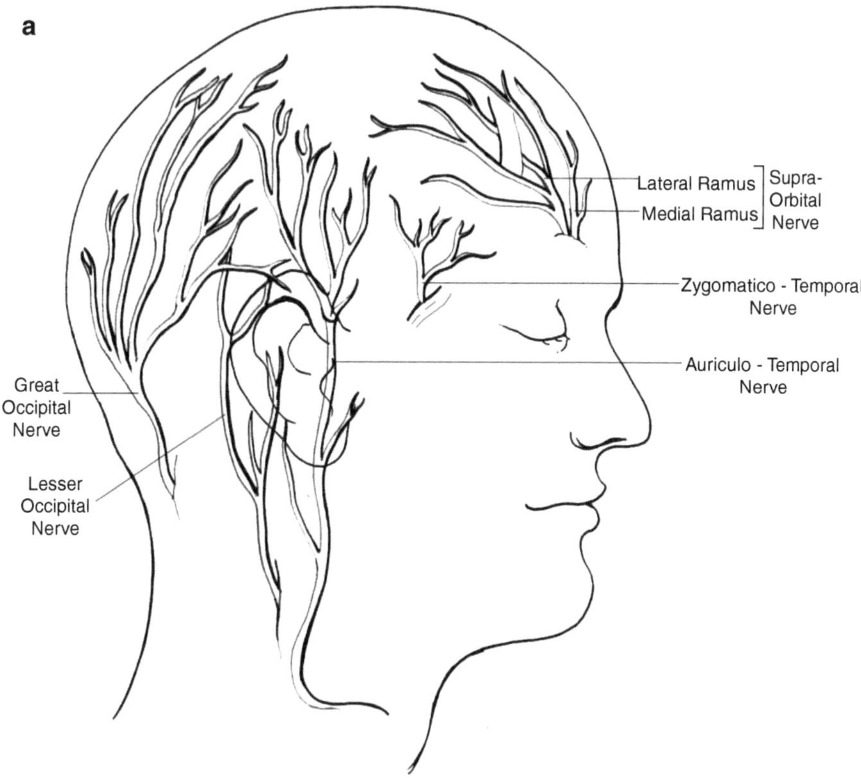

Fig. 3.1 The sites of injection for blockade of scalp nerves with local anesthetic. Illustrations depicting (**a**) the anatomical routes of the nerves innervating the scalp on the right side of the head, (**b**) the sites at which the injections of local anesthesia are conducted in order to achieve sensory blockades of the regional areal innervations of the nerves, and (**c**) the expansion of the area covered with local anesthesia by alterations in the position of the needle during the injection, thus using only the single puncture of the scalp (Redrawn, with permission, from Girvin (1986a))

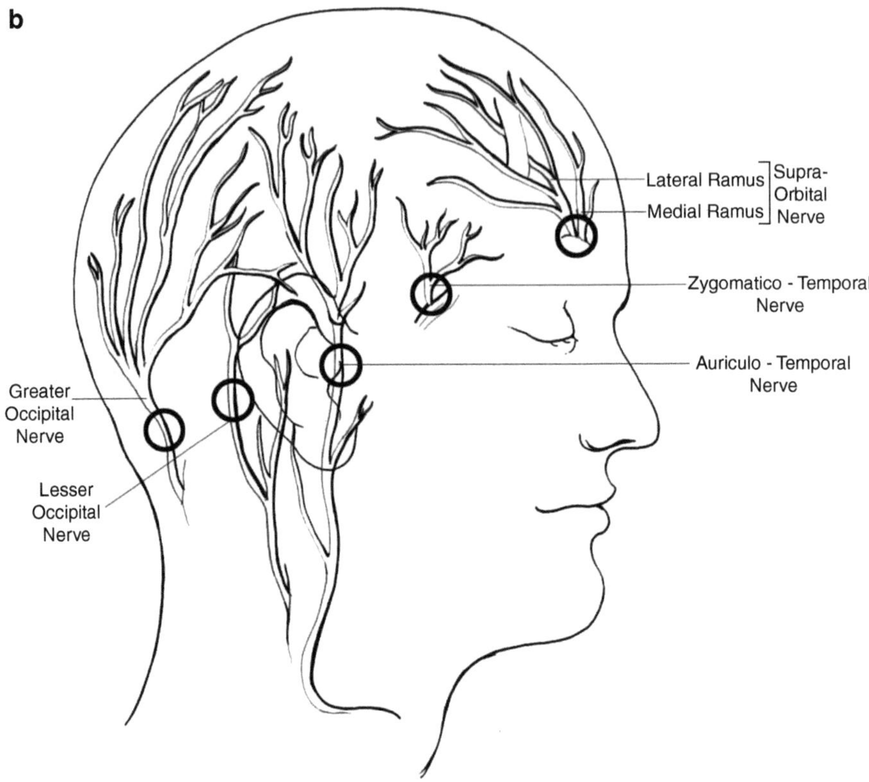

Fig. 3.1 (continued)

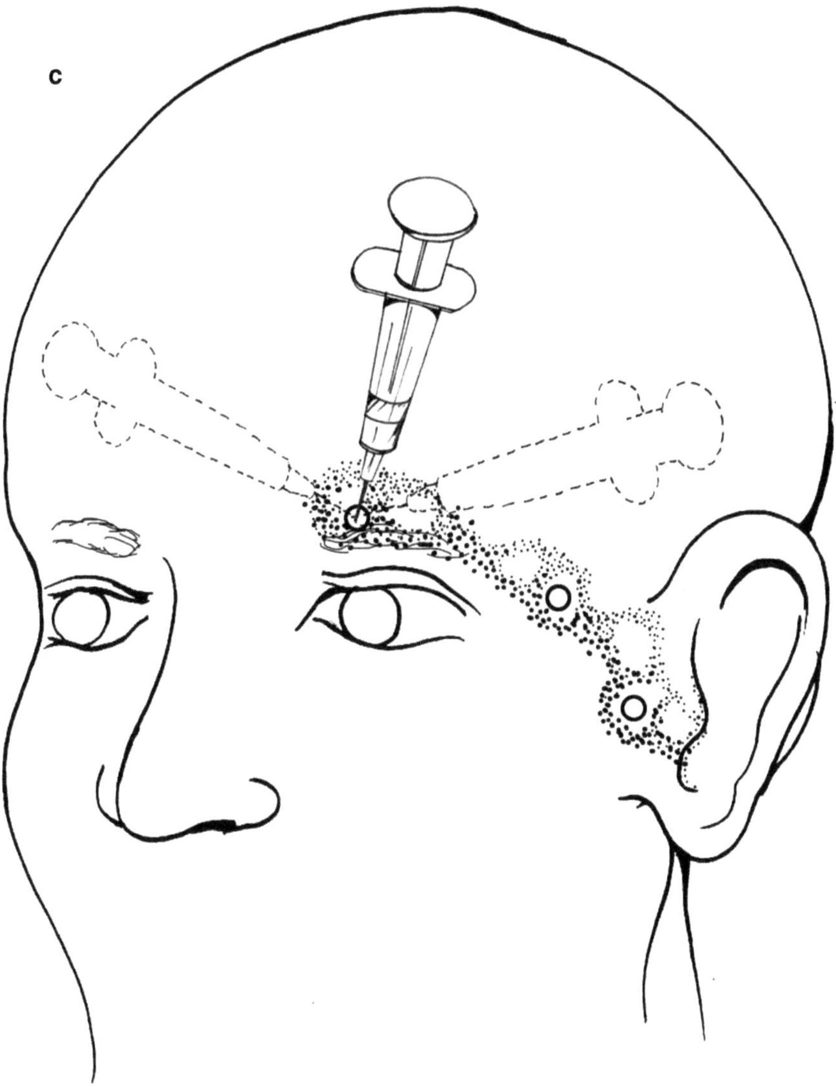

Fig. 3.1 (continued)

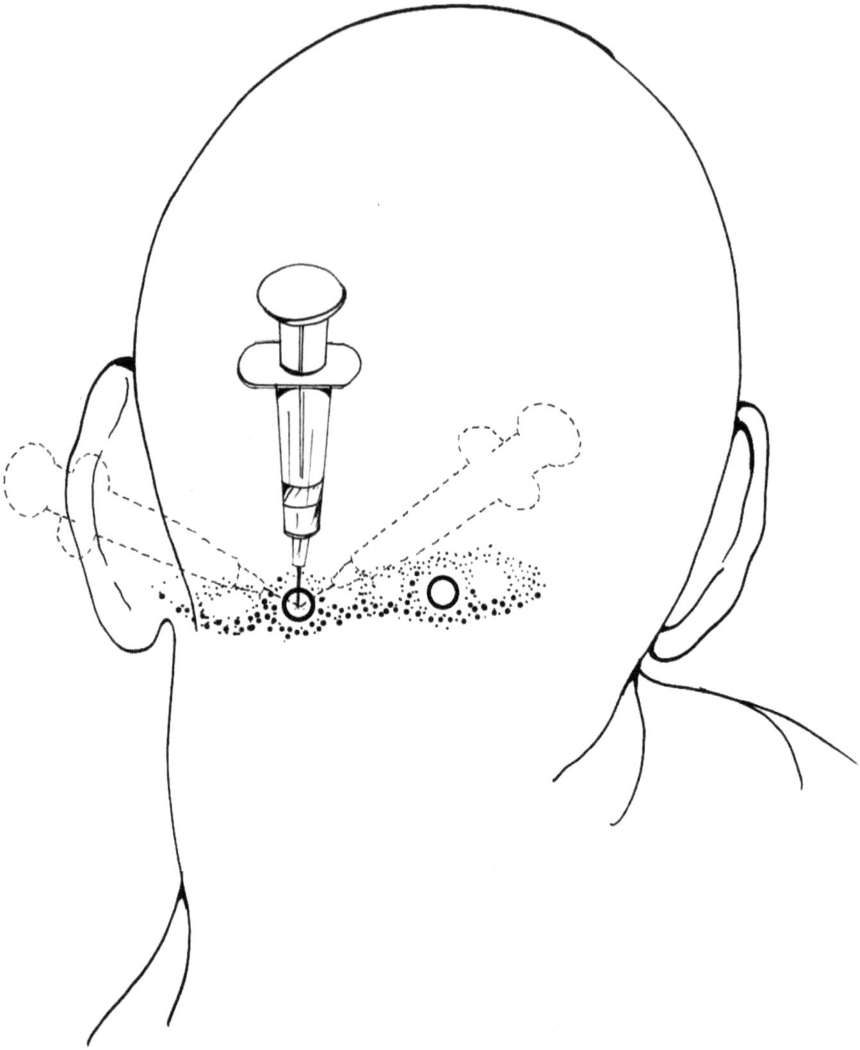

Fig. 3.1 (continued)

The *lesser occipital n.* and its branch, the *posterior auricular n.*, are located about 1 cm behind the base of the pinna. The anesthetic is injected in this location and then more anteriorly onto the base of the pinna.

The *auriculotemporal n.* is blocked by an injection just in front of the tragus of the ear. The primary site is on or just immediately above the zygoma and 0.5–1 cm in front of the tragus. It is one of the more painful injections, and the discomfort is reduced, as in most injections, by a very slow injection.

The *supraorbital n.* is just above the supraorbital notch of the orbital rim. It is left to the last, or nearly the last, of the injections, as it is perhaps the most painful of the group of nerves. Once again better anesthetization is likely with alteration of the needle end laterally and medially, in addition to the primary site of injection.

The *zygomaticotemporal n.* is not uniformly situated such that it can be recognized easily. Further, it may be composed of a variety of smaller branches. It is effectively anesthetized by inserting the needle midway between the site of injection of the auriculotemporal n. and the lateral aspect of the orbital rim. Injections into the subcutaneous tissue and perhaps some temporalis musculature, which can be achieved by a single scalp puncture and the needle being directed as far as possible both posteriorly and anteriorly during the injection, result in satisfactory anesthesia. This injection is most important in the case of surgery of the temporal lobe. Further, this is supplemented when injecting the scalp incision (see Sect. 3.3.4).

I am also of the belief that movement of the small needle around, through the same scalp puncture, during the delivery of the anesthetic in *all* of the injection sites is associated with a more satisfactory anesthetic blockade, as shown in Fig. 3.1c. This is particularly the case for the zygomaticotemporal nerve, as this tends to be more diffuse and more difficult to localize, but perhaps of more importance it tends to innervate the base of the scalp that is to be reflected.

My preference with respect to the order of the conduct of the various nerve blocks is starting with the least painful blocks. While there is nearly no discomfort using the small #25 gauge needle, there is discomfort associated with the flow of the anesthetic agent into the subcutaneous tissues. Thus, beginning with the injection, which is the least likely to produce pain, is easiest for the patient. Interestingly, once they are told and realize that they do not feel the needle puncture, they then nearly always have less concern when they learn that it is the anesthetic that produces the discomfort. Why does the patient react in this way? I have no idea, but it is true! Thus, for example, in the local anesthesia for an aTLY (anterior temporal lobectomy), my routine has been to block the greater occipital nerve first and to then move forward through the lesser occipital, auriculotemporal, and zygomaticotemporal nerves and lastly the supraorbital nerve.

It might also be mentioned that in most cases where the times of the lengths of operations are much less than 8–10 h, the local regional blocks are usually still complete into the early postoperative period and thus provide analgesia in that period, in addition to whatever further local anesthesia is utilized during the operative procedure.

3.3.3 The Local Anesthetic Blockade of Individual Scalp Nerves

Table 3.2 outlines the nerves, the blockades of which may be necessary for satisfactory anesthetization of the various craniotomy operative sites. For any given craniotomy, those nerves to be blocked with local anesthetic depend upon the location of the craniotomy site. The table outlines in the initial column the various craniotomy sites and in the middle column is a list of those ipsilateral nerves that usually require blockade for satisfactory narcotization of the scalp that is to be incised for the

Table 3.2 The nerves requiring anesthetic blockade for different craniotomies

	Nerves to be blocked (local anesthetic)	
Site of craniotomy	Ipsilateral	Contralateral
Frontal	Supraorbital Auriculotemporal	? Supraorbital
Temporal	Supraorbital Auriculotemporal Zygomaticotemporal Lesser occipital ? Greater occipital	–
Parasagittal	Supraorbital Greater occipital	Supraorbital Greater occipital
Central (Rolandic)	Supraorbital Greater occipital ? Auriculotemporal ? Greater occipital	? Supraorbital ? Greater occipital
Occipital	Greater occipital Lesser occipital	Greater occipital

craniotomy in question. In the far right column is a list of the nerves on the other (contralateral) side of the head that might require narcotization even though not on the side of the identified craniotomy (see question marks).

In the case of craniotomies that might require some visualization of midline parenchyma, e.g., frontal, occipital, superior central, or parasagittal craniotomies, both sides of the midline usually require anesthetization. Question marks are placed in front of those nerves which may or may not be required in a given craniotomy incision, depending upon its size and the extent of its periphery. For example, in the case of the frontotemporal craniotomy, one may choose to use a scalp flap, which is taken posteriorly above the ear, in which case the lesser occipital nerve will require anesthetic blockade and even possibly the greater occipital nerve if the whole of the temporal lobe is to be exposed, e.g., to 9 cm behind the pole of the lobe. Similarly, the frontotemporal craniotomy may require exposure of the parasagittal parenchyma, thus requiring anesthetization of the contralateral supraorbital nerve. Another pertinent example is the case of the *central* (Rolandic) craniotomy, requiring only exposure of the Rolandic cortex of the head and arm area. In this case, often the auriculotemporal and lesser occipital nerves do not require blocking, and only very rarely would there be a necessity to block the contralateral nerves, e.g., the medial part of the craniotomy is usually well below (lateral to) the midline.

3.3.4 The Anesthetic Blockade of the Scalp Incision

It has been the routine of this author to use bupivacaine in the proposed scalp incision once the latter has been sterilized with povidone-iodine, i.e., *prior to the final surgical draping*. Using the pinprick exploration of the craniotomy site with a fine

Table 3.3 The amount of local anesthesia used for the blockade of the scalp nerves

Blockade (bupivacaine HCl)	%	Volume (ml)	Amount (mg)
Regional nerves	0.5	20	100
Scalp incision	0.33	60	~200
Total	–		300

hypodermic needle will verify the extent of the earlier preoperative regional blocks and will provide the opportunity to recognize scalp that is incompletely narcotized and to complete the remainder of the preoperative injections of the local anesthetic in the incision line. It is easier to do it at this stage, when the appropriate surface is most easily visualized. Additionally, it allows time for the bupivacaine hydrochloride (1) to diffuse in the tissues before the scalp incision is actually made, (2) to exert its vasoconstrictive effect before the incision of the scalp, and (3) to be injected into the surrounding scalp into which sutures are used to sew the drapes in place. In the normal adult, 60 ml of a 0.33 % solution with 1:200,000 adrenaline is used in the scalp.

3.3.5 The Quantity of Local Anesthetic Used

Table 3.3 outlines the quantity and concentrations that I have used since the introduction of bupivacaine hydrochloride. There is rarely a necessity for the use of more than these suggested values of the anesthetic agent, but based on my own personal experience, there is certainly a significant safety factor in using more than these quantities, which, incidentally, adds to the advantage of carrying out the regional blockades 2–3 h before the scheduled onset of the operation.

The use of 0.33 % solution for the scalp narcotization is purely arbitrary. It was made up of two (20 ml) bottles of 0.25 % and one bottle of 0.5 % bupivacaine hydrochloride, all with 1:200,000 epinephrine. I started using this solution of Marcaine purely arbitrarily when it was first introduced and since I found it to be so satisfactory, and without ever having experienced any adverse side effects, I have not altered the concentrations, in spite of the fact that I suspect that the use of a 0.25 % solution may be just as efficient.

3.4 Draping of the Patient

The patient is placed on a bed of pillows, or on a very thick mattress of good-quality sponge rubber, in the lateral position on the operating table for most operations. The head is placed on a good adjustable sponge rubber headrest. Additional pillows are placed behind the patient, wedged in between the fixed, restraining fence of the table and between the patient's knees. Often a further one to two pillows are placed in front of the patient such that the upside arm can be comfortably rested on them during the procedure. This is illustrated in Fig. 3.2.

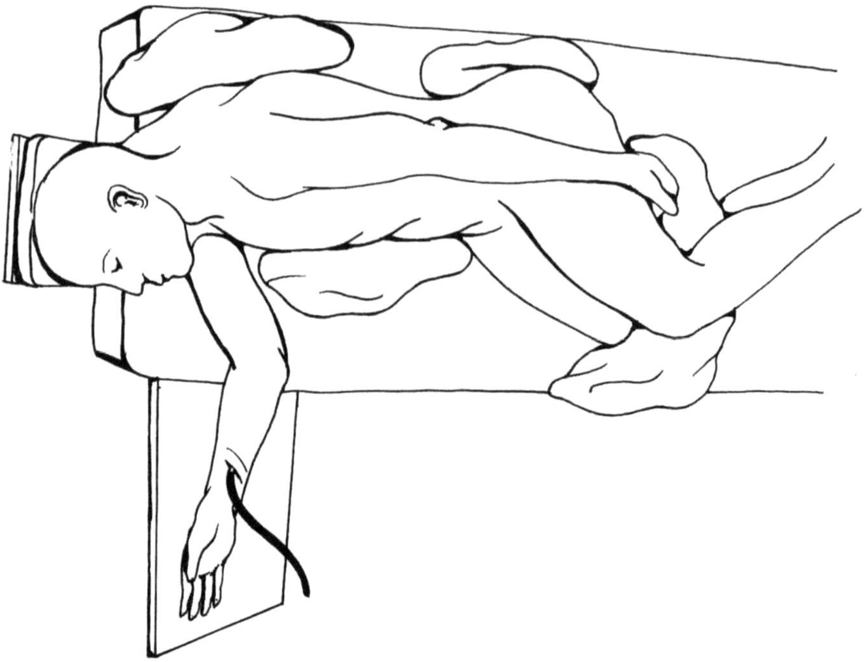

Fig. 3.2 Illustration of a *pillowed* position, which provides satisfactory comfort for patients under local anesthesia. Illustrates the lateral *pillowed* position of the patient on the operating table

The appropriate draping of the patient may in fact play the most important role, or even a more important role than the pillows, in achieving a comfortable and cooperative patient. The drapes should be positioned such as to provide the greatest view out into the operating room (see Fig. 3.3). The actual view, per se, is not as important as the *size* of the view, i.e., the window of outlook or what I call the *port*, and the proximity of it to the patient's face; both are important in precluding an enhancement of any claustrophobic tendency. Claustrophobic patients, hidden under drapes, in dark holes, with little *breathing room* are patients whose operations have a high likelihood of not only being very unsatisfactory events but also of being discontinued under local anesthesia, which under some circumstances may lead to the discontinuation of the surgery, i.e., by the patient because of anxiety and claustrophobia or by the surgeon because of the necessity of the operation being carried out in an awake patient. Further, such robust window (*port*) facilitates the ease of communication between the operating room staff and the patient. There is nothing more distressing to the whole operating room team than to see such a patient in irreconcilable, irreversible claustrophobic panic. To continue the proposed operation under these circumstances, it can take as much as 30–60 min of readjusting the drapes and consoling and reassuring the patient, and in many cases, the local anesthesia, of necessity, has to be replaced with general anesthesia. Thus, the more the patient is *in* the operating room and feels part of the room, as opposed to simply presuming that the little bit of light that is seen at the end of a dark tunnel is the room, the more at ease will he/she be.

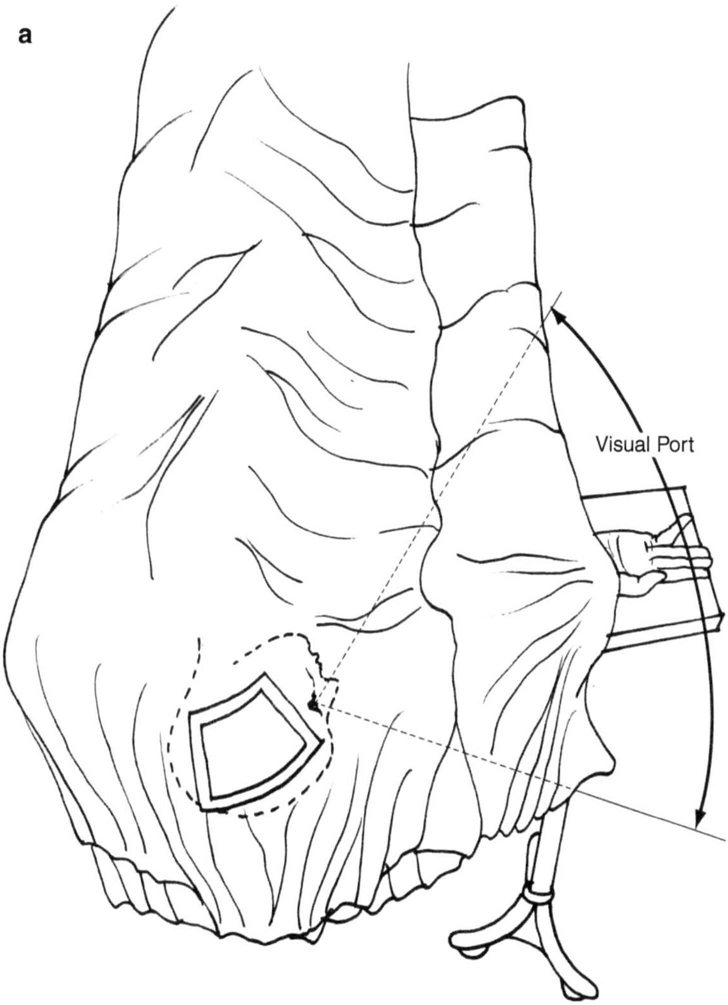

Fig. 3.3 The optimal visual port (window) under local anesthesia. (**a**) An illustration of an ideal *port*, or view, through which the patient can see after being draped for an operation under local anesthesia. The angle of the port should be made as wide (open) as possible, thus reducing the possibility of the patient experiencing *any* significant anxiety or claustrophobia. (**b**) An illustration of the *window* of the port through which the patient can see and communicate with the operating room staff

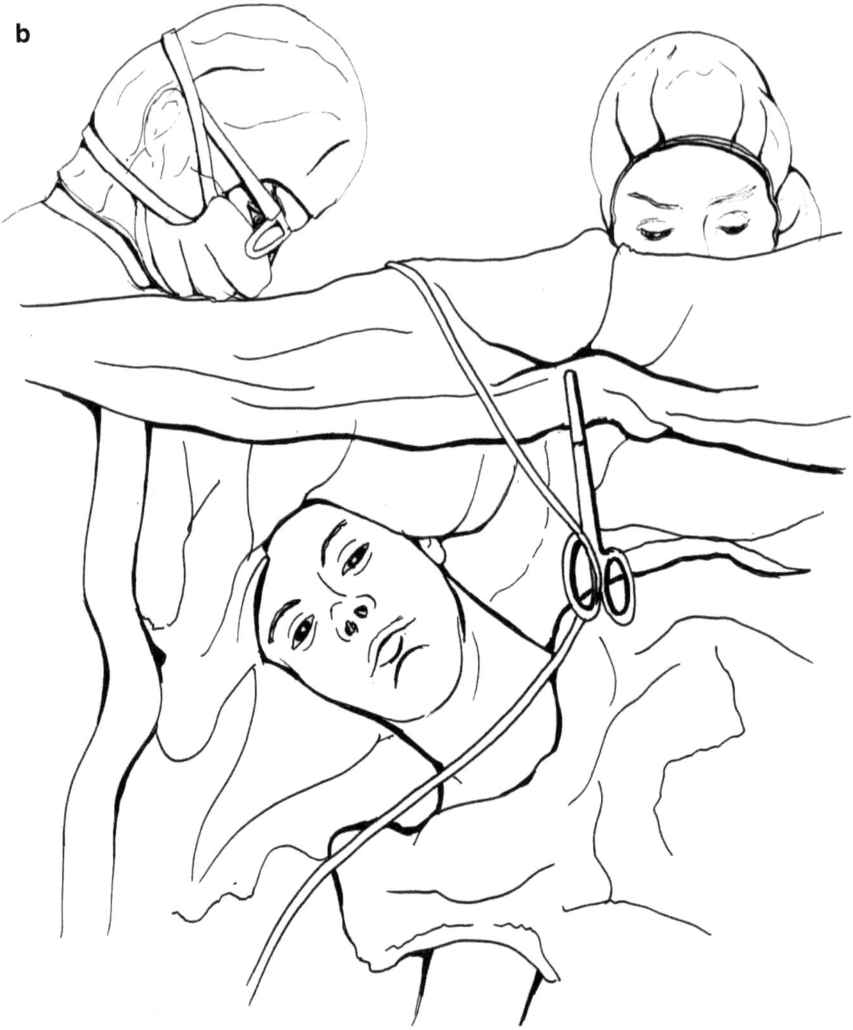

Fig. 3.3 (continued)

3.5 Intraoperative Comfort of the Patient

3.5.1 The Communication of the Operating Room Staff

The importance of the sensitivity of the whole operating room staff, including the surgeons, anesthetists, nurses, and technicians, cannot be overemphasized. The appreciation that all of the staff forms a communicative and collegial team provides confidence to the patient. This is particularly important in the case of the anesthetist, who is so very involved with the patient from moment to moment throughout the operation. The responsibility of the anesthetist is much more consuming under local anesthesia than under general anesthesia, which can lead to discomfort on the part of some anesthetists to engage in operations conducted under local anesthesia and neuroleptanalgesia. It is the frequent, sensitive, and casual communication of the team with the patient that makes the latter comfortable and with a sense of belonging. These may seem like perfectly natural and expected responsibilities. Indeed they are, but it is the experience of the staff as a result of the frequent use of local anesthesia that is so clearly evident and better, in contrast to literally similar individuals that have infrequent exposure to the same situations.

3.5.2 The Questionable Use of Urinary Catheters

Initially, my own practice was to insert a urinary catheter in all patients. After a few years and a few cases of cystitis, attributable to the catheterization, it was dropped in male patients, with the view that it was a simple matter of handing the male patient in the operating room a urinal. The very infrequent necessity to do this in the male patients led, after a few more years, to the practice of not catheterizing any patients. Indeed, after decades of this practice, there were no incidents that made us feel that one of the earlier practices should have been reinstituted. That is to say, it was only very, very infrequently that any patient, male or female, required the use of a urinal or bedpan. Part of the reason is likely also attributable to the fact that over time the usual operation was gradually shortened, ending up at 3–4 h.

3.5.3 The Use of Intraoperative Local Anesthesia

I suspect that any local anesthetic can be used intraoperatively between the leaflets of the dura mater. I initially used a mixture of 50 % each of 2 % Xylocaine (for immediate anesthetization) and 0.25 % bupivacaine. Because of the concern about getting epinephrine on the brain, I initially did not use epinephrine in the *intra*operative local anesthesia. I no longer believe that this rationale has any particular merit. The amount of anesthetic agent that will invariably get on the brain during the course of a temporal craniotomy is either sufficiently small or has no effect, as I have never witnessed anything that was of concern.

3.5.4 The Recognition of Intracranial Sources of Pain

The papers from the Montreal Neurological Institute represent very solid observations regarding the sources of pain that the surgeon may encounter in dealing with the intracranial contents in the awake patient (Penfield 1934, 1954; McNaughton 1937; Penfield and McNaughton 1940; Feindel 1954; Feindel et al. 1960). These are very helpful in the important understanding of the types of pain that might be described by patients and where the injections of the dura are likely to be most beneficial in reducing or abolishing the reported pain. There is uniform endorsement of the fact that pain is commonly associated with various types of injury when applied to the dura, e.g., heat, coagulation, electrical stimulation, stretching, etc. Penfield implied that stimulation or manipulation of the middle cerebral artery or its branches not infrequently resulted in pain (1954). While apparently others have witnessed this, I have *never*, in my own experience, *clearly* encountered such a response. On a couple of occasions, I have encountered what I thought might indeed have been discomfort from stimulation of large MCA branches, but it could not be predictably repeated (also *vide infra*, Sect. 3.5.4.1).

3.5.4.1 Questionable Pain from Cerebral Substance

Can pain be produced from injurious stimuli to the cerebral parenchyma? Penfield indicated that the insular cortex was the only area of which pial stimulation was painful, in approximately 50 % of patients, which he attributed to the branches of the middle cerebral artery (1954). Again, I must reiterate that this has certainly not been my personal experience. I believe that *in general* pain associated with stimulation of cerebral tissue, per se, does not occur. However, within this context, I have to once again note that on one or two instances, out of the conduction of thousands of such stimuli, I would have to challenge my dogma in this regard! In both cases, which resulted in significantly severe pain from electrocortical stimulation, using the routine stimulus parameters, e.g., frequency of 25–50 Hz, pulse durations of 500 μs, and train durations of 1–3 s. The initial observation of this was during the course of a dominant lateral occipital corticectomy. Stimulation was carried out in order to outline any primary occipital cortex that might be in the field of the demonstrated epileptogenic cortex. The stimulation over a very restricted area, approximately 1 spherical centimeter, resulted in the perception of rather intense pain in this very stoic individual. The response was reliably repeatable, easily separated from sham stimulations, only able to be produced from this very small area of the cortex, and unassociated with any vasculature under the stimulating electrode. In my view, this observation defied any intuitive, anatomical, or physiological bases of understanding. The other such case was similar.

3.5.4.2 Pain Innervation of the Basal Dura

Feindel, Penfield, and McNaughton in 1960 carried out an anatomical study of nerves innervating the dura in postmortem specimens and correlated these findings with observations of the clinical results of their local anesthetic blockades in patients undergoing surgery under local anesthesia (see also Penfield 1954). These observations have provided the most important information regarding the innervation of the dura. Nearly all the dura is innervated by the ophthalmic division of the trigeminal nerve, most certainly that dura with which the neurosurgeon might most likely be concerned, i.e., that of the supratentorial compartment. They described two sets of nerves—the *meningeal nerves* and the *tentorial nerves*. The former—the *meningeal nerves*—arise from the first division of the trigeminal nerve and follow the course of the middle meningeal arteries as perivascular plexuses. The latter—the *tentorial nerves*, so named by Arnold—also arise from the ophthalmic division of the trigeminal nerve and travel between the leaflets of the dura, forming a diffuse

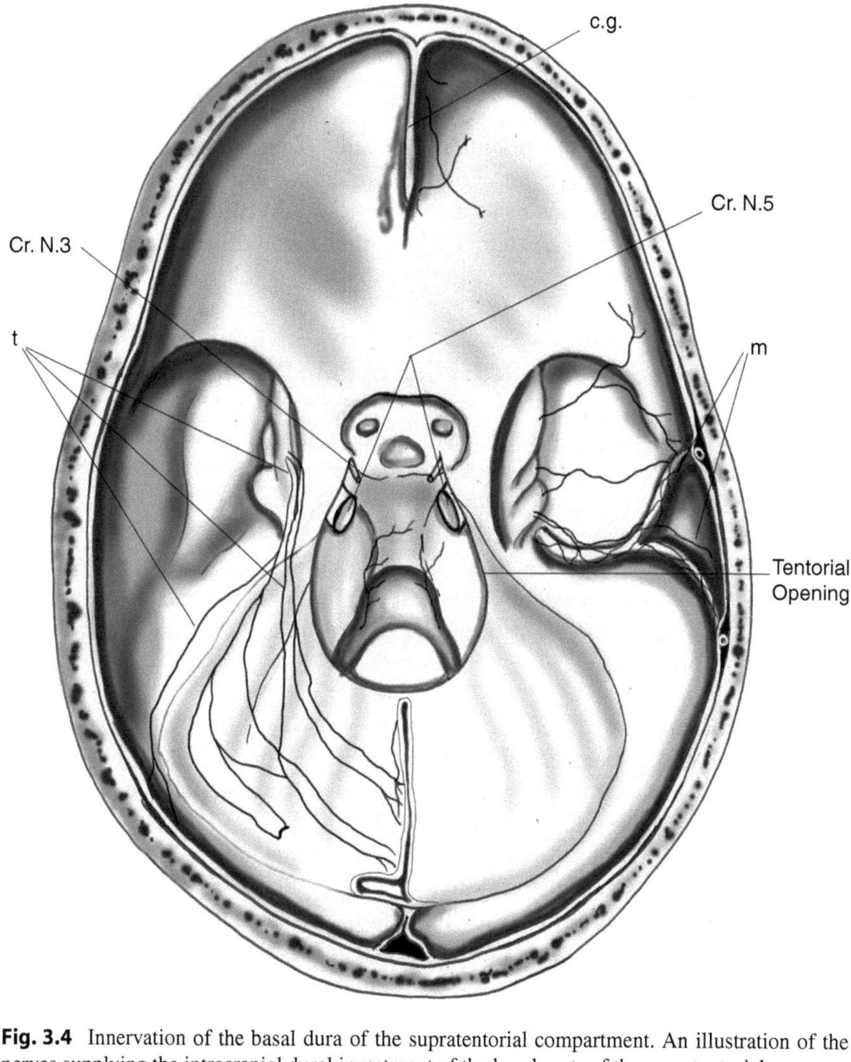

Fig. 3.4 Innervation of the basal dura of the supratentorial compartment. An illustration of the nerves supplying the intracranial dural investment of the basal parts of the supratentorial compartment of the cranium (see text). *c.g.* crista galli, *Cr.N.3* oculomotor nerve, *Cr.N.5* trigeminal nerve, *m* meningeal nerves, forming perivascular plexuses in association with the middle meningeal arterial vasculature, *t* tentorial nerves, forming a diffuse plexus within the dura (Redrawn, with permission, from Feindel et al. (1960))

plexiform innervation, coursing posteriorly and ending in large parts of the walls of the lateral and superior longitudinal dural sinuses, with particularly rich innervations around the terminal junctions of their cerebral venous contributions. Upon leaving the tentorium posteriorly, they course anteriorly in the falx cerebri, to at least the junction of its anterior and middle thirds. They also spread very meagerly over the dorsolateral dura where there is overlapping with the innervation of the meningeal nerves. These anatomical features are illustrated in Fig. 3.4.

Feindel and colleagues (1960) provided the clinical counterparts of their postmortem studies, which largely confirmed the predictions that might have been made from the anatomical observations. That is to say, injections of local anesthetic into areas proximal to the more distal areas of nervous innervation resulted in the abolition of the pain that prior to the injections could be produced by electrical and/or mechanical stimulation. From this reference and Fig. 3.4, the surgeon can visualize where injections of local anesthetic would be necessary in order to anesthetize the area of the basal dura that might be involved in different operative sites.

3.5.5 The Intraoperative Reduction of Pain During Craniotomy

The preoperative regional nerve blocks, the local infiltration of the craniotomy incision, the importance of appropriate draping of the patient, and the absolute necessity of continually talking to the patient have all been noted in the foregoing discussion. Any introduction of a consideration of reducing a patient's pain during the course of a craniotomy under local anesthesia should address all of these important preoperative and early intraoperative cares. They all reduce anxiety, which is a precursor to an uncomfortable patient, an eventual lack of cooperation, or even a state of claustrophobia.

3.5.5.1 Introduction

It is important to remember the generalization that dural pain is most likely encountered in the vicinity of the cranial base and the major venous sinuses (Penfield 1954). Within this generalization, there are some regional differences. The dura near the cranial base of the anterior part of the middle fossa at the sphenoid wing is the most sensitive region of the intracranial dura. This is depicted in Fig. 3.5 where the density of the stippling is proportional to the density of the pain endings and, consequently, the severity of the pain resulting from its electrical or mechanical stimulation. This area of which the pain endings are derived from the *meningeal nerves* associated with the meningeal arterial irrigation (perfusion) of the dura is much more extensive than the areas next to the venous sinuses. This is a most important recognition in the case of the craniotomy for a temporal lobectomy.

Thus, in the case of craniotomies in awake patients under local anesthesia, it is those closest to these anatomical structures that are most likely to require the most attention. This *attention* pertains to the continual awareness of the potential of the patient perceiving pain and the *necessity of talking to and warning* the patient with each maneuver associated with the removal of bone. Contrariwise, this same generalization is reflected in the fact that the typical *central* (Rolandic) craniotomy, involving only the middle of the dorsolateral dura, is the least painful of the whole group of craniotomies, i.e., it is relatively remote from *any* of the major venous

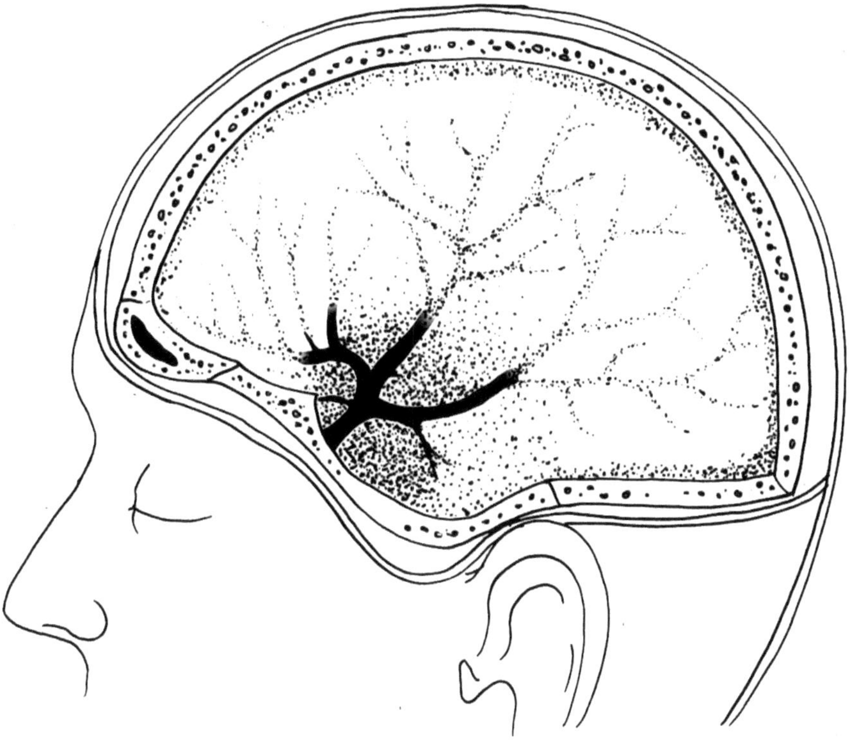

Fig. 3.5 Sources of dural pain (temporal region). Illustration of the sources of dural pain over the inferior aspect of the lateral temporal dura. The potential production of pain by electrical or mechanical stimulation of the dura is proportional to the darkness of the stippling. In contrast to the *tentorial* nerves, this is typical of the distribution of innervation of pain fibers from the *meningeal* nerves, i.e., the concentration of the innervation is inversely proportional to the distance from the artery (Redrawn, with permission, from Girvin (1986a))

sinuses, the base of the supratentorial compartment, and the vicinity of the major meningeal arteries.

3.5.5.2 Dural Injection Sites for Reducing Pain

Figure 3.6 is a series of diagrams that illustrate a series of clinical observations, demonstrating locations where electrical and/or mechanical stimulation (●●●) resulted in the production of pain and sites of injection of local anesthetic (✲✲), which abolished the pain. Knowledge of the innervation of the basal dura clearly allows the predictability of where local injections of anesthetic will most likely abolish pain from various sites, as noted in the paper of Feindel et al. (1960). Figure 3.6a, b shows examples taken directly from the observations of Feindel et al. Fig. 3.6c is simply an extension of what would be predicted from Fig. 38 (vide supra).

3.5.5.3 Referred Pain from Dural Stimulation

Knowledge of where pain, remote from the location of the dural stimulus, might be perceived is often helpful in determining the location from which it is arising (Penfield 1954). This is particularly the case when the pain occurs in the absence of specifically applied stimuli. For example, the actual location of referred pain arising as a result of specifically localizable stimuli is primarily academic, as its precise location allows the relatively easily recognized area to which application of local

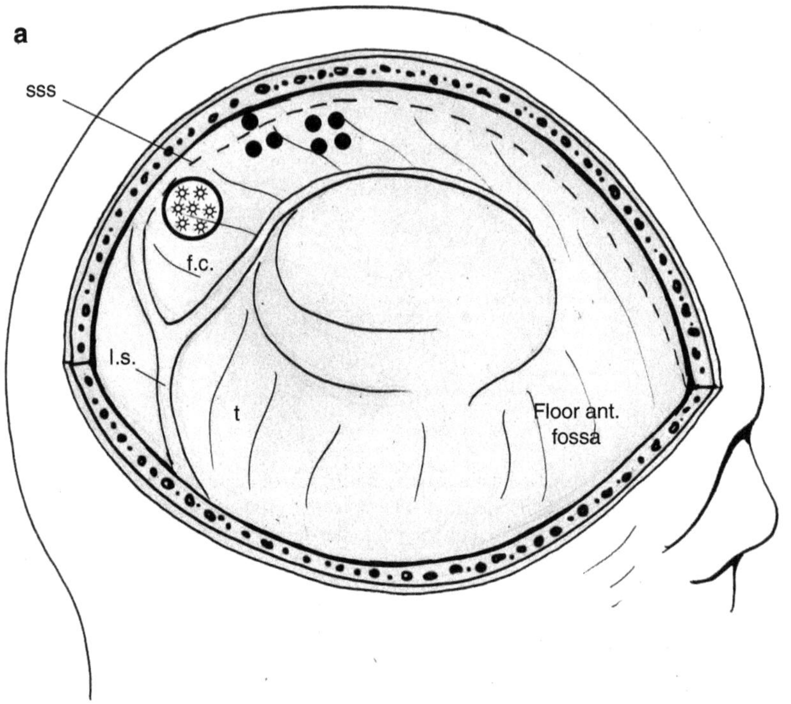

Fig. 3.6 Dural locations where physical/electrical stimuli may result in pain and the areas where injections of local anesthesia will abolish the pain. Illustration of locations where pain is produced by mechanical or electrical stimulation of the dura and those sites where the injection of local anesthesia is most likely to abolish the pain. (**a**) An example of pain produced by stimulation in the middle (anteroposterior) of the falx and abolished by anesthetization applied more posteriorly in the falx (Redrawn from Feindel et al. (1960)). (**b**) An example of the production of pain from stimulation in the area of transverse sinus and occipital dura and abolition of it by injections of local anesthetic in the posterior part of the falx and tentorium cerebelli. (**c**) An example of pain in the lower part of the dura of the temporal region, above the middle meningeal arterial vasculature, and abolition of the pain by local anesthesia injected into the base of the more inferior dura around the periphery of the middle meningeal artery. ● ● ●, locations where the application of injurious stimuli results in the production of pain; ✲ ✲ ✲, sites where the injection of local anesthetic results in the abolition of the pain; *f.c.* falx cerebri, *l.s.* lateral sinus, *m.m.a.* middle meningeal artery, *sss* superior sagittal sinus, *t* tentorium cerebelli (Redrawn, with permission, from Feindel et al. (1960))

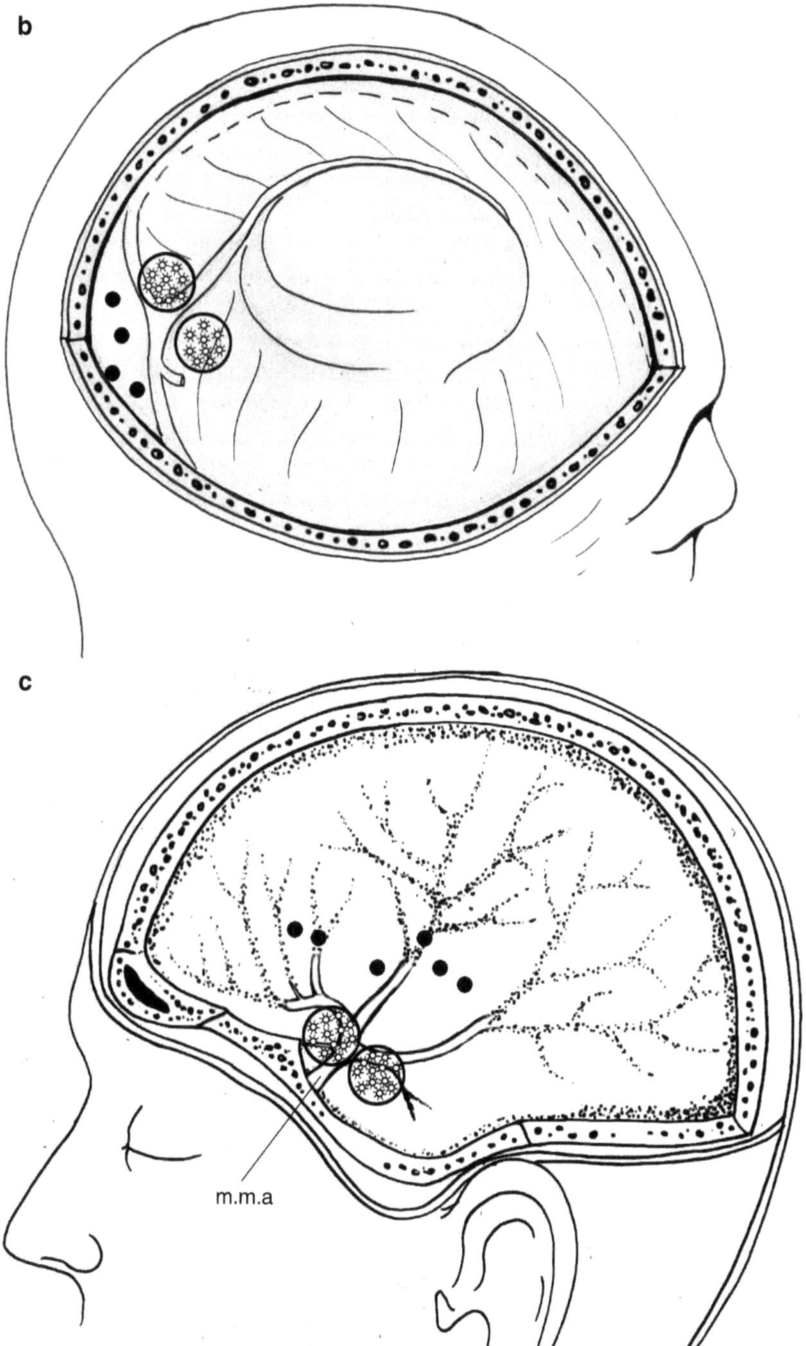

Fig. 3.6 (continued)

anesthesia will lead to its abolition. On the other hand, pain may be the result of irrigation under pressure, irrigation with solution of potentially injurious temperatures, traction on a lobe of the brain, or the wearing off of previously applied dural anesthesia. The localization of the origin of these pains is frequently unknown. However, in such instances the clinically determined physical (anatomical) distribution of the pain may be helpful in the prediction of its anatomical origin and thus the area where narcotization is likely to abolish it.

The literature addressing the issue of the anatomical locations to which pain is referred from various intracranial structures, often as a result of observations made with respect to the primary objective of determining the intracranial origins of clinical headaches, was particularly prevalent in the early part of the last century (Penfield 1934; McNaughton 1937; Penfield and McNaughton 1940; Ray and Wolff 1940; Wolff 1948; Feindel 1954). Figure 3.7 is redrawn from Penfield and McNaughton (1940) and indicates the dural locations, the stimulations of which result in referred pain and the places in the head where the referred pain is perceived by the patients. From this, one can obtain from a patient's perceived location of her/his pain as to where its origin might be in the dura. Perhaps, the most common

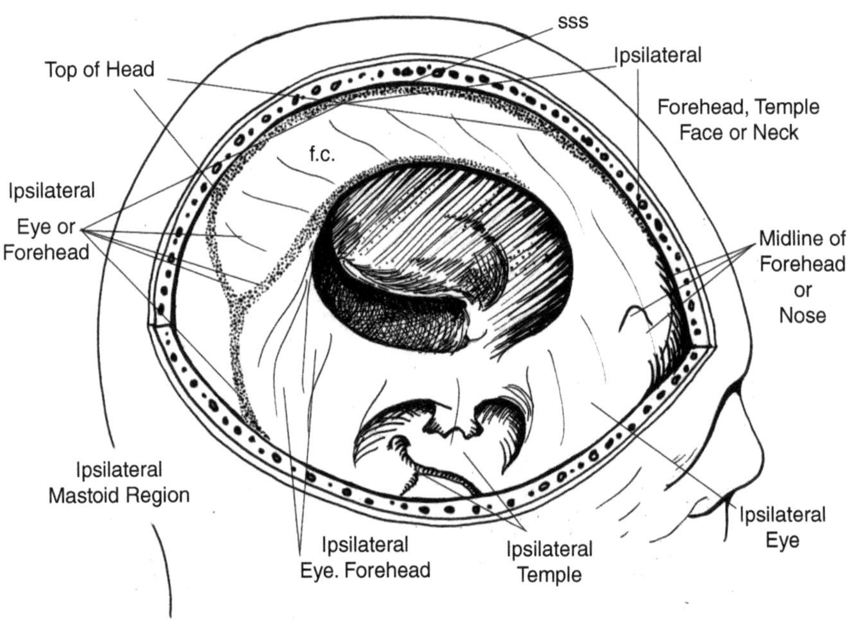

Fig. 3.7 Illustration of clinical sites of referred pain from dural stimulation. An illustration of the clinical sites to which pain is referred from electrical or mechanical stimulation (see text). *f.c.* falx cerebri, *sss* superior sagittal sinus (Redrawn, with permission, from Penfield and McNaughton (1940))

observation in my own experience is the perception by the patient of pain in the temporal area during the course of an aTLY (anterior temporal lobectomy), well into the operative procedure, e.g., >1–2 h. This is nearly always the result of surgery that has reached the basal dura/tentorium cerebelli over the floor of the middle fossa or the local anesthetic effect on the lateral temporal dura having lessened; in the case of the latter, the pain is likely due to traction on the dura, as a result of the elastic bands used to reflect it.

As a medical student, one typically learns that referred pain, usually with origins in the abdominal organs, is often diffuse, deeply situated, and poorly localized. While this may be true in the case of referred pain from intra-abdominal structures, nevertheless, as has been noted in the foregoing, referred pain from intracranial structures often is rather strikingly localized in the head. This was never more instructional than my memory of a case of a young man upon whom I was carrying out a left inferior posterior temporo-occipital corticectomy for epilepsy in 1983 in whom *any* mechanical stimulus in the immediate vicinity of the lateral sinus produced a remarkably well-localized headache in the ipsilateral forehead over roughly a 2 cm spherical area. The unusual features, from my perspective, consisted of the absence of *any* discomfort whatsoever in the left temporal or posterior auricular/mastoid region, which stood in rather marked contrast to the severity of the very, very discrete localized pain in the ipsilateral frontal (forehead) region. The area of the referred pain is in keeping with the referred pain responses shown by Penfield and McNaughton (1940) in the posterior part of the tentorium (redrawn in Fig. 3.7). Often there is some suggestion of local discomfort, which in this case was totally absent.

3.5.5.4 Intradural Injection of Local Anesthetic

The easiest method for the injection of local anesthetic between the dural leaflets in tight bony restricted areas is with the use of an insulin syringe, the needle of which is bent at an angle somewhere between about a 45 and 90°, such that the bevel is parallel to the dural surface, with the bevel (containing the exit hole) facing inferiorly. The bend is best made a millimeter or so from the tip of the hypodermic needle and then inserted *intra*durally between the leaflets of the dura (see Fig. 3.8a). Figure 3.8b is the same as a, but with a small bubble of injected local anesthetic in an unaltered normal base of a burr hole. At times this can be difficult because of the *tightness* of the surrounding bone. This in turn can be significantly improved by the removal of some of the surrounding bone, as shown in Fig. 3.8c (see also Fig. 3.9b and its associated text).

If the bevel is positioned satisfactorily between the dural leaflets, then the injection will be appreciated physically by a resistance when injecting and visually by a *bubble* appearing in the dura as a result of the expansion of the potential space between the leaflets, as illustrated in Fig. 3.8c. Only 0.1–0.2 ml of anesthetic is required at this point for adequate narcotization. This is sufficient also if the primary source of pain is associated with an artery, as once it has been anesthetized, further close-by separation of dura from the cranium can be undertaken without significant discomfort. If there is no resistance appreciated with the injection, then one can presume, with reasonable predictability, that the injection was not intradural. Thus, the syringe should be reloaded with local anesthetic, and a further attempt is made to find a satisfactory *intra*dural injection. If the situation is pertaining to a burr hole and there are a number of repeated failures, then some bone should be gently curetted in order to enlarge the base of the burr hole, as illustrated in Figs. 3.9b and 3.8b, in the direction most compatible with achieving the most satisfactory anesthetization of the exposed dura, i.e., in the most proximal available course of the innervating nerves.

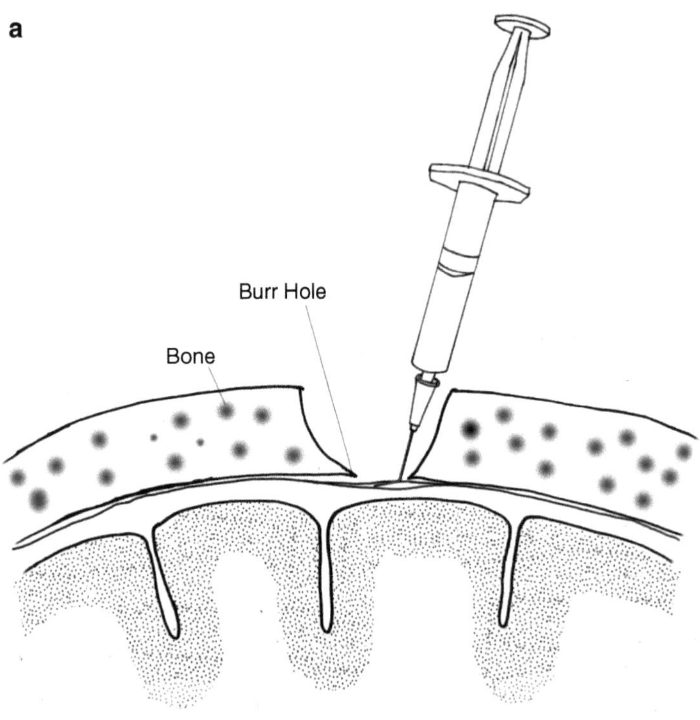

Fig. 3.8 Intradural (between dural leaflets) injection of local anesthetic. (**a**) The use of a syringe with a very fine needle, which is bent at about an angle of 45–90°, such that the bevel is facing downwards and parallel to the dural surface. (**b**) This depicts the injection of some local anesthetic between the leaflets, i.e., *intra*dural, of dura in the depth of a normal, unaltered burr hole. (**c**) This is the very same figure as Fig. 3.9b, which demonstrates the enlarged space over the dura at the bottom of a burr hole after removal of some bone (see text associated with Fig. 3.9). *b bubble* of injected local anesthetic

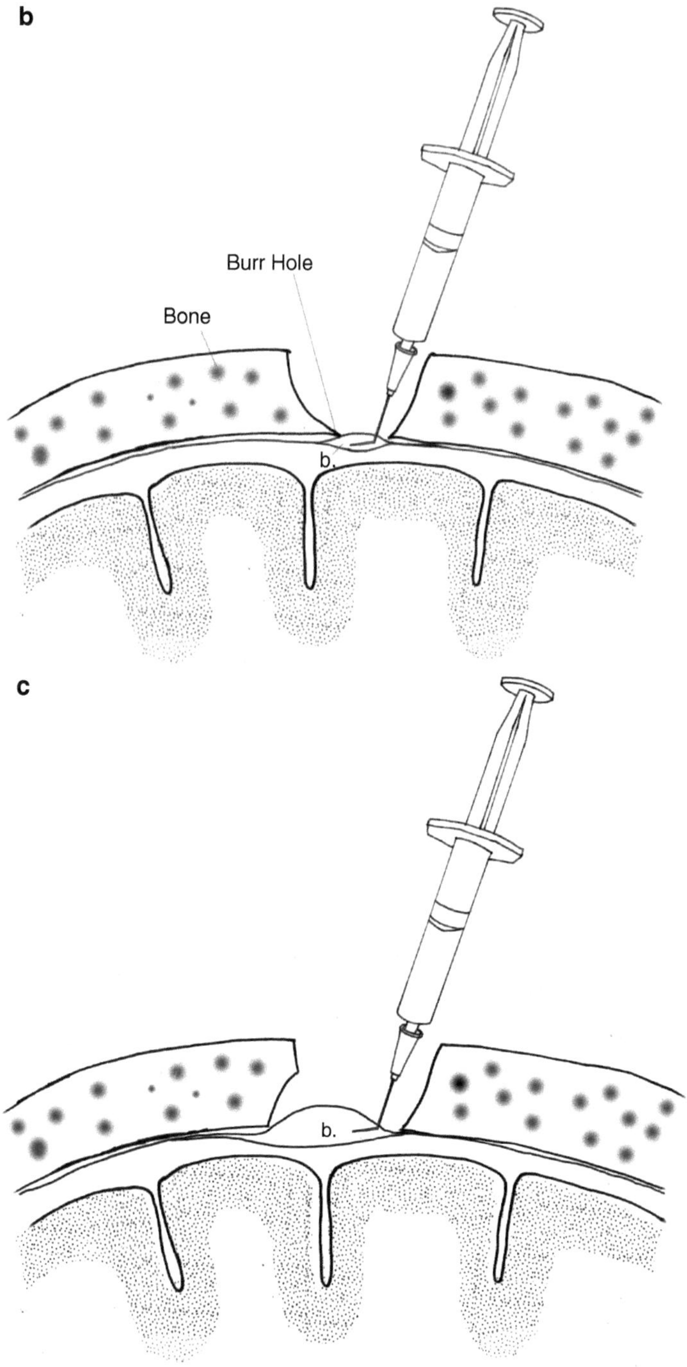

Fig. 3.8 (continued)

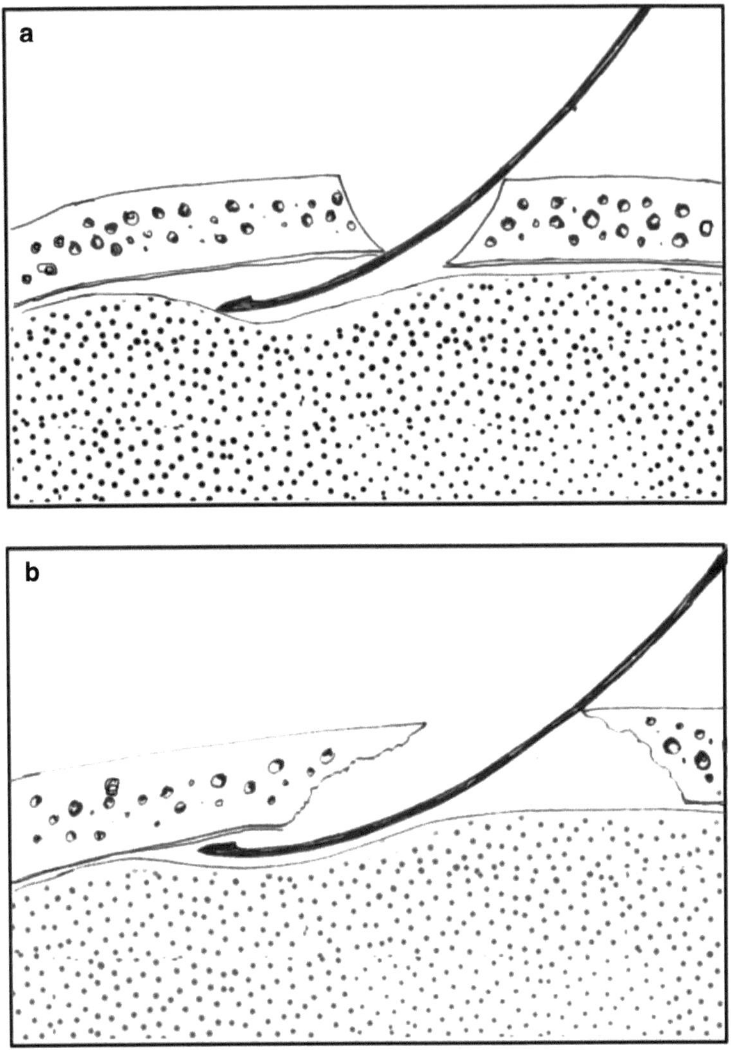

Fig. 3.9 Mechanism of avoiding pain in removal of dura from the cranium. The separation of dura from the inner table of the cranium without (**a**) and with (**b**) the removal of part of the inner table with a curette. Note the much smaller distance of the separation of the dural membrane off the undersurface of the cranium, with the use of the Gigli saw guide, than in the case of illustration (**a**) (Redrawn, with permission, from Girvin (1986a))

3.6 Craniotomy (Under Local Anesthesia)

3.6.1 Introduction

It is worth pointing out the features that best facilitate operations under local anesthesia. As with all neurosurgical practices, most surgeons individualize not only their clinical methods of practice but also their surgical techniques. In the process of learning, in large part through exposure to the individual preferences or biases of mentors in residencies, fellowships, and early consultant practice, one gradually puts together those characteristics of surgery, which seem best and with which one feels comfortable. This gradual process continues throughout a career and, in fact, represents the so-called continuing medical education, even though it is not necessarily learned in a conference or lecture room! That is to say, the *gradual process* may be the result of formal education (e.g., lectures, conferences, hands-on opportunities), communicating with colleagues, etc., but the largest part often originates from one's own continuing search of trials of improvement, discarding those that seemingly exhibit insufficient improvement while keeping those that result in improvements, adding them to ongoing characteristics of practice. This section is a rehash of the characteristics of surgery under local anesthesia that represent my current biases!

3.6.2 Preoperative Scalp Preparation

The patient is brought into the operating room and is usually placed in the lateral position, if the operation is under local anesthesia. The proposed scalp incision is then outlined with an indelible pen. The operative area is sterilized with whatever antiseptic protocol is used in the institution. The use of a very fine sharp point, e.g., # 25 hypodermic needle, will allow pinprick exploration of the region of the scalp incision that will, in turn, allow the assessment of the quality of the previously administered local anesthetic blockades of the regional scalp nerves. This will simply provide the surgeon with information about the places where slower injections of the 0.33 % bupivacaine hydrochloride solution, as outlined in Sect. 3.3.4, in the incision are recommended, i.e., in those areas where the prior blockades are less complete. The advantage of anesthetizing the scalp prior to draping the patient is that often the drapes are sewn in place with sutures or anchored with tissue clamps. Either of these produces pain in the unanesthetized scalp and should be avoided. As emphasized so many times earlier in this monograph, the avoidance of pain, especially without warning, is liable to result in a stressed, anxious, and eventually uncooperative patient (see Sect. 3.2), especially if failure of this part of the protocol occurs early in the operative procedure. This will not happen, once the scalp is properly anesthetized.

In temporal craniotomies, it is *mandatory* to inject at least 5–10 ml of the anesthetic in multiple deep injections into the base of the temporalis muscle in the vicinity of the zygoma. If this is not done, then pain will often occur when the muscle is being removed from the temporal bone with the periosteal elevator. Good analgesia is extremely important at this juncture and will preclude discomfort occurring with the surgery at this point. The patient is then surgically draped, as outlined in Sect. 3.4.

3.6.3 Scalp Flap

The scalp is raised without the use of any clamping of the scalp. Hemostasis is achieved with bipolar coagulation of obviously bleeding vessels, which are gently packed with peroxide gauze. The necessity of hemostasis is largely avoided if the scalp incision is made with a cautery knife. However, the use of peroxide gauze to cover the scalp incisions provides good moisture, as well as reasonable hemostasis. Certainly, the edges seem much healthier when clamps are not used, but perhaps the greatest advantage of the use of only the peroxide gauze is that there is little or no bleeding when, at the termination of the operation, the incisions are uncovered, preparatory to closing the scalp. (The use of peroxide gauze in this manner is something I picked up from Richard Perrin (1970 and 1971), when I was operating with him in aiding his development of an surgical epilepsy program in Toronto in the early 1970s; I have faithfully used only peroxide gauze overlying the edge of the flap ever since.)

3.6.4 Instrumentation

The instrumentation, which a given surgeon decides upon for use under local anesthesia, may be quite different than that used under general anesthesia. Many years ago, I had the rather disappointing and distressing experience of attempting to insert burr holes with the craniotome in a young woman under local anesthesia. I only once attempted it again. Since both attempts were met with not so much pain, but rather with nearly pathologically stressful anxiety for the patient, I felt that the better choice was simply to abandon the use of the air-powered craniotome. From that time onwards, I used the old-fashioned brace and burr bits to manually make the burr holes and the old Gigli saw to incise the cranium. I felt that the decision to not use the craniotome at that time (early 1970s) was justified at the time. There have been a number of improvements in the craniotome in recent years that might well make it perfectly satisfactory to use now. On the other hand, I went on to believe that there is little difference between the time taken to use the craniotome and the use of old-time tradition. Further, I fail to have ever witnessed the loss of the dura in so doing!

On the other side of the coin, I have always utilized the simple air (Hall) drill for making perforations in the bone for sutures and with ball burrs for removing bone. The diamond burrs are indisputably of higher quality than non-diamond burrs for drilling away bone. Not only are they less likely to result in tears in the dural membrane, but they also are much less likely to result in the production of pain, the reason for which I have no explanation! (I have often wondered whether it is a simple example of heat production by the non-diamond drill, as a result of a longer period of removal of the same volume of bone than would be required with the diamond drill.)

3.6.5 Reduction of Pain Associated with Burr Holes

The most helpful knowledge in predicting and assessing the likelihood of associated pain when making burr holes is that relating to the distribution of pain fibers within the dura. These were outlined in Sects. 3.5.4 and 3.5.5. When the burr holes are to be placed in an area of dense dural innervation with pain fibers, e.g., inferior temporal region, one can be certain of the necessity of injecting anesthetic into the dura at the base of the burr holes.

The perception of pain while burring through the bone, prior to reaching the dural surface, is extremely uncommon, except in those areas where arterial vessels are likely to be embedded in the undersurface of the bone or actually within the bone. This is not uncommonly found in the inferior temporal area around the area of the sphenoid wing when the middle meningeal arterial vasculature may be found in the deeper reaches of the bone. If the parent artery is in the bone, there may be significant momentary discomfort. Thus, it is important to advise the patient of the possibility of this occurrence.

When pain is experienced while making a burr hole, then it usually signifies that the dura has been reached. When the burr does contact the dural surface in those areas identified previously as heavily innervated with pain fibers, then the resulting pain may be significant, especially if it is directly over an underlying meningeal vessel. This is most likely to occur with the inferior burr holes in a temporal craniotomy. Once again, it is emphasized that in these particular situations it is *mandatory* to continually indicate to the patient at each point of the surgery that he/she might experience potential discomfort. If discomfort occurs, then it is worthwhile injecting a small amount of local anesthetic between the leaflets of the dura at this point. The more severe and the more abrupt the appearance of pain, the greater is the likelihood that the burr is in contact with a meningeal vessel at the base of the burr hole. If for any reason there is too small a bony opening to provide for a sufficient local anesthetic injection, then the opening can be expanded with the use of a fine bone curette, as demonstrated in Figs. 3.8c and 3.9b, which allows the relatively painless removal of the edges of the bone at the bases, belonging to the inner table of the cranium. These injections should be made in the inferior part of the burr hole, particularly if an underlying artery is identified, as these vessels will most likely have superior courses.

3.6.6 Separation of Dura from Inner Table of Cranium

When pain is encountered in the depth of a burr hole, then the process of anesthetization of the dura to be exposed is initiated at this point, as noted in the immediate foregoing. If pain is not encountered at this point, then the dura is very gradually separated in the directions of the planned bony craniotomy opening. Some curved instrument, e.g., Penfield # 3 dissector or a curved subperiosteal dissector, will most easily achieve this separation. If the amplitude of the separation can be kept to a minimum, then potential pain can be minimized. In the immediate foregoing, it was noted that small amounts of curettage of the base of the burr hole enlarge it such that the injection of the local anesthetic is facilitated (Fig. 3.8c). This very same curettage in greater amounts is recommended in *all* burr holes in craniotomies under local anesthesia, in the directions of the proposed lines of the craniotomy, i.e., those projecting from one burr hole to another. This very significantly reduces the potential discomfort that is produced by the traction placed on the dura with the separation of the dura from the cranium between burr holes, which may be over many centimeters. Figure 3.9a demonstrates the separation of the dura from the cranium around a burr hole when there is no enlargement of the base of the burr hole. In this case, the dura is separated from the inner cranial table by a dissector of some type; it can even be the Gigli saw guide. In order to achieve sufficient separation, there is most often significant traction on the dura, i.e., enough to produce discomfort. This can be avoided by a significant enlargement of the base of the burr hole through the use of vigorous curettage of the inner cranium, as illustrated in Fig. 3.9b, which, by the way, is painless, if conducted properly! This is simply an extension of the bony removal that was illustrated in Fig. 3.8c, which facilitated the injection of local anesthetic. The extension is easily achieved with the use of a cup curette and/or a pair of rongeurs, depending upon the thickness of the bone.

Once the dura around the base of the burr hole has been anesthetized, further separation of the dura from the underside of the cranium can usually be achieved without further significant discomfort, especially if it is done slowly and gently. However, even without discomfort initially around a burr hole the continued separation from one burr hole to the next, using the chosen dissector, may still, albeit uncommonly, give rise to discomfort; in this case, a very gentle intermittent advancement of the dissector alternately from the two burr holes allows satisfactory separation, especially if the curettage of the base of the burr holes is extensive. It is only very infrequently that this is not satisfactory, i.e., the discomfort is sufficient that the full extent of the required separation cannot be satisfactorily achieved. If there really is a problem, it may be remedied under these circumstances with the use of a small infusion of intravenous neuroleptanalgesia or anesthesia or a gradual piecemeal removal of bone in the tract with rongeurs. In the latter case, serial injections of intradural anesthesia following each stepwise piecemeal removal of bone will often allow identification of the source of pain, after which the dura can be separated satisfactorily without further discomfort.

3.6.7 Anterior Middle Fossa Exposures

Given a perusal of Figs. 3.5, 3.8, and 3.9, it is predictable that the craniotomy for an anterior temporal lobectomy (aTLY) is associated with the most potential discomfort of the routine craniotomies utilized for epilepsy surgical exposures. The requirement for the removal of bone inferiorly, including the outer part of the sphenoid wing, is more extensive than what can be accomplished by linearly cutting the bone, e.g., with the Gigli saw, between the two inferior burr holes. In addition, the bony removal in this location is over the most significantly pain-sensitive dura. Finally, the innervation of nearly all of the dura that is reflected for an aTLY originates in the inferior dura. Thus, for all these reasons, it is the inferior removal of bone which should be undertaken initially, as once the bone has been removed and the dura anesthetized, the remaining conduct of the craniotomy is truly relatively painless.

Over the course of a number of years and in spite of my initial concern about the use of the craniotome, nevertheless I have found that the use of a simple air drill with various sizes of diamond burrs is the most satisfactory method of removing the inferior temporal bone, along with cervical rongeurs. In this way, the outer part of the sphenoid wing is preserved as part of the craniotomy flap, and, as a by-product, there is *no* postoperative cutaneous depression (indentation) in the anterior temporal area—a most important aspect to some patients, most particularly young women. The remainder of the description of this craniotomy (for the aTLY) will be noted in Chap. 6, including the anesthetization of the trigeminal nervous input to the dura.

3.6.8 Closure of the Craniotomy

The closure of the craniotomy can be carried out in whatever is the practice of the operating surgeon. If the practice of the surgeon is to fill the cavity under pressure with the irrigating solution, which I do routinely, after the dura is closed, then one should be aware that this usually causes the patient transient discomfort in the form of headache. Presumably this results from stretching of pain-sensitive elements of the dura. Sometimes this can be alarming to the patient, but both the avoidance of extremes of temperature of the irrigating fluid and the appropriate proactive communication with the patient to the effect that there may be some discomfort associated with this will abolish any alarm in most circumstances. It will *never* be alarming to the patient if continual warning by the surgeon of possible potential discomfort is given to him/her!

3.7 Alternative Strategies to the Traditional Method of Achieving Awake Patients During Craniotomy

3.7.1 Introduction

As noted earlier in this chapter, there have been many advances, which have led to altered requirements with respect to the importance of, or the requirements for, having patients awake in certain craniotomies. As a result, there are surgeons who feel that with the aid of the more recently introduced very short-acting anesthetic agents, more satisfactory and comfortable local anesthesia strategies are preferable to what I have referred to as the historically *traditional* method of achieving satisfactory craniotomies with patients fully conscious.

3.7.2 The Traditional Wake-Up Procedure

The so-called *wake-up* procedure was introduced and utilized historically in centers where the use of local anesthesia and neuroleptanalgesia was not in common usage and where its use, usually occurring only very infrequently, was found to be unsatisfactory. It consists of initiating the operative procedure general anesthesia, until such time as it is required for the patient to be awake. The general anesthesia at this point is then discontinued, and the patient is allowed to wake up. This proved to be satisfactory in some cases, but this was not the rule. It is well known that most anesthetic agents enter the extravascular compartments and then are exponentially released from these compartments in accordance with their partition coefficients. Based on this, the agents may be sorted into ultrashort-, short-, medium-, or long-lasting anesthetic groups. The achievement of a satisfactory, alert, awake patient in the so-called wake-up procedure is dependent upon a significant clearance of anesthetic from the neurons in the substrate that maintains the alert, awake state. In cases where prolonged operative times preceded the period of wake-up, there were still sufficiently significant amounts of anesthetic agent in the extravascular spaces (including neurons). Under these circumstances, the patients did not in fact *wake up* satisfactorily and hence were too drowsy and/or confused in order to achieve the objectives of the fully conscious state. Pasquet doesn't necessarily refer to *wake-up* procedures, but does discuss the use of general anesthesia as a potential *intermittent necessity*, when using local anesthesia (1954).

3.7.3 The Use of New Short-Acting Anesthetic Agents

The recent introduction of very short-acting general anesthetics has greatly facilitated the objectives of the wake-up procedures. Sodium pentothal, a short-acting barbiturate, was commonly used in the early *wake-up* procedures, along with various general anesthetic and neuroleptic agents. The combinations of these agents varied a great deal and were most commonly chosen on the basis of the familiarity of their uses by the involved anesthetists. The current agent in use for this purpose is propofol, which was introduced in 1986. Propofol is a short-acting, nonbarbiturate sedative drug, with a very short time of diffusion out of the extravascular tissues. It allows the achievement of a satisfactorily deep general anesthesia and, upon its discontinuance, a reasonably quick return to an alert, fully conscious state. With the use of propofol, the local anesthetic blocks of the nerves innervating the scalp, the *pinning* of the head in a head holder, the application of local anesthesia in the proposed scalp incision, the craniotomy exposure, and the intraoperative anesthesia of the dura can all be achieved under general anesthesia. The then quick wake-up of the patient allows a much more satisfactorily awake patient for achieving both the length and the purpose of the surgery.

3.8 The Associated Neuroleptanalgesia

The discussion of craniotomies under local anesthesia would be incomplete without the recognition of the extreme importance of the use of various neuroleptanalgesic agents. In many earlier notes, the importance of the anesthetist in cases of operations under local anesthesia has been emphasized, and it will be reiterated again that this importance cannot be overemphasized. One of the key functions of the anesthetist looking after patients under local anesthesia is the determination of when and how much of a neuroleptanalgesic agent should be administered. In the eventuality of a novitiate operating room team, the anesthetist and surgeon often make the determination of the use of a neuroleptanalgesic agent collaboratively. However, that decision falls entirely in the domain of an experienced anesthetist.

It is beyond the scope of this monograph to discuss the variety of neuroleptanalgesic agents. For a comprehensive review of the subject, the reader is referred to Pasquet's discussion of various ways of dealing with the anesthetic requirements for such operations (1954), which was again repeated in the International Anesthesiology Clinics in 1986.

3.9 A Consideration of the Operating Room Times for the Conduction of Operations Under Local Anesthesia

Is there a differential in the times required for carrying out operations under local anesthesia as compared to general anesthesia? There is no doubt that the answer is *yes* to this question, in the case of a young surgeon undertaking her/his first operation under local anesthesia. However, there is a dramatic reduction in operating times with increasing experience—a reduction that is dependent upon the increasing experience of the *whole* operating team. I only have included this consideration because of the number of times I have been asked that question. My own experience was that it was halved over the course of time. Over the last years, a typical aTLY, including pre-resection ECoG recording of at least 30 min, involved 3.5–4 h. In spite of this, when I have gone to other hospitals with colleagues who are not accustomed to operating under local anesthesia, the time can still be 2–3 h longer—the best example that it is the whole team that contributes to the shortening of operating times!

References

Burns BD. Some properties of isolated cerebral cortex in the unanaesthetized cat. J Physiol. 1951;112:156–75.

Feindel W. The nervi tentorii and intracranial pain. Anat Rec. 1954;118:298.

Feindel W, Penfield W, McNaughton F. The tentorial nerves and localization of intracranial pain in man. Neurology. 1960;10:555–63.

Foerster O, Penfield W. The structural basis of traumatic epilepsy and results of radical operation. Brain. 1930;53:99–120.

Girvin JP. Neurosurgical considerations and general methods for craniotomy under local anesthesia. Int Anesthesiol Clin. 1986a;24:89–114.

Girvin JP. Resection of intracranial lesions under local anesthesia. Int Anesthesiol Clin. 1986b;24:133–55.

McNaughton FL. The innervation of the intracranial blood vessels and dural sinuses. ARNMD. 1937;18:178–200.

Pasquet A. Combined regional and general anesthesia for craniotomy and cortical exploration. Part II. Anesthetic considerations. Curr Res Anesth Analg. 1954;33:156–64.

Penfield W. A contribution to the mechanism of intracranial pain. ARNMD Proc. 1934;15:399–416.

Penfield W. Combined regional and general anesthesia for craniotomy and cortical exploration. Part I. Neurosurgical considerations. Curr Res Anesth Analg. 1954;33:145–55.

Penfield W, McNaughton F. Dural headache and innervation of the dura mater. Arch Neurol Psychiatry. 1940;44:43–75.

Penfield W, Roberts L. Speech and brain-mechanisms. Princeton: Princeton University Press; 1959. p. 286.

Ray BS, Wolff HG. Experimental studies on headache—pain-sensitive structures of the head and their significance in headache. Arch Surg. 1940;41:813–56.

Wolff HG. Headache and other head pain. Oxford: Oxford University Press; 1948.

Wyler AR, Hermann BP. Comparative results of temporal lobectomy under local or general anesthesia: seizure outcome. J Epilepsy. 1988;1:121–5.

Electrocortical (Cerebral) Stimulation

4

4.1 General Considerations

Electrocortical stimulation of the human neocortex in patients under local anesthesia has now been practiced for over a century, beginning around the turn of the nineteenth to twentieth century, in Britain (Horsley 1886, 1887) and Germany (Krause 1924; Foerster 1926, 1929a, b, 1936a, b; Krause and Schum 1931; Urban 1937). In the middle of the twentieth century, Dr. Wilder Penfield of the Montreal school used the training he had learned from Professor Otfrid Foerster in the use of such stimulation to explore the functional localization of the human cortex in patients who were undergoing surgery for the relief of epilepsy under local anesthesia. His observations and the observations of those whom he trained and who followed him at the Montreal Neurological Hospital and Institute form the most extensive systematic exploration of cortical function in human patients. Their observations still provide the most important contributions to the understanding of the localization of function in the human brain.

Electrocortical stimulatory exploration was established as the gold standard for identifying functional areas within the human cortex and has provided important information to neurosurgeons regarding the safe limits of cortical resection. Outcomes of surgical resections have added to that field, but the progressively increasing sophistication of medical imaging of the brain is now providing a most important array of observational data, which, much more noninvasively, is adding significantly to our understanding of the function of many areas of the brain, especially those areas which have been naively labeled by some as the "non-eloquent" cortex, e.g., that without any obviously apparent clinically important function. For purposes of brevity, the term "eloquent cortex" will be used to indicate the cortex, the stimulation of which produces a clearly identifiable clinical function. However, this use should not be construed to infer that the "non-eloquent" cortex is indeed without any clinical significance.

Electrical stimulation of every area of the human cerebral cortex and in every human being is capable of resulting in the production of an epileptic seizure, even

J.P. Girvin, *Operative Techniques in Epilepsy*,
DOI 10.1007/978-3-319-10921-3_4

in the hands of experienced individuals who adopt carefully regulated stimulation protocols. Interestingly, the experienced neurosurgeon can often appreciate more early the onset of a seizure compared to less experienced operating room staff that may actually be watching the patient. This may result from some subtle alteration in speech, a motor movement that is below the visual threshold, or some other ill-understood experiential background. Nevertheless, this observation is a very frequent occurrence! It is unimportant as to how a potential seizure is perceived or by whom it is perceived, but it is extremely important to recognize the onset of a seizure as early as possible, in order to ward off a simple partial seizure progressing to a secondary generalization, which can destroy the reasons for operations under local anesthesia, e.g., the presence of a fully alert patient. If the surgeon is aware early on of a beginning seizure and the anesthetist warned about it, then, if necessary, the anesthetist's preoperatively prepared syringe of the appropriate agent, now most likely propofol, can be injected to abolish it. I have had the experience of such generalization of a seizure occurring when operating in the posterior aspect of the Sylvian fissure *before* the temporoparietal speech area was appreciably outlined; it took the patient 1 h to wake up, at which point we continued!

Under ideal circumstances the surgeon, in any given operation, can usually gain all the observational data that are required of the stimulation in a matter of tens of minutes. That is to say, 10–20 min of stimulation may be all that is required to obtain the localization of the functional cortex, or the lack of function within the cortex, under observation. In more complex situations this may rise to 30–60 min. During this time, it is important to minimize the risk of creating an epileptic seizure. A very focal seizure may be only a nuisance. However, a generalized seizure, which is allowed to undergo its full course, can result in a postictal altered conscious level that precludes any useful stimulation for an hour or more and indeed occasionally may preclude *any* further useful stimulation in the operation. This can be catastrophic under some circumstances, including the one I noted in the preceding paragraph.

There are other methods for the "mapping" of cortical function, including the use of evoked potentials, sometimes the satisfactory use of surface stimulation of the motor cortex under general anesthesia, and perhaps eventually the use of the ever improving fMRI imaging. These will not be discussed further.

4.2 Physical and Electrical Characteristics of Stimulation

4.2.1 Stimulus Pulse Waveform

Lilly and his colleagues ushered in a new era of understanding the basis of safe stimulation of the brain in the middle of the last century with the systematic investigation of various aspects of biological stimulation (Lilly et al. 1952, 1955a, b; Lilly 1961). Their primary contribution was a demonstration of the injurious effects of long-term monophasic waveform stimulation of brain tissue. They suggested that the injury was the result of the total charge content of the train of monophasic

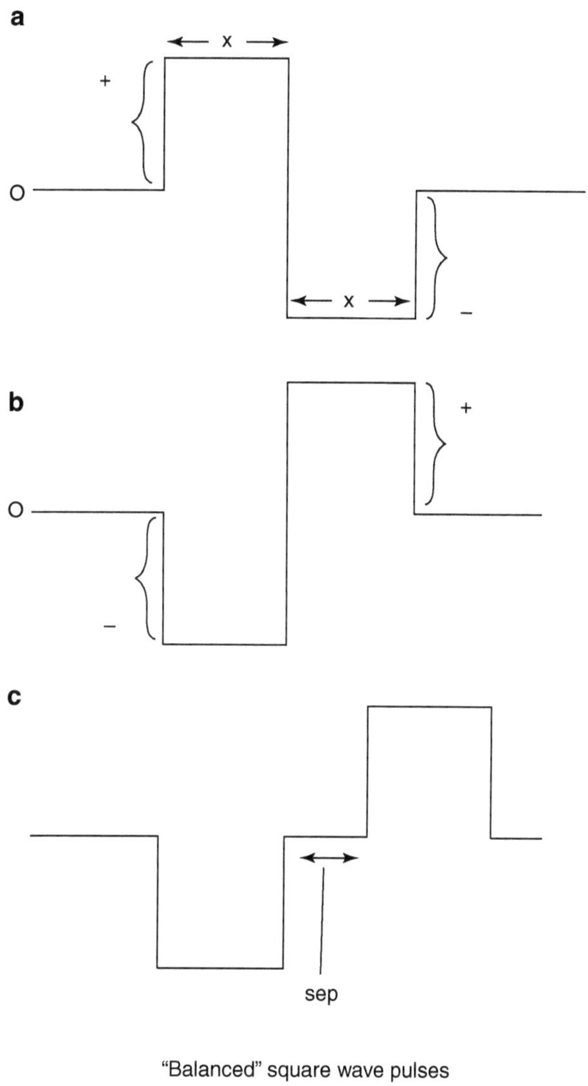

Fig. 4.1 The balanced waveform pulse of electrical stimulation. The so-called balanced waveforms, i.e., the charges of the two phases are equal and opposite, result in no *net* transfer of charge to the tissue being stimulated. This is shown as a rectilinear (*square wave*) pulse, but the "balance" can be achieved with *any* waveform, quite irrespective of its shape. (**a**) The leading phase is the anodal wave; (**b**) The leading phase is the cathodal wave. (**c**) The same stimulating pulses of figure (**b**), but with separation (time) between the two pulses. *sep* separation (time interval) between the two pulses, *x* the width (time) of the pulse, {— the current of the pulse

pulses, as opposed to the peak current of the train. They felt that the very high peak current required for stimulation, when using very brief pulses, could cause thermal injury, while on the other hand, excessively long pulses could result in sufficient transfer of charge over the pulse duration to cause electrolytic injury. They experimented with biphasic waveforms that were "balanced" about zero, thus giving rise to no net transfer of charge (Fig. 4.1). These were shown to cause no tissue damage. This waveform has become known as the "Lilly," "balanced," "bidirectional," or "biphasic" waveform. Further, they demonstrated that the threshold for the production of movement from the motor cortex stimulation was lower with anodal monophasic waveform pulses than with cathodal monophasic pulses, and they further demonstrated that the balanced waveform gave the same thresholds as the anodal pulses. Experimenting with separations (intervals) between the two phases of the waveform of less than 100 μs was attended by higher thresholds, and they finally concluded that ideal stimulation with bidirectional pulses consisted of the two phases of the pulses separated by approximately 100 μs.

While the balanced waveform is not necessarily important in short periods of acute stimulation, nevertheless, it has led to the preferred use of balanced waveforms in any chronic biological stimulation. MacIntyre et al. (1959, 1960) showed that any lack of balance between the two phases of a bidirectional pulse increased the size of potential lesions at the electrode sites, but demonstrated no lesional effects of separations of the two phases over the range of 0–150 ms (see Fig. 4.1c). They further showed that *any* waveform, if balanced, gave similar results, e.g., sinusoidal discharges, rectangular discharges, condenser discharges, etc. (see review by Girvin 1978).

4.2.2 Stimulus Parameters

Mihailović and Delgado systematically investigated the parameters of stimulation, applied to the monkey motor cortex, resulting in the threshold of movements, and concluded that biphasic pulses of 0.1–0.2 ms, at 60–150 Hz, were optimal (1956). Lilly and colleagues arrived at similar conclusions with respect to ideal parameters of stimulation, e.g., pulse durations between 0.1 and 1.0 ms and frequencies of about 60 Hz. Libet and colleagues studied the parameters of stimulation in the human somatosensory cortex under local anesthesia and similarly concluded that optimal parameters included train durations of about 1 s, pulse durations of 0.5–1 ms, and frequencies in the range of 15–100 Hz (1959, 1961, 1964, Libet 1973).

The Montreal school used relatively constant parameters of stimulation over the years. These consisted of ~2 ms pulses, at a frequency of 60 Hz, with variable train durations of a few seconds and current strengths produced by outputs of 1–4 V (Penfield and Jasper 1954, pp. 761–2; Rasmussen and Milner 1975). My own preference has been the use of 200–500 μs pulses, at frequencies of 10–50 Hz, train durations of a few seconds, and currents of 1–5 mA. In the stimulation of the cortex, looking for motor responses, I have found that the use of a frequency below that of the fusion frequency of muscle contraction is beneficial, i.e., in frequencies less than 10 Hz. It allows one to observe very fine movements in muscle, which may not be seen at threshold when using higher frequencies and low current; that is to say, it may be disguised by the fusion of subtle contractions.

My own experience has been the same, although much less extensive as the Montreal school in that there has been no specific parameter of stimulation, upon which "the nature of the response is… dependent on any of the parameters tested to date" (Rasmussen and Milner 1975, p. 240).

4.2.3 Electrode Composition

Electrode arrays contain at least two components—the metallic material of the electrodes and the substrate which is carrying the electrodes or in which the electrodes are embedded. In the case of a simple single stimulating electrode, the latter substrate is not terribly important. It has been known for some time that not all electrode metals and substrate components have the same biocompatibility (Dymond et al. 1970). The flow of current from an electrode into biological tissue requires a transformation of the electrical current passing through the stimulating electrode into an ionic (electrolytic) current passing through the excitable tissue. The choice of electrode metal is optimal when the required levels of stimulating current are well below those that cause significant dissolution of the chosen metal.

MacIntyre et al. (1960) demonstrated the striking difference in lesion sizes occurring as a result of the very same stimulation when using copper in comparison to stainless steel electrodes. Those in the former were much more striking. There have been many investigations involving the use of electrodes of varying composition. Many of the observations arising from these studies are anecdotal in that the purpose of the investigations was not directed to a systematic comparison of the metals. Certainly metals such as cobalt, copper, lead, mercury, and silver have all been shown to be significantly toxic to biological tissues. In general, the noble metals have shown much greater biocompatibility. Platinum (Pt) or the much more mechanically strong alloy of platinum and iridium (Pt-Ir) has been accepted as the most biocompatible electrode metal. However, even Pt has been shown to result in tissue damage in experimental animals with excessive stimulation (Agnew et al. 1975, 1977, 1983).

4.3 Variables in Electrical Stimulation of the Human Cortex

4.3.1 Introduction

From most textbook descriptions of stimulation, the reader cannot help but be left with the impression that cortical stimulation and the interpretation of the responses to that stimulation are perfectly straightforward. It is true that in the majority of stimulations, such may be the case. However, there are variations, which can occur and which lend difficulty to interpretations, especially in the initial observations of a novitiate. Some knowledge of these is important in those practices where cortical mapping will be widely utilized. These variations usually can be grouped under certain categories, including (1) stimulus output, (2) unifocal versus bifocal stimulation, (3) responses to threshold versus suprathreshold stimulation, (4) regional differences in threshold, and (5) the potential variability in the reliability and repeatability of cortical responses. All of these require at least mention.

4.3.2 Stimulus Output

It is the flow of current that brings about the stimulation of excitable tissue. Thus, at least intuitively, a constant current stimulator has the best output for such stimulation. However, if the impedance of the stimulating electrode is constant, or relatively constant, then a constant voltage stimulator is just as efficacious in putting out constant current for a given voltage. Over the last century the constant voltage stimulator was much more available than the constant current stimulator, and hence, most of the stimulation studies used the former. This was certainly true until the last quarter of the twentieth century.

4.3.3 Unifocal Versus Bifocal, Stimulating Electrodes

Stimulation can be carried out using a single point of stimulation, referred usually to a large independent electrode remote from the point of stimulation on the cortex, or using two points of stimulation. While these two methods have often been referred to as unipolar and bipolar stimulation, the terms unifocal and bifocal are really more accurate in describing the stimulation, as there are *always* two poles to the stimulus and thus theoretically *all* stimuli are bipolar! Unifocal stimulation implies a current density, which is maximal at a single point, i.e., the point of application of a single stimulating electrode. It is characterized by stimulation through an electrode on the cortex with the current path being completed by an indifferent electrode placed elsewhere, e.g., cranium, large areas of exposed tissue in the craniotomy site, areas of the body, etc. In this instance the stimulating current is delivered through the cortex at this single point alone (Fig. 4.2a). The amount of stimulated cortex will be a function of a number of variables, including the strength of the stimulus, the impedance and size of the electrode, and very occasionally to some extent the location of the remotely placed indifferent electrode.

In the case of bifocal stimulation, there are two electrodes on the cortex, usually close to one another, e.g., units of millimeters, and usually they are equal in size, construction (metal and substrate), and connecting wires. Thus, the current flow through the two electrodes is equal, and other than being in opposite directions, e.g., anodal and cathodal, the electrodes have the same charge characteristics and current densities. The current pathways are illustrated in Fig. 4.2b.

What is the difference between the two varieties of stimulating electrodes? Either of the two different electrodes can be used effectively. Generally the preference comes down to that with which the surgeon is most familiar, or with which he/she was trained. The bifocal electrode has two points of stimulation, e.g., both the cathode and anode. As outlined in the foregoing text, anodal stimulation usually has a lower threshold than cathodal for the elicitation of responses from the cerebral cortex. While one may not be certain as to which of the electrodes might be responsible for the response, in most cases this is not important, especially when the two electrode points are very close together, as the area stimulated is in the area under and between the two electrode contacts on the surface of the cortex (Fig. 4.2b). Because

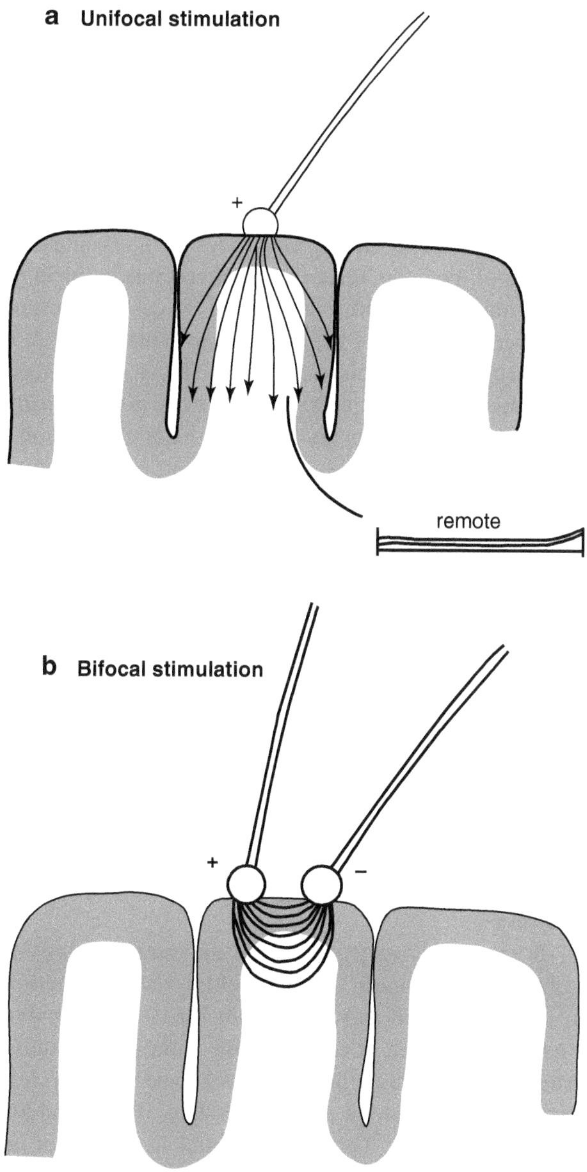

Fig. 4.2 Current pathways in electrocortical stimulation. An illustration of the current pathways associated with stimulation of the cortex. (**a**) Unifocal stimulation, in which the current is delivered through a single electrode, with the return pathway being that of a significantly larger, remotely placed electrode. (**b**) Bifocal stimulation, in which the current is delivered through one of a pair of small electrodes, at any given time, with the return path being that of the other electrode. + anode, — cathode

of the fact that the actual area of the cortex stimulated can perhaps be more easily ascertained, there has been a prevailing view that the bifocal stimulation is more localized, i.e., more discrete. I am not convinced of this.

I have always preferred the use of the unifocal electrode for a number of reasons. (Yes, it is the electrode upon which I was brought up and with which I am the most familiar!) Having used both types of electrodes, I do not feel that the discreteness of stimulation is an issue. It is interesting that the Montreal school initially used "a bipolar electrode made of two small platinum ball tips placed 2–3 mm. apart," but "more recently we have found it preferable to employ a monopolar electrode with an indifferent contact strapped to the leg" (Penfield and Jasper 1954, p. 761). I believe that there are a number of advantages of the unifocal electrode. It provides less variation in responses to a given stimulation. I have found it easier to place a single electrode in contact with the cortical surface than in placing two electrodes on the cortex such that the pressures and the areas of the electrode contacts are always the same in the two electrodes from one site of stimulation to another. In the absence of the latter, there can be alterations in the impedance and the amplitude of the stimulating current, especially in the case of constant voltage stimulators, which can alter the results of the stimulation. This latter can be altered to some extent by the use of a more mechanically flexible pair of electrodes, but usually this results in a potential difference in the interelectrode distance with varying degrees of pressure of application and thereby again with some variation in the characteristics of the stimuli. Finally, perhaps of most importance is that the single electrode is much more easily placed satisfactorily on an area of the cortex.

4.3.4 Threshold Stimulation

The basic studies involving stimulation of both experimental animals and human patients utilize threshold (T) or "just threshold" stimulation. Using the least amount of stimulating current to cause an effect, i.e., threshold current, is the safest current, for many reasons which will be discussed. Within that context, once a threshold has been determined, there is enough variability in response that each "threshold" (T) stimulus may fail to duplicate exactly the same response from one stimulation to the next. For this reason it is not uncommon to use some stimulus that is just above T, e.g., 1.25 T (25 % above threshold), which generally provides for more stable responses.

It was shown very early on in the cortex of dogs that repeated subliminal, i.e., subthreshold, stimuli, if placed close enough together, may result in a threshold response (Bubnoff and Heidenhain 1881). This phenomenon has become known as *summation*. From electrocortical stimulation studies in subhuman primates, Sherrington and his colleagues recognized what was referred to as "functional instability of cortical motor points" (Graham Brown and Sherrington 1912; Leyton and Sherrington 1917). They disclosed that as a result of preceding stimulation applied in the same vicinity of the cortex, there could be different responses, which they divided into three categories, (1) facilitation of response, (2) reverse of response, and (3) deviation of response. That is to say, the influence of prior stimulation was able to give rise to a variety of alterations in the normal response to stimulation of the succeeding response; variations did not occur if sufficient time was allowed between the successive stimulations. Penfield and Rasmussen (1968) referred to this variability as "instability of a motor point," noting the work of Sherrington and his colleagues. Facilitation has been used to describe the summation noted above, i.e., the phenomenon of two successive subliminal responses reaching a threshold response (Grünbaum and Sherrington 1901, 1903). It has also been shown that similar repeated stimulation, at rather longer intervals, may lead to a reduction in response, a phenomenon referred to as *extinction* (McCulloch and Dusser de Barenne 1935).

4.3.4.1 Regional Differences in Threshold

There are regional differences in threshold estimations. Some of such differences are predictable, while others are less so. The thresholds for the elicitation of motor responses from the motor cortex or somatic sensory responses from the sensory cortex are generally accepted as the lowest cortical thresholds. This has given rise to the common practice of initially determining the threshold of the Rolandic cortex, if it is exposed in the craniotomy, in order to obtain what might likely be a safe level of stimulation in which to initiate an exploratory stimulation. It is particularly important to get some idea of a reasonable threshold stimulation when the exploratory stimulation is to involve the cortex which may not result in clinically recognizable responses, e.g., thus giving rise to the possibility of the use of excessive current strengths resulting in seizures.

Perhaps one of the best examples of regional, or areal, differences in thresholds is that pertaining to the anterior and posterior speech areas. The threshold for the stimulation-induced interference of speech from Broca's and Wernicke's areas is higher than that of the Rolandic cortex. The difference may be as high as five- to tenfold. Usually the threshold for such dysfunction in Broca's area is lower than that in Wernicke's, but, on the other hand, in any given patient the thresholds may vary widely and in fact the threshold in the cortex of Wernicke's speech area may even be lower than that in Broca's area in the odd case.

In some experimentation of penicillin convulsions in monkey cortex, Walker and colleagues concluded that the "reactivity to Penicillin follows closely the electrical excitability of the cortex" (1945), simply reflecting different properties in different areas of the cortex. Similar observations have been made by French and colleagues (1956).

4.3.4.2 Why Are There Regional Differences in Thresholds?

There are many neurophysiological explanations for differences in thresholds from one area of the cortex to another. These are intrinsic properties, which are not pertinent to this discussion. What are pertinent, however, are considerations related to the stimulating equipment, per se, on the one hand and, on the other hand, anatomical variations in the localization of the functional cortex being stimulated. With respect to the former, it is most important that the hardware being used is maintained in satisfactory condition, as this is not something that should ever have to be sorted out in the operating room! However, it is worth noting that commonly the dials on the stimulator are not sterile, in which case it is common for some other member of the operating room staff to be responsible for altering the parameters of stimulation and the strength of stimulation. If this member does not have a reasonable familiarity with the apparatus, the dials associated with the stimulation parameters (pulse waveform, pulse duration, frequency, and in some, train duration), and particularly the current strength, then there can be variations in stimulation and areal thresholds that are not interpreted accurately because of errors in the appropriate settings of the output stimulation—the resulting interpretations therefore being "apparent," not real.

What can lead to erroneous interpretations in thresholds is the lack of uniformity of the electrical characteristics of the actual cortical surfaces being stimulated. It is important to keep the cortical surface as uniformly moist (saline) as possible, thus keeping to a minimum the possibilities that threshold differences are reflected simply in differences in the impedances of the stimulating electrode, which may be significant when moisture is not present, or contrariwise if there is too much irrigating fluid present. This is particularly important when using a constant voltage stimulator.

Perhaps the most important true alterations in apparent thresholds are due to anatomical variations in the locale of the eloquent cortex. This will be addressed in Sect. 4.5.

4.3.5 The Afterdischarge of Electrocortical Stimulation

Ever since the introduction of electrical stimulation of the mammalian cortex, it has been recognized that if the strength of such stimulation is raised sufficiently, seizures can nearly always be produced. The ECoG (electrocorticogram) in the region of the stimulation (or the ECoG if the stimulation is that from an earlier placed subdural array of electrodes) allows the observation of the cortical electrical activity and any alteration of the activity resulting from the stimulation. Under this circumstance, "after-discharges", which consist of post-stimulus, e.g., beyond the cessation of stimulation, abnormal electrical activity in the area of stimulation may be observed. Afterdischarge very rarely might occur with near-threshold stimulation, but with increasing strengths of stimulation, the probability of occurrence of afterdischarges rises. Some type of afterdischarge nearly always precedes seizures produced by electrocortical stimulation. This afterdischarge may assume a variety of morphologies, e.g., rhythmic waves, polyspike bursts, sequential waves etc., which may be seen with one another, may change from one to another, and may be observed in any part of the area surrounding the point of stimulation (see Blume et al. 2004).

As indicated in the foregoing, under the usual circumstances of subthreshold or just at threshold stimulation, there is nearly never stimulation-induced electrical activity outlasting the actual period of stimulation. This is demonstrated in Fig. 4.3a. The recording of the cortical activity is lost during the artifact of the stimulation, per se, as well as its following brief blockage of the recording apparatus, but following this the recording is re-established. When the strength of stimulation is elevated above threshold, especially when excessive, the appearance of abnormal artifactual electrical activity may be seen in the stimulated cortex and outlasting the period of stimulation. Since rhythmic activity is the commonest abnormality seen in the afterdischarge, this will be illustrated in Fig. 4.3b, c. Afterdischarge, occurring in eloquent cortex, may be associated with a clinical abnormality, e.g., the interference,

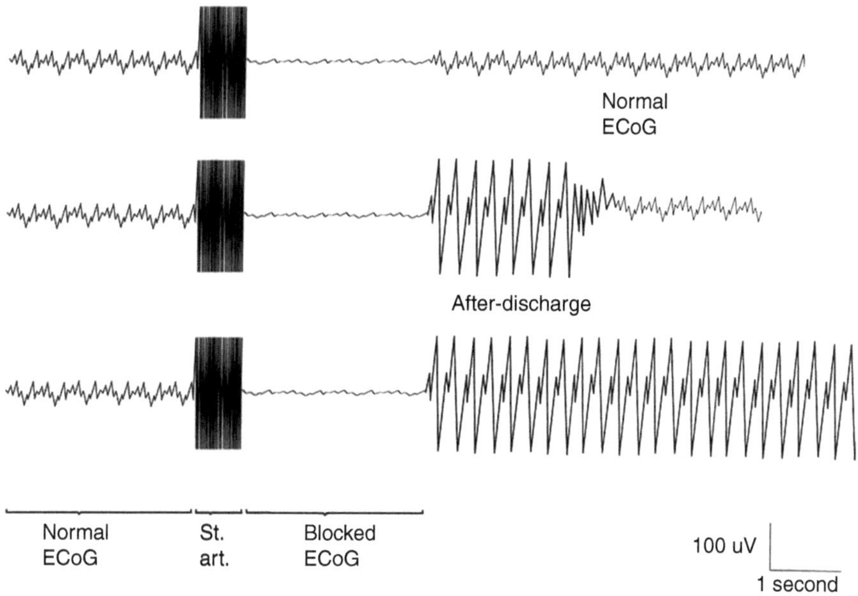

Fig. 4.3 Afterdischarge following electrocortical stimulation. (**a–c**) each discloses the initial normal electrical activity (ECoG) of a region of the cerebral cortex and the alterations that occur in the ECoG as a result of increasing strengths of applied electrical stimulation. Each of the figures demonstrates the initial normal ECoG, the marked abnormal artifact from the 0.5 s electrocortical stimulation, followed by a ~1–2 s of no electrical activity as a result of the transient blockage of the ECoG by the stimulation. Following these three fixed alterations are different responses, as a result of increasing strength of the current of the stimulation. (**a**) depicts the result of a stimulus at threshold, which does not alter the normal activity, i.e., it is not associated with any abnormal discharge *after* the termination of the effect (artifact and ECoG blockage) of the cortical stimulation. (**b**) illustrates the result of an increase in the current of the stimulation, such that it leads to a transient self-sustained, self-limited, afterdischarge. (**c**) illustrates a further increase in the stimulation current that is strong enough to produce a self-sustained afterdischarge, which progresses and spreads to the nearby cortex and often eventually results in an epileptic seizure. *μV* microvolts, *st. art.* stimulation artifact

positively or negatively, with the clinical function of the area. While this afterdischarge is self-sustained, it is usually transient with small increases in stimulation current (see Fig. 4.3b). That is to say, the afterdischarge is self-limited and thus whatever clinical alteration might have occurred will similarly be self-limited as well. In this circumstance the electrocortical abnormality will be localized, primarily to the area of the stimulated cortex. As higher stimulus strengths are applied, the afterdischarge may become fully self-sustained, as shown in Fig. 4.3c. Under this circumstance the electrical activity may spread to the adjacent cortex, may be associated with more vigorous electrographic epileptic activity (see Erikson 1940), and may exhibit evidence of clinical epileptic activity that is likely related to the functional cortical area being stimulated. As indicated earlier, this very same sequence may be seen from stimulation of the non-eloquent cortex, the clinical epileptic activity either starting locally, as a result of the spread of the afterdischarge to a nearby area of the eloquent cortex, or even in the form of a typical generalized grand mal seizure. If the seizure is not stopped by the administration of anesthetic or pharmacologic means, when it is clearly progressing, then it will usually end up in a generalized full-blown convulsion.

Walker (1949a, b) found that the lowest thresholds for the production of afterdischarges were associated with those areas of the cortex in and about epileptic foci in patients with intractable seizures. He referred to this cortex as "hyperirritable" or "hyperexcitable." Putting aside the foregoing it must be remembered that with sufficient electrical stimulation, nearly *any* area of the cortex can be made to give rise to afterdischarges and epileptic seizures.

Just as there are regional variations in threshold responses in the eloquent cortex to electrocortical stimulation, there are variations in the thresholds for the production of afterdischarges. For example, the threshold for the production of the latter is much lower for the Rolandic cortex than for the non-eloquent cortex such as that in the anterior temporal and frontopolar regions. The characteristics of the afterdischarge, e.g., asynchronism, synchronism, rhythmicity, types and frequency of waveforms, etc., may vary widely from one area of the cortex to another.

To summarize, once afterdischarge occurs, it may (1) be a self-limited discharge, disappearing in a matter of a few to tens of seconds; (2) remain very localized, transient, and stationary for a significant period and even in this state can demonstrate clear focal epileptic discharge and associated clinical focal seizure activity; (3) spread and again terminate in a self-limited fashion; or (4) spread, in association with spreading clinical epileptic activity, which terminates in a full-blown generalized seizure. Penfield and Jasper (1954) have also shown that remote afterdischarge can occur, e.g., afterdischarge that may be some centimeters away from the stimulated area. This is not seen often and is not really very well understood. As outlined in the foregoing section on threshold stimulation (Sect. 4.3.4), subthreshold stimulation, rapidly repeated, can lead to summation, evidenced by the appearance of a threshold response, even though the stimulus, which finally elicited it, was subthreshold. This same phenomenon of summation may occur with afterdischarges. Thus, a series of subthreshold stimuli, repeated sufficiently close together, can result not only in a threshold response but even in the summation of afterdischarges, which, like any afterdischarge, may reach sufficient strength to be associated with an epileptic seizure.

I would be remiss in not indicating that in practice the majority of careful stimulations are not associated with any afterdischarges and that when they do occur they are self-limited and without an accompanying ECoG abnormal activity; the surgeon would be unaware of any abnormality. However, during sessions of electrocortical stimulation, the surgeon must continually bear in mind the possibility that afterdischarge may be continually produced and thus be prepared, along with the anesthetist in charge, to take whatever precautions that are necessary to avoid the production of seizures, especially generalized seizures (*vide infra*), which can interfere with the gathering of the information, which was the primary objective of the use of local anesthesia.

4.3.6 Isolation of Current Input

Isolation of the stimulus input to human tissue is required in most jurisdictions. This has become more important down through the years to the point that now some stimulators have the isolation available within the stimulator per se. Isolation may be carried out in a number of ways, e.g., transformer, capacitor, optical, etc. There is no necessity to describe the various strategies in detail. The importance of this can be found in the literature (Dobelle and Mladejovsky 1974; Dobelle et al. 1974).

4.4 The Conduct of Exploratory Stimulation

4.4.1 Introduction

Exploratory stimulation really applies to the initiation of the objective of mapping the cortex in question in order to determine the localization of function within that cortex. It will be the knowledge of where this function is located, which will allow the surgeon to determine the safe limits of resection in and about its location. An associated objective of the exploration is the mandatory precaution of minimizing the likelihood of the production of seizures from the stimulation.

It is important at the outset of the exploration to explain to the patient that the stimulation of the cerebral cortex is not painful. Many patients who hear that they are to undergo a stimulation consisting of "electrical" stimuli immediately interpret the stimulation as being associated with a number of electric shocks. A more relaxed patient will be achieved by making certain that such an interpretation is precluded.

Communicating with the patient such that she/he knows when the stimulus is being applied is perhaps the most important methodological issue to be addressed in routine mapping of the functional cortex. The patient must know *exactly* when the stimulus is being applied. Failure to satisfy this feature of stimulation leaves responses which are usually associated with tremendous uncertainty. I have usually used the word "now" in some context. Commonly, I will say something to the effect that "the stimulus is coming …. now," but nearly always end up simply saying "coming …. *Now*," applying the electrode to the cortex exactly coincident with the "now."

4.4.2 Minimizing the Likelihood of Stimulus-Induced Seizures

As noted in the foregoing, it is most important to avoid the production of generalized seizures. Thus, it is the prophylaxis, rather than the management, of these seizures that should be the foremost strategy. Prophylactic initiatives include (1) the use of low currents of stimulation, (2) the employment of random spatial stimulation, (3) optimal temporal spacing of successive stimuli, (4) the "no-return-to-a-previously-delineated-area" policy, (5) the use of ECoG monitoring, and (6) anesthesia-on-the-ready.

4.4.2.1 The Use of Low Stimulus Currents

The initial stimulating currents used in exploration should be very small. One of the practices with the greatest risk of producing seizures is that of simply initiating the exploration at a stimulating current, which is simply too high. As noted in Sect. 4.3.5 afterdischarges may be seen following stimulation of the cerebral cortex. Such discharge may become self-sustained and end up in the production of a generalized tonic-clonic seizure. The appearance and severity of afterdischarges increase with increasing strengths of stimulation. Thus, the initial stimuli in the exploration should be as low as that compatible with the production of clinical responses. This will be based upon the experience of the surgeon with the stimulator at hand. It would be expected in the range of 0.5–1 mA in the case of constant current stimulators or in the range of 2–5 V in the case of constant voltage stimulators.

If the Rolandic cortex is exposed, then the exploration is best started in its vicinity. Since it has the lowest threshold responses, one can be certain that once a threshold is found in the Rolandic cortex, then using this current strength for the initial exploration in other cortical areas, there is little likelihood of producing seizures. If currents over 3–4 mA are not capable of bringing about responses from the stimulation of the Rolandic cortex, then usually either the stimulation apparatus is faulty, the Rolandic cortex is damaged, or it is not the Rolandic cortex that is being stimulated. Most of the other so-called eloquent areas of the cortex will have thresholds at least two to three times greater than that found in the Rolandic area. Thus, once a Rolandic cortical threshold is obtained, the surgeon can proceed with much more confidence with the remainder of the exploratory phase of the stimulation. If there is further necessity to explore the Rolandic cortex, then the threshold, which has been achieved, need not be altered a great deal in order to outline further Rolandic cortical function.

If the primary objective is to make certain that the cortex outside of the Rolandic cortex is not indeed the functional cortex that cannot be sacrificed in the resection that is proposed and the Rolandic cortex is not available for the determination of its threshold characteristics, then the exploration is initiated at small currents (e.g., 0.5–1.0 mA). The stimulus current is then raised in steps until there is relative certainty that it is not the eloquent cortex. It may be necessary to use currents up to tenfold greater than what might have been required to establish the thresholds in the Rolandic region, e.g., as high as ~10 mA.

If there are no responses at these currents, then there is either malfunctioning of the stimulator or the cortex being stimulated is not the cortex that is clinically eloquent.

4.4.2.2 The Use of Random Spatial Stimulation

In Sect. 4.3.5 the point was made that summation of afterdischarges may occur when the following stimulations of the same area are made before the afterdischarge from the previous stimulation has not ceased. Thus, even if such discharges are normally mild, rather insignificant, self-sustaining discharges, nevertheless if a number of them arise from close intervals of stimulation and sum, they may give rise to a fully self-sustained, spreading discharge that may terminate in the production of a generalized seizure. As noted earlier most afterdischarges are very focal, arising beneath the stimulating electrode and usually remaining in this location. Thus, when stimulating a given cortical area, the potential summation of afterdischarges can be reduced or abolished by randomly stimulating different areas, distant from one another, with the application of successive stimuli. Therefore, the safest strategy of stimulation, achieved in the shortest period of time when a given area is to be explored, is by randomly stimulating the area such that successive stimulations are as spatially distant from one another as possible.

4.4.2.3 Optimal Temporal Spacing of Successive Stimuli

Reference to the foregoing paragraph notes the summation, which can occur with the afterdischarges following electrical stimuli. In Sect. 4.3.5 it was noted that most stimuli-induced afterdischarges are self-limited. That is to say, they arise, and within some period of time, usually a few seconds, they wane and disappear. To reiterate, if in such circumstances the time between the applications of successive stimuli is greater than the period required for the complete waning of the afterdischarge of the preceding stimulus, then summation cannot occur. Thus, if it is necessary to apply successive stimuli to the same point on the cortex, then increased safety from the production of a generalized seizure can be achieved by simply increasing the time between the applied stimuli. If this a significant problem, for whatever reason, then the monitoring of the afterdischarge by the simultaneous use of an ECoG is useful.

4.4.2.4 The "No-Return-to-a-Previously-Delineated-Area" Policy

Once an area of the cortex has been satisfactorily defined with respect to its function, then it should not be returned to as the stimulus strength is raised in order to define the functional aspects of other cortex requiring exploration. The only exception to this strategy is the case where there is uncertainty as to whether the observed response is indeed accurate. In this case the exploration is best undertaken with the same stimulus strength, which gave rise to the initial response. If uncertainty remains, then a slightly stronger stimulus should suffice to sort out the uncertainty. However, once a clearly defined response is obtained, then one should not return to the same point with stronger stimuli, in order to avoid creating a significant afterdischarge and possible seizure.

4.4.2.5 The Use of ECoG Monitoring

If one wishes to explore the characteristics of electrocortical stimulation more fully and an ECoG is readily available, then its use as an accompanying monitor of the electrical activity in the vicinity of the stimulation is helpful. This will allow the determination of when afterdischarges are produced from the stimulation and at the same time allow the identification of the characteristics of the progression of such electrical discharge. An associated ECoG is particularly helpful to the members of an operating team that is in the early stages of developing an expertise in the use of local anesthesia and electrocortical mapping. The educational appreciation of the phenomenon of afterdischarges is much greater when visualizing it than simply hearing about it and even more so than seeing examples in a journal. A good ECoG allows one to recognize not only the post-stimulatory afterdischarge but also the nature and extent of its spread and (hopefully not often) the association of the electrical ECoG abnormalities and clinical events.

4.4.2.6 Anesthesia-on-the-Ready

It pays handsome dividends to notify the anesthetist at the initiation of the exploratory stimulation, especially in the case of an anesthetist who might be relatively new to the practice, of the importance of having an antiepileptic agent loaded in a syringe before the onset of exploratory stimulation. Our anesthetists always have some propofol ready in a syringe, such that when there is suspicion of progression of focal epileptic activity into a generalized seizure, the propofol may be injected intravenously. The appropriate administration of some propofol will result in the reduction of the tendency to generalization on the one hand and on the other hand will be insufficient to produce general anesthesia.

With increasing experience, the team, led by the anesthetist and the surgeon, can judge at what point to administer intravenous propofol during the course of an initial focal seizure. It must be kept in mind that the majority of focal seizures will *not* go on to generalization. Hence, simply being "on-the-ready" will allow early appreciation of potential spread of the focal seizure, which then calls forth the likelihood of the requirement for the administration of propofol.

4.4.3 The Use of Sham Stimulation

There are frequently points during the stimulation when it is difficult to be sure that the responses are truly bona fide responses. If *any* uncertainty exists, then sham stimulations should be applied. As noted in Sect. 3.2, related to surgery in the awake patient and earlier in this Section (Sect. 4.4.1), the surgeon is responsible for making certain that the patient is fully aware beforehand of any maneuvers being undertaken as part of the conduct of the operation, which might be new or different, particularly those that might be the least bit potentially frightening. Thus, ordinarily the patient is notified of each stimulation of the cortex by the surgeon uttering "coming .... *Now*," at the time of delivery of the stimulus. When there is a concern about whether the patient is accurate in the appreciation and description of a given stimulus, sham stimuli should be mixed with the bone fide stimuli, i.e., the "coming .... *now*" is used for them, in the absence of associated stimuli. If the application of the stimulation is perceived because of some discomfort, a very uncommon situation, which is nearly always associated with excessively high strengths of current, then the stimulus can be applied to some other point that is known to be unexcitable. If the same discomfort is perceived, then it is the result of the current of the stimulating apparatus.

There is no shame in using as many sham stimuli as may be required to sort out the certainty of responses! It takes very little time and the benefit far outweighs the small commitment to a bit of extra time.

4.5 The Interpretation of Responses to Electrocortical Stimulation

4.5.1 "Inhibitory" Stimulation

It was Penfield who first pointed out that stimulation can in fact interfere with the function of the normal cortex, even to the point of suppressing normal responses (1958), e.g., speech arrest with stimulation of Broca's area. This was initially observed in the sensory cortex and was interpreted as possibly due to the transient loss of normal perception of peripheral stimuli during the cortical stimulation. This has to be seen on the background of the acceptance that cortical stimulation never reproduces perfectly natural sensory experience (Penfield 1958). Usually Penfield's "inhibitory stimulation" can be appreciated as an "interference" with the normal function of the cortical area being stimulated, as opposed to an "absence" of response.

From a purely neurophysiological consideration, if the frequency of stimulation is sufficiently high, it may not allow the cortex sufficient time, between the stimuli, to declare the clinical function that is localized in the cortex being stimulated.

4.5.2 The Absence of Responses to Stimulation

As outlined in the foregoing, the absence of responses to stimulation can occur from (1) faulty (nonfunctioning) stimulation equipment and (2) the cortex from which the stimulation will not provide clinically identifiable responses, e.g., the "non-eloquent" cortex. In addition to these there are other circumstances, which may result in the apparent absence of responses, especially at low strengths of stimulation. One such example is the case in which the functional cortex being looked for is in the depth of a sulcus. The human cortex is a gyrencephalic cortex. That is to say, as the phylogenetic scale is ascended, there is, within the mammalian species, an increasing infolding of the cerebral cortex. As a result there are increasing numbers of gyri and increasing depth to the sulci that separate them. This leads to much of the cortex being "buried," as it were, in the depths of sulci. Such cortex cannot be visualized on the surface, nor is it as amenable to surface stimulation. A good example of this can be appreciated in the human primary visual cortex, in which approximately 67 % is within the depths of the calcarine sulcus and its sulcal branches (Stensaas et al. 1974). There is no need for elaboration of the fact that, when subjected to electrocortical stimulation on the surface, an area of the eloquent cortex located in the depth of a sulcus will have a significantly higher, albeit "apparent," threshold than the same neurophysiological cortex situated on the surface of a gyrus. Further, if it is at the very depth of the sulcus, the surface stimulation may not be strong enough to elicit *any* response.

While the recognition of this is straightforward, the omnipresent importance of this recognition cannot be overemphasized during the course of stimulation, the objective of which is the delineation of the eloquent from the non-eloquent cortex

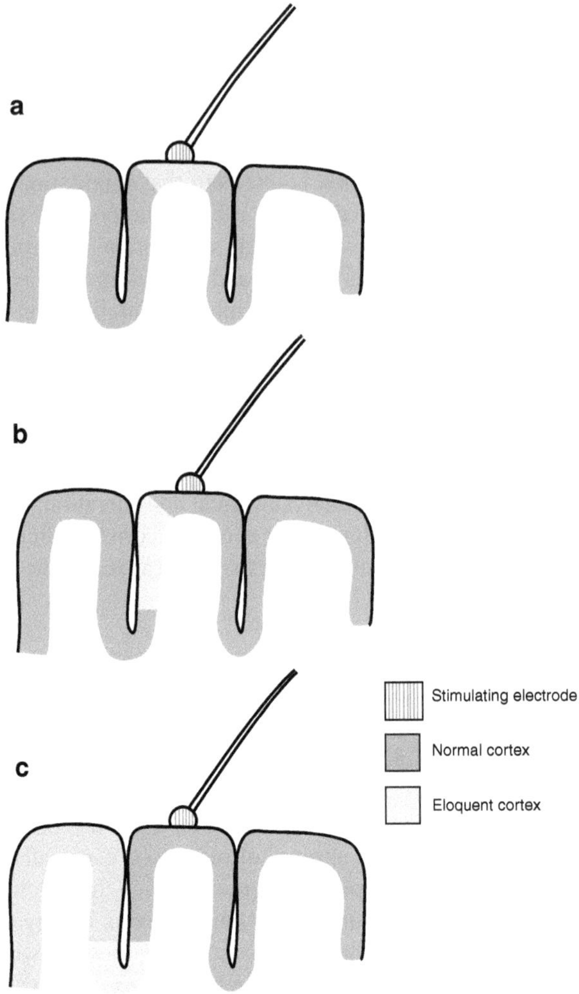

Fig. 4.4 Stimulation of the "eloquent" cortex in various locations in the gyri. An illustration of three different cortical positions of the eloquent cortex, each subjected to exploratory surface stimulation, while looking for specific clinical responses to its stimulation, preparatory to surgical resection in the area. (**a**) The anatomical location of the eloquent cortex, e.g., speech, visual, motor, or sensory, on the surface beneath the stimulating electrode; (**b**) the anatomical variation in which the eloquent cortex is "hidden" or "buried," e.g., within the sulcus; and (**c**) the anatomical variation in which the eloquent cortex is "buried" in the very depth of a sulcus (see text)

for the purposes of outlining the dimensions of a corticectomy. The question of the term "eloquent" to describe a cortical segment will be iterated, as it was in Sect. 4.1. The eloquent cortex is cortex the stimulation of which results in a clinically identifiable alteration, while the non-eloquent cortex is that which is unassociated with any clinical event. The stimulation of an eloquent area of the cortex in the upper part of a sulcus may simply give rise to higher threshold, than it would on the surface of a gyri. This circumstance is not liable to result in a significant error in the determination of resectability. On the other hand, if the cortex is sufficiently "buried," such that no response is obtained and the interpretation is that the eloquent cortex is not present, then it may indeed give rise to a catastrophic error in resection.

The potential circumstances outlined in the foregoing are illustrated in Fig. 4.4. Figure 4.4a demonstrates an example of the easy localization of the area of the eloquent cortex being investigated, e.g., speech, visual, motor, and/or sensory, in which the area is on the surface beneath the stimulating electrode. The threshold will be low and the area relatively well localized, such that the movement of the electrode a short distance away will result in the lack of a response, an alteration in the response, or the requirement of a significantly raised stimulating current in order to reach threshold. Figure 4.4b demonstrates the variation in which the functional cortical area is situated *below* the *surface* of the cortex, in the more superficial cortex within the sulcus. In this case the stimulation must travel through more cerebral parenchyma, with the consequence of a pathway with greater electrical resistance and hence the requirement for a larger current than that in Fig. 4.4a, in order to reach its threshold. There is also a greater likelihood of somewhat poorer localization, i.e., the electrode may be moved around a greater area with smaller changes in response than in Fig. 4.4a. Finally, in Fig. 4.4c the area of the eloquent cortex is located in the depth of the sulcus and hence is significantly below the surface of the cortex and the stimulating electrode. Thus, the pathway is still longer and has greater electrical resistance than even that in Fig. 4.4b, and thus it will likely have a significantly greater threshold, or there may be no response at all to the stimulation on the surface. If there is a response, it may change very little with significant movement of the electrode before there is any change in the response. This would be a very, very unusual situation. However, if there is suspicion that the buried eloquent cortex might be in the depth of the sulcus, then the surgery around that sulcus should be carried out slowly, under local anesthesia, and clinically monitored.

The greatest concern in using cortical stimulation is that an erroneous interpretation might lead to the removal of the eloquent cortex, which is not appreciated. Some of the reasons for this have been previously addressed. However, the greatest possibility of error arising from the anatomical variation is outlined in Fig. 4.4c. It is because of this potential eventuality that the stimulus strength must be raised significantly before declaring that the stimulated cortex is not eloquent and therefore can be removed.

4.5.3 The Variability in the Reliability and Repeatability of Responses

Variation in responses to the application of a given (constant) stimulus to a given point on the cerebral cortical surface does occur. However, having stated that, it must be acknowledged that variations are not the rule, but rather the exception. Wide variations are very, very uncommon. On the other hand, minor variations can occur. If the impedance of the stimulating electrode varies, then there will be a variation in the amount of current delivered to the cortex, if all other parameters are the same. If this difference in the delivery of current between successive stimuli is significant, then variability in the responses obtained may be significant, especially when stimulating the Rolandic cortex. This was briefly referred to in Sect. 4.3.3. It usually results from variations in either the amount of cortical surface contacted by the electrode or the amount of moisture in the environment of the electrode. It is more likely to occur when the electrode is being applied by hand, in which case it can usually be corrected by simply paying close attention to the placement of it on the cortex. It is also less likely to occur (1) with a constant current stimulator, in contrast to a constant voltage stimulator; (2) through the use of a mechanical electrode holder; or (3) through the use of a fine saline spray for keeping constant moisture of the cortex.

Variations in responses may occur as a result of an overzealous method of conducting the exploratory stimulation. These have been discussed earlier. Variations are more likely if the stimulating current is right at threshold (T) for the response, especially when stimulating the Rolandic cortex. This was discussed in Sect. 4.3.4, where it was suggested that the use of a stimulus just above threshold, e.g., 1.25 T, might well abolish this as a cause of variation in responses. In Sect. 4.3.5 the phenomenon of afterdischarges immediately following the stimulus and their contributions to possible errors in interpretation were noted. If there is an accompanying ECoG, this will be evident. If not, then the appropriate spatial separation (see Sub-sect. 4.4.2.2) and/or temporal separation (see Sub-sect. 4.4.2.3) of stimuli will preclude this cause of variation.

When all the foregoing potential causes of variations in responses are attended to, then the artificial, non-physiological causes of variation should be significantly reduced or abolished. What does this leave? If variations continue to occur, then one must accept that these variations are examples of neurophysiological origin, presumably associated with fluctuations in the excitability of the underlying neural networks.

4.6 Responses to Stimulation of Specific Functional (Eloquent) Cortical Areas

4.6.1 Speech

There are two traditionally recognized speech areas—Broca's and Wernicke's. Historically these have been identified as involving expressive and receptive aspects of speech, respectively. However, there have certainly been observations that have failed to follow the initial traditional view of pure expressive and pure receptive functions in the two areas in that a mixture deficits may be observed from an injury to only one of the areas. Thus, this distinction is not as clear-cut as one might predict from medical school education. This will not be discussed in any detail, but awareness of the lack of such exact divisions is important. This will become more apparent in references to observations of the transient deficits, which may follow frontal or temporal corticectomies of the dominant hemisphere.

Electrical stimulation of the speech areas *never* produces speech and, in fact, never produces *any* type of vocalization, in contrast to stimulation of the supplementary motor area (SMA) or the inferior Rolandic cortex of either hemisphere (Rasmussen and Milner 1975, p. 239). Stimulation of a speech area in a patient who is not speaking at the time results in no subjective perception of the stimulation.

This is in contrast to stimulation of the lower Rolandic area (*vide infra*, Sect. 4.6.2), in which motor movements or abnormal sensory perceptions will be perceived. Responses of patients who are speaking when the threshold stimulation is applied may result in a variety of perceptions, which provide evidence of interference with speech. The commonest observation is an arrest of speech, but other variations include hesitancy, intermittent repetitions, or something akin to stuttering, dysphasia, or a slow, overly premeditated speech. These latter alterations are more commonly observed when the stimulus strength is very, very gradually raised. Thus, when they appear they represent threshold responses as opposed to arrests of speech. If arrest of speech is not the threshold response, then with very little increase in the strength of the stimulus, arrest will be observed. When the patients are asked "what happened" or "why did you stop speaking," they usually utter something to the effect that they do not know, e.g., "I don't know…," or "I don't know… I guess I just stopped," or "I don't know… it just happened," or "I couldn't think of the right word," or "I'm not sure."

Interestingly, not dissimilar responses may be *observed* from stimulation of the lower Rolandic area, especially the precentral (motor) gyrus, while patients are speaking. However, the differentiation between the two responses can be determined by asking the patients what they feel was responsible for the speech abnormality, by stimulating the areas when there is no ongoing speech. Under this circumstance, stimulation of the speech areas results nearly always in the patients being completely unaware of any abnormal perception. On the other hand, the abnormalities from stimulation of the Rolandic area are recognized by motor movements, often reported as an awareness of "something" wrong, often with the reference that it is appreciated at "the back of my throat," or some type of abnormal sensory perception. If asked directly, they usually confirm that it has something to do with an altered articulation. If there is difficulty in differentiating the responses from stimulation of Broca's and inferior Rolandic areas, the most rapid method of sorting it out is to have the patient protrude his/her tongue. Stimulation of the Rolandic area will be associated with contralateral deviation of the tongue (e.g., in the operating room it is deviation towards the floor), while that of Broca's area results in no motor response. Another strategy is that of stimulating at frequencies below that which produces fusion of skeletal muscle, e.g., <10 Hz. In this case the individual movements from Rolandic motor stimulation can be seen easily or appreciated in speech at roughly the same frequency as the stimulation frequency when stimulating the motor cortex.

4.6.1.1 Broca's Area

Broca's area is the area of the neocortex, in the dominant frontal operculum, immediately anterior to the inferior motor (Rolandic) cortex. The area may consist of the immediately anterior gyrus, alone, or the two gyri immediately anterior to the precentral sulcus (Broca 1861). There have been cases where "a silent gyrus" exists, not associated with speech, between the precentral gyrus and a more anterior opercular gyrus, the stimulation of which is clearly identified as Broca's area (Rasmussen and Milner 1975, pp. 240–1 and Fig. 4.5). However, this indeed is the exception to

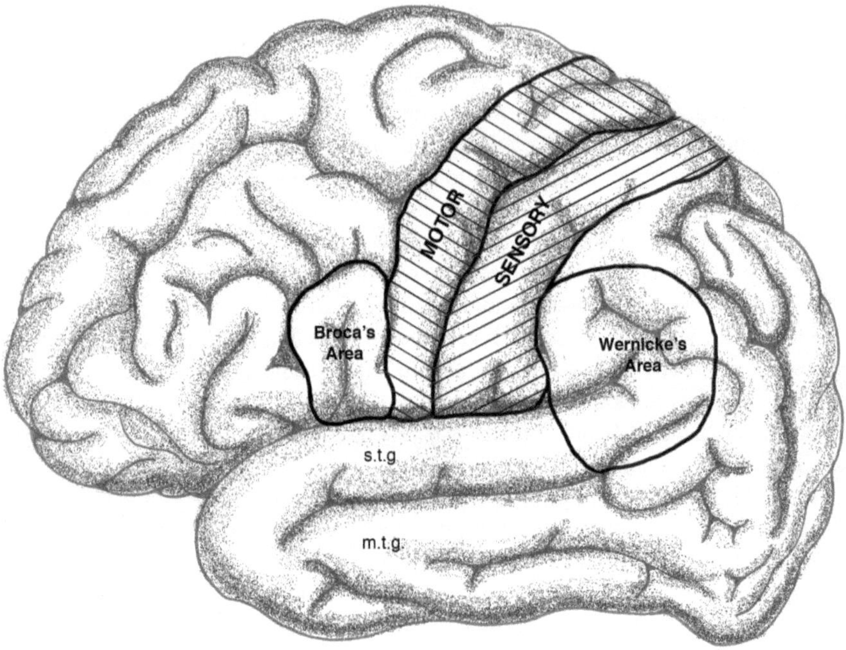

Fig. 4.5 Functional cortical localization, left cerebral hemisphere. Functional areas of the cortex of the left hemisphere, which have been delineated through many observations made from electrocortical stimulatory mapping. *m.t.g* middle temporal gyrus, *s.t.g* superior temporal gyrus

the rule that it is the gyrus that is immediately anterior to the precentral sulcus in the dominant operculum, which is Broca's speech area (see Fig. 4.5).

The threshold of Broca's cortex is usually higher than that of the Rolandic region. Usually it is in the neighborhood of two to three times the Rolandic threshold, i.e., ~2–3 T, but indeed may be only very slightly higher or significantly higher, e.g., up to 5–10 T. Finally, a discussion of stimulation of the cortex which is assumed to be Broca's area, e.g., in the presumed location of Broca's area, would not be complete without indicating that infrequently there may be no evidence whatsoever of an alteration in speech, even in the circumstances where the stimulation strength is raised so high that stimulatory responses from the Rolandic cortex cannot be avoided. One is always concerned about the latter, in that with higher stimulation strengths the concern about producing seizures rises significantly. What is the interpretation of such absences of responses? I cannot answer this query. However, if there are no extenuating circumstances, pointing to another more likely reason, my tentative interpretation is that the area is located somewhere in the hidden, or buried, cortex. I have never required the removal of this area, under these circumstances. However, if I were in the position of having to remove this cortex, for whatever reason, I would certainly choose to carry out the resection under local anesthesia, if the responses had been obtained preoperatively (on the ward) through subdural stimulating electrodes. Further, the resection should be carried out slowly, using stimulation and with a continual associated clinical examination of speech.

4.6.1.2 Wernicke's Area

Wernicke's area is much larger and is not so predictably localized as Broca's area. It is located in the vicinity of the dominant posterior perisylvian fissure, involving the middle to posterior temporal cortex and the juxtaposed cortex of the parietal operculum (see Fig. 4.5). The temporal cortical portion of the area involves the superior and middle temporal gyri. The anterior part of this involved temporal cortex is posterior to Heschl's gyrus and usually at or posterior to the postcentral sulcus. Rasmussen noted that it was "mainly [in] the second [middle] temporal gyrus behind the level of the postcentral sulcus and extending posteriorly for 2–3 cm and [in] the adjacent convolution above, behind the transverse gyri of Heschl" (Rasmussen and Milner 1975, p. 241). It *never* involves the inferior temporal gyrus. The characteristic stimulation thresholds and responses are similar to those found on stimulation of Broca's area.

The parietal cortical representation of the area is located in the immediate suprasylvian parietal cortex and behind the postcentral sulcus. Unlike Broca's area, which is nearly always juxtaposed to the face area of the precentral gyrus across the precentral sulcus, the parietal cortex of Wernicke's area may be much further behind the postcentral sulcus. It may also extend as far as 3–4 cm above the Sylvian fissure. In shorter Sylvian fissures the center "wraps around," if you will, the posterior end of the fissure.

There is a higher percentage of absence of responses from Wernicke's area than Broca's area, and this is even in the face of the much higher strengths of stimulation that can be applied, without the appearance of the effects of associated adjacent Rolandic stimulation. It is perhaps the latter which leads one to interpret that this temporoparietal cortex is one of the less excitable cortices, with respect to the production of post-stimulatory afterdischarges and/or cerebral seizures.

4.6.1.3 Preoperative Speech Testing

Juhn Wada introduced what has become known as "the Wada test" or the "intracarotid amytal test," which consists of the intracarotid injection of sodium amytal that causes a transient dysfunction of the cortex of the ipsilateral hemisphere, which is narcotized by the injection (1949). Its introduction was primarily designed to allow determination of the hemispheric dominance for speech (Wada 1949, 1982; Wada and Rasmussen 1960; Branch et al. 1964; Rasmussen and Milner 1975). The procedure is widely used and until the recent introduction of functional magnetic resonance imaging (fMRI) was really the only valid method of preoperatively establishing the dominant hemisphere for speech. It has, since its introduction, been used for various other functional determinations.

4.6.2 Motor

As alluded to earlier (Sub-sect. 4.3.4.1) the Rolandic cortex is the most excitable human cortex. The Penfield homunculus is the best guide to the approximate locations and proximities of the various segments of motor behavior (Penfield and Boldrey 1937). The parameters of stimulation were discussed briefly earlier

(Sect. 4.2.2). The electrode impedance of most stimulating electrodes is in the range of 2–5 kΩ. Thus, when using the parameters noted earlier (Sect. 4.2.2) and a constant voltage stimulator, Rolandic thresholds will be approximately 2–5 V and in the case of a constant current stimulator approximately 0.5–1.0 mA. Once threshold (T) is established, a greater stability in responses is achieved with slightly higher thresholds (*vide supra*, Sect. 4.3.4), e.g., 1.25 T. Although responses may vary widely with small alterations in the stimulus strength around threshold, nevertheless with a constant strength, a bit above threshold, a relatively reliable repeatability of responses can be achieved. However, it is worth being aware that reports of "instability" can occur with no change in the point of stimulation and no change in stimulation parameters (Brown and Sherrington 1912).

As noted in the foregoing (Sect. 4.6.1), vocalization may be produced by stimulation of the face area of either hemisphere. The vocalization is not like normal speech, but rather guttural, inarticulate, and with unfamiliar sounds. If the patient is speaking, then the common response to stimulation is a type of dysarthria, e.g., distorted speech, as a result of a variation of slurring. However, this type of speech is usually understandable, even though with some difficulty.

Any frequency of stimulation may be used. However, I again reiterate that the use of lower frequencies is often more advantageous when stimulating the motor cortex in that in frequencies less than the fusion frequency of muscle contraction, e.g., 5–10 Hz, very subtle contractions may be able to be discerned visually, especially in the case of naïve observers. This was also noted by Liddell and Phillips (1950). In some cases this may be more accurate than the subjective perception of the patient who is drowsy.

A typical example of the escalating responses that may accompany small variations in stimulus strength, using the stimulus parameters of 40 Hz, 500 μs pulses, and 1–2 s train durations, delivered to the same point on the Rolandic motor cortex, resulted in a threshold of 6.25 V. At threshold there was extension of the little finger. When the voltage was raised to 7.5 V and then to 8.25 V, forearm pronation and flexion of the elbow, respectively, were observed. A naïve observer, who recorded, quite accurately, the major movements from the stimulations, noted all of these responses. However, the importance of recognizing the response at threshold, in cases such as this example, cannot be overemphasized, as it is the response at threshold, in this case extension of the little finger, which denotes the accurate segment of the homunculus that has been stimulated.

Interestingly, Cushing, many years ago, felt that "It may be noted that the motor area of the epileptic's brain seems to be unduly excitable to electrical stimulation, and that focal or general seizures can be elicited on faradization more easily than from the normal cortex" (1910, p. 245).

4.6.3 Sensory

The sensory cortex has the typically lower thresholds of the Rolandic cortex. However, unlike stimulation of the motor cortex, when both the observer and the patient may perceive responses, the responses to stimulation of the somatosensory cortex are dependent entirely upon the perception of the patient. As noted earlier, with both speech and with the somatosensory (Rolandic) cortex, natural, e.g., clinically normal, responses are never obtained. Thus, normal sensations, such as light touch, temperature alterations, proprioceptive movements, pressure, etc., are not perceived. When asking patients to describe what might be the closest familiar sensory perception to what they experience to the stimulations, there is usually clearly expressed uncertainty in answering the question. "I don't know" is a common response. Often there is a "I feel something…" and the "something" may be further elucidated by "like… Buzzing," or "some kind of a funny feeling," "most like tingling," or….

While a patient may have great difficulty in describing the *quality* of the responses to Rolandic sensory cortical stimulation, no such difficulty is encountered in describing the *localization* of the response. The responses can usually be localized very accurately and they are usually reliably repeatable.

There is no reason to utilize low frequencies of stimulation, and in fact I think that the higher frequencies within the 10–50 Hz range are more liable to result in more stable responses than the lower frequencies.

Motor responses may be produced when the strength of stimulation is raised significantly above threshold levels, even occasionally vocalizations.

4.6.4 Vision

Penfield and Rasmussen stimulated the visual areas of many patients and never reproduced any complex visual hallucinations (1968). Rather, their stimulations produced "elementary" hallucinatory activity, which included unformed images of spots, wheels, stars, balls, or flashes of light, darkness, and/or color, which may be stationary, flashing, or moving in the contralateral visual field. They considered that stimulation of all three Brodmann's areas, 17–19, probably gives rise to these hallucinatory images and that there was no clear evidence to suggest that there were any differentiating characteristics between the three areas.

In the early part of the twentieth century, German neurosurgeons noted the appearance of dots of light in the contralateral visual field in response to punctuate occipital cortical stimulation (Krause 1924; Foerster 1929a, b; Krause and Schum 1931; Urban 1937). More recent stimulation of the visual cortex has confirmed that in the absence of head movement these dots of light are motionless, usually white, but may have many different hues and are in the contralateral visual field. These dots have become designated as "phosphenes" (Brindley 1973; Brindley and Lewin 1968). Movement of the eyes results in the movement of the phosphenes in the same direction, in much the same fashion as the movement of retinal afterimages. Phosphenes may be seen in hemianopic fields or even in blindness, but *only if* the patients have visual memory. In other words, those blind from birth do not seemingly perceive phosphenes to stimulation nor any other evidence of something that might be interpreted as visual in origin.

The plotting of a phosphene visual field follows, within gross limits, the Holmesian retino-cortical map disclosed in the early part of the twentieth century (Holmes 1918, 1919, 1931, 1945; Holmes and Lister 1916) and in recent stimulation studies (Brindley and Lewin 1968; Dobelle et al. 1974, 1979). The occipital cortical area, from which phosphenes may be produced by stimulation, includes the medial cortex of the occipital lobe and less predictably a small narrow portion of the immediate parasagittal part of its dorsolateral cortex.

4.6.5 Memory

Unlike the foregoing considerations, whose neural substrate is the *neo*cortex, the most important cortex subserving memory is the *allo*cortex of the hippocampus. While it is not common to stimulate the hippocampus intraoperatively, nevertheless, it is a strategy that may be of use in unusual circumstances, e.g., cases in which there is some uncertainty as to whether the hippocampus can be removed without a resultant postoperative memory deficit.

The initial strategy of the investigation of the quality of memory in each of the temporal lobes was initiated by Milner and her colleagues (1962). She took advantage of the technique introduced by Wada to determine the cerebral dominance of speech (Wada 1949; Wada and Rasmussen 1960). In this test, intracarotid amytal procedure (ICAP) is utilized for memory evaluation, e.g., the intracarotid amytal procedure for memory (ICAP-M); in this test sodium amytal is injected into one carotid artery, thus narcotizing one temporal lobe. In the latter it is assumed that the effect of the amytal on the hippocampus of the injected side is a transient abolition of its function. During the period of narcosis, a few minutes, the patient is presented material and asked to remember it. After the narcosis has worn off, e.g., ~10–15 min, if the patient is unable to recall the previously presented material or to recognize it from among the presentation of a larger amount of material in which it is included, then the ICAP-M is said to have been a "failed" test. That is to say, the interpretation is that patient was unable to remember the presented material when the function of the injected (amytal) hippocampus was considered to be absent and thus the patient's memory is dependent upon that hippocampus. In other words, it is concluded that the injected hippocampus is mandatory for the patient's normal memory and that, therefore, it cannot be surgically removed. When a patient failed the ICAP-M on both sides, it was traditionally considered that neither hippocampus could be removed.

In the 1980s we theorized that it was unlikely that the failed ICAP-M bilaterally really was compatible with the notion that both hippocampi were necessary for a patient's normal memory. The methodology for investigating this hypothesis, through intraoperative electrical stimulation, which will be outlined in the following, was used for establishing the fact that bilateral failure of significant memory, as determined by the bilateral intracarotid amytal procedure for memory (ICAP-M), was not a contraindication to the performance of an anterior temporal lobectomy (aTLY) on either side (Girvin et al. 1987; Kubu et al. 2000). This same methodology may be, and indeed has been, used intraoperatively in other circumstances in which preoperative assessment of the integrity of the hippocampus for memory was unable to be determined otherwise with certainty.

The *intra*operative testing of memory, when required, can really only be achieved with confidence by surface stimulation of the hippocampus (HPC). In fact, the primary reason for the testing would be in cases where some type of temporal lobe surgery was being undertaken, usually for the removal of an epileptic focus, where there was some uncertainty as to whether the HPC could be removed without producing a memory deficit. I have not used the technique in an operation, which consisted of the smaller (less invasive) procedure of amygdalohippocampectomy, but it should be able to be used in that operation as well as the more standard aTLY in which the initial neocortical removal leaves clear visual access to the majority of the surface of the HPC.

The technique, in short, consists of serially stimulating contiguous segments of the HPC, with associated serial removals of the segments, the stimulations of which fail to indicate that they are necessary for memory. An example of this arbitrary division of the hippocampus into segments is depicted in Fig. 4.6a. It is known that excessive stimulation of the cerebral cortex may render it functionless during the period of stimulation, i.e., "The invariable effect… is to produce interference

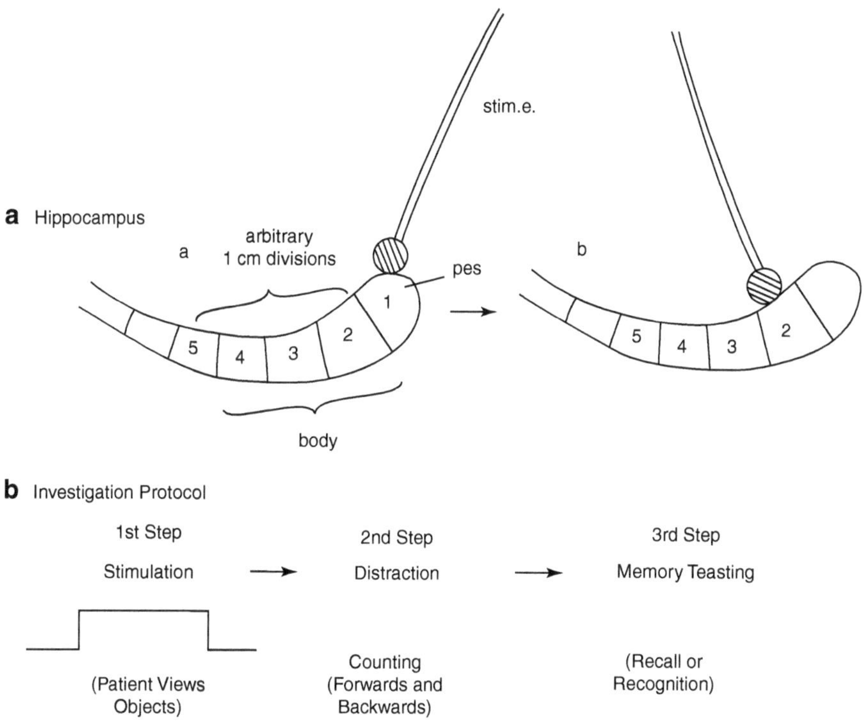

Fig. 4.6 Electrical stimulation of the hippocampus for the determination of the presence of satisfactory memory. The illustration of the stimulation protocol and methodology for the intraoperative investigation of the integrity of the hippocampus for memory function. (**a**) An illustration of the hippocampus and its *arbitrary* divisions into a number of 1 cm segments for stimulation; (a) initial stimulation of segment 1; (b) stimulation of the second segment, after removal of initial (first) segment. (**b**) The clinical protocol, outlining the events involved in the investigation of each of the hippocampal "segmental" stimulations. *1, 2, -5* arbitrary 1 cm divisions of the hippocampal body, *body* body of the hippocampus, *pes* pes (head) hippocampus, *stim.e.* stimulating electrode

with the normal employment of the area affected by the electrical current" (Rasmussen and Milner 1975, p. 238). The validity of the technique depended upon our empirical assumption of the strategy that the use of transient trains of suprathreshold stimulation pulses on arbitrarily designated 1 cm segments of the HPC would result in the transient abolition of function of those segments during the course of the stimulations. Thus, it is not dissimilar to the effect of the injection of amytal in the ICAP-M. The difference is simply that the latter is *assumed* to abolish the whole of the hippocampal function during the few minutes after the injection of amytal, whereas in our investigation we *assumed* that suprathreshold, high-frequency stimulation would produce neural dysfunction involving at least the cubic centimeter of the HPC beneath the stimulating electrode. The strength of the stimulation was a multiple of the threshold that was determined in the stimulation of the Rolandic cortex of the same patient. The usual current strength that we used was five times the threshold (T) for responses from the Rolandic cortex, i.e., 5 T. The other parameters of stimulation were 50 Hz, 0.2 ms pulses, and train durations of 2–5 s.

The ability of the patient to identify various materials presented by our neuropsychologist is assessed prior to the application of stimuli, usually both on the day before the operation and then during the course of the surgery, just before the stimulation. Once such an assessment is considered satisfactory, investigation of the patient's memory is initiated. The investigative procedure is outlined in Fig. 4.6b, which is divided into three steps. The initial (first) step consists of the ~5 s period of the stimulation of segment 1 (see Fig. 4.6Aa). Immediately after the onset of the stimulation, the neuropsychologist presents pictures of objects, often verbalizing their names, after which the stimulation is turned off. Thus, the presentation of the material is only *during* the course of the stimulation. Shortly after the cessation of the stimulation, the second step, distraction, is begun, consisting of a few minutes during which the neuropsychologist talks to the patient for a few minutes with simple distracting stimuli, featured particularly counting forwards and backwards. It might also include the presentation of irrelevant material and the engagement in unrelated conversation. After this the third step, memory testing, is initiated. The patient is asked to name the pictures that had been presented during the stimulation. If they recalled the pictures accurately, then it was assumed that our initial assumption was correct, i.e., that that stimulated segment was not required for their memory. If they did not remember the pictures, de novo, then they were presented a series of pictures, which included those shown during the stimulation, and the patient was requested to identify (i.e., recall) the pictures that had been shown during the stimulation. If the patient was able to accurately recognize the previously presented pictures from the series, then once again the stimulated segment of the HPC was considered expendable. Under these circumstances the stimulated segment was resected. Figure 4.6Ab illustrates the removal of the first segment and the stimulating electrode placed on the second segment. The very same series of undertakings relating to segment 1 is simply repeated with respect to segment 2. The series is continued, if each stimulated segment fails to have difficulty recalling or recognizing the presented objects, until the hippocampus is removed.

The operation is terminated under one of two circumstances. On the one hand, if the patient was unable to recall or to recognize the presented material on repeated occasions, there was no consideration of resection. On the other hand, if memory was continually intact, then the stimulated segments were serially resected until the hippocampus was removed.

4.7 The Altered Interpretations of Electrocortical Stimulation That May Occur in the Presence of Congenital Lesions

It is a well-known fact that the presence of *congenital lesions* may displace the eloquent cortex, if they are situated in the normal cortical areas associated with predictable functional localization. The commonest lesions to do this are large arteriovenous malformations (AVMs). These lesions can result in the transfer of speech centers to the opposite (nondominant) hemispheres and the transfer of the Rolandic cortex anteriorly or posteriorly in the dorsolateral hemispheric cortex. In my own experience, if there is no deficit of any kind that could be attributable to the lesion as viewed in the imaging studies, then the likelihood is that there has been some kind of movement (transfer) of the functional cortex to a non-lesional area, i.e., in the normal or more normal cortex away from the lesion, around the periphery, or, in the case of speech, to the contralateral hemisphere.

The foregoing may also be observed in the case of speech in *acquired lesions*, especially traumatic, before the age of 5–8. That is to say, significant trauma to the speech center of a child under the age of 6 (common range is 5–8) will result, after a period of a few weeks of dysphasia or a very few months, in its transfer to the contralateral hemisphere (see Branch et al. 1964; and especially Rasmussen and Milner 1975).

The foregoing becomes of significance if surgical management of epilepsy foci or AVMs is considered in these eloquent areas. While the use of functional magnetic resonance imaging (fMRI) is now at the outset of potentially beginning to replace the use of the intracarotid amytal test in the lateralization of speech and the assessment of hippocampal function, nevertheless, there are still instances where such imaging is not satisfactory. In these cases the traditional intracarotid amytal procedure may be used. However, its use in the cases of high-flow AVMs is very suspect, as the amytal may largely flow through the AVM, rather than the cortex associated with it; therefore, the function of that cortex cannot be evaluated through fMRI nor the ICAP. Thus, in the face of "negative" tests, i.e., those in which the amytal results in no neurological change, very little is learned from the tests. In the case of speech, the contralateral ICAP may give important information. In spite of the ICAP and the fMRI assessments, in the face of AVMs in eloquent areas, there is still often the necessity of operating on such patients under local anesthesia, when electrocortical stimulation mapping really remains the gold standard.

4.8 Operative Record of Cortical Sites of Importance

For those who wish to retain evidence of operations in which areas of cortical functional localization have been observed, it is very worthwhile to achieve some type of archival recording. I have used simple alphanumerical symbols to place on the areas of cortex that I wish to retain and use photographs of the areas to archive them. The symbols are illustrated in Fig. 4.7. This is simply a photograph consisting of a number of letters, numerals, arrows, and distances that I used for years. It is sterilized and the scrub nurse simply cuts off whatever pieces of information are used at the time. My own protocol was to use the numbers as designations of the recording electrode numbers, the letters reflecting various responses to stimulation, and the combination of arrows and numbers to designate the distance (in millimeters) from one place to another, usually that from the pole of a lobe.

After the completion of the application of the tickets to the cortical sites, a photograph of them provides a permanent record, which can be used for reference in the

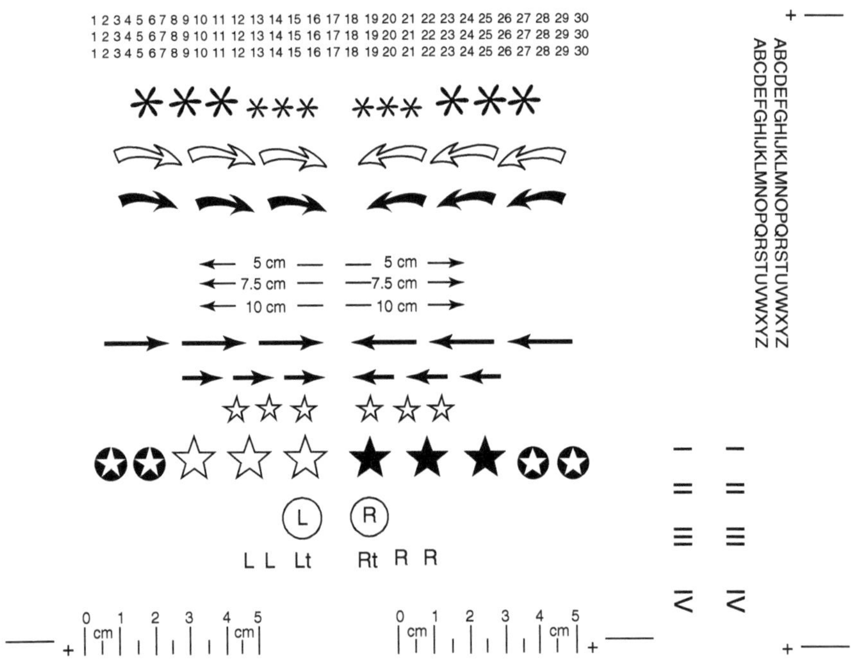

Fig. 4.7 Illustration of symbols and alphanumerical designations, useful in marking the cortex for photography. An illustration of a photograph of symbols and alphanumerical designations, utilized to outline various sites on the cortex, which can be photographed for permanent archives (see text)

event of another operation at the same site or more importantly for retrospective research analyses associated with cortical functional localization, assessment of electrocorticographic abnormalities, and numerous correlations.

References

Agnew WF, Yuen GH, Pudenz RH, Bullara LA. Electrical stimulation of the brain. IV. Ultrastructural studies. Surg Neurol. 1975;5:438–48.

Agnew WF, Yuen TGH, Pudenz RH. Neuropathological effects of intracerebral platinum salt injections. J Neuropathol Exp Neurol. 1977;36:533–46.

Agnew WF, Yuen TGF, McCreery DB. Morphologic changes after prolonged electrical stimulation of the cat's cortex at defined charge densities. Exp Neurol. 1983;79:397–411.

Blume WT, Jones DC, Pathak P. Properties of after-discharges from cortical electrical stimulation in focal epilepsies. Clin Neurophysiol. 2004;115:982–9.

Branch C, Milner B, Rasmussen T. Intracarotid sodium amytal for the lateralization of cerebral speech dominance: observations on 123 patients. J Neurosurg. 1964;21:399–405.

Brindley GS. Sensory effects of electrical stimulation of the visual and paravisual cortex in man. In: Jung J, editor. Handbook of sensory physiology, vol VII/3B, Central Processing of Visual Information. New York/Berlin/Heidelberg: Springer-Verlag; 1973. pp. 583–94.

Brindley GS, Lewin WD. The sensations produced by electrical stimulation of the visual cortex. J Physiol. 1968;196:479–93.

Broca P. Sur la siège de la faculté du language articulé. Bull Soc Anat (Paris). 1861;6(2 Série):355.

Brown TG, Sherrington CS. On the instability of a cortical point. Proc R Soc. 1912;85:250–77.

Bubnoff N, Heidenhain R. Ueber Erregungs- und Hemmungs-orgänge innerhalb der motorischen Hirncentren. Arch Ges Physiol. 1881;26:137–200. English translation: von Bonin, McCulloch WS. In: Bucy PC, editor. The precentral motor cortex. Urbana: University of Illinois Press. Chapter VII. p. 173–210.

Cushing H. Chapter XXXVI. Surgery of the head. In: Keen WW, editor. Surgery: its principles and practice, vol. III. Philadelphia: W.B. Saunders Company; 1910. p. 245.

Dobelle WH, Mladejovsky M. Phosphenes produced by electrical stimulation of human occipital cortex, and their application to the development of a prosthesis for the blind. J Physiol. 1974;243:553–76.

Dobelle WH, Mladejovsky MG, Girvin JP. Artificial vision for the blind: electrical stimulation of visual cortex offers hope for a functional prosthesis. Science. 1974;183:440–4.

Dobelle WH, Turkel J, Henderson DC, Evans JR. Mapping the representation of the visual field by electrical stimulation of human visual cortex. Am J Ophthalmol. 1979;88:727–35.

Dymond AM, Kaechle LE, Jurist JM, Crandall PH. Brain tissue reaction to some chronically implanted metals. J Neurosurg. 1970;33:574–80.

Erickson TE. Spread of epileptic discharge: an experimental study of the after-discharge induced by electrical stimulation of the cerebral cortex. Arch Neurol Psychiatr. 1940;43:429–52.

Foerster O. Zur operativen Behandlung der Epilspsie. Dtsch Z Nervenh. 1926;89:137–47.

Foerster O. Sur Pathogenese und chirurgischen Behandlung der Epilepsie. Zentralbl Chir. 1929a;52:531–49.

Foerster O. Beiträge zur Pathophysiologie der Sehbahn und der Schsphäre. J Psychol Neurol Lpz. 1929b;39:463–85.

Foerster O. Sensible corticale Felder. In: Bumke O, Foerster O, editors. Handbuch der Neurologie, vol. 6. Berlin: Springer; 1936a. p. 1–448.

Foerster O. The motor cortex in man in the light of Hughling Jackson's doctrines. Brain. 1936b;59:135–59.

French JD, Gernandt BE, Livingston RB. Regional differences in seizure susceptibility in monkey cortex. AMA Arch Neurol Psychiatr. 1956;75:260–74.

Girvin JP. Basic aspects of chronic stimulation of excitable tissue. In: Cooper IS, editor. Chronic cerebellar stimulation. New York: Raven; 1978. p. 1–12.

Girvin JP, McGlone J, McLachlan RS, Blume WT. Validity of the sodium amobarbital test for memory in selected patients [abstract]. Epilepsia. 1987;28:636.

Graham Brown T, Sherrington CS. On the instability of a cortical point. Proc R Soc. 1912;85B:250–77.

Grünbaum ASF, Sherrington C. Observations on physiology of the cerebral cortex of some of the higher apes. Proc R Soc Lond. 1901;69:206–9.

Grunbaum ASF, Sherrington C. Observations on the physiology of the cerebral cortex of the anthropoid apes. Proc R Soc. 1903;72:152–5.

Holmes G. Disturbances of vision by cerebral lesions. Br J Ophthalmol. 1918;2:353–84, 449–68, 506–16.

Holmes G. The cortical localization of vision. Br Med J. 1919;2:193–9.

Holmes G. A contribution to the cortical representation of vision. Brain. 1931;54:470–9.

Holmes G. The organization of the visual cortex in man. Proc R Soc Lond. 1945;132:348–61.

Holmes G, Lister WT. Disturbances of vision from cerebral lesions, with special reference to the cortical representation of the macula. Brain. 1916;39:34–73.

Horsley V. Brain-surgery. Br Med J. 1886;2:670–5.

Horsley V. Ten consecutive cases of operation upon the brain and cranial cavity to illustrate the details and safety of the method employed. Br Med J. 1887;1:863–5.

Krause F. Die Sehbahnen in chirurgischer Beziehung und die faradische Reizung des Sehzentrums. Klin Wochenschr. 1924;3:1260–5.

Krause F, Schum H. Die spezielle Chirugie der Gehirnkrankheiten. In: Kuttner H, editor. Neue Deutsche Chirugie, 3 Bände. II. Band. Die epileptischen Erkrankungen. Enke, Stuttgart; 1931. 49a:482–6.

Kubu CS, Girvin JP, McLachlan RS, Pavol M, Harnadek MCS. Does the intracarotid amobarbital procedure predict global amnesia after temporal lobectomy? Epilepsia. 2000;41:1321–9.

Leyton ASF, Sherrington CS. Observations on the excitable cortex of the chimpanzee, orang-utan, and gorilla. Q J Exp Physiol. 1917;11:135–222.

Libet B. Chapter 19. Electrical stimulation of cortex in human subjects and conscious sensory aspects. In: Iggo A, editor. Handbook of sensory physiology, vol. II. Somatosensory system. Berlin-Heidleberg: Springer-Verlag; 1973. pp. 743–90.

Libet B, Alberts WW, Wright EW, Levin G, Feinstein B. Sensory perception by direct stimulation of human cerebral cortex: stimulus parameters. Fed Proc. 1959;18:92.

Libet B, Alberts WW, Wright EW, Levin G, Feinstein B. Direct excitation of human somatosensory cortex. Electroencephalogr Clin Neurophysiol. 1961;13:498.

Libet B, Alberts WW, Wright EW, Delattre LD, Levin G, Feinstein B. Production of threshold levels of conscious sensation by electrical stimulation of human somato-sensory cortex. J Neurophysiol. 1964;27:546–78.

Liddell EGT, Phillips CG. Thresholds of cortical representation. Brain. 1950;73:125–40.

Lilly JC. Injury and excitation by electric currents: the balanced pulse-pair waveform. In: Sheer DE, editor. Electrical stimulation of the brain. Austin: University of Texas Press; 1961. p. 60–4.

Lilly JC, Austin GM, Chambers WM. Threshold movements produced by excitation of cerebral cortex and efferent fibers with some parametric regions of rectangular current pulses (cats and monkeys). J Neurophysiol. 1952;15:319–41.

Lilly JC, Hughes JR, Alvord EC, Galkin TW. Brief, non-injurious electric wave form for stimulation of the brain. Science. 1955a;121:468–9.

Lilly JC, Hughes JR, Galkin TW, Alvord EC. Production and avoidance of injury to brain tissue by electrical current and threshold values. EEG Clin Neurophysiol. 1955b;7:458–9.

MacIntyre WJ, Bidder TG, Rowland V. The production of brain lesions with electric currents. Proc Nat Biophys Conf (1st, 1957). 1959. pp. 723–32.

MacIntyre WJ, Bidder TG, Rowland V. Effect of electric currents on brain tissue: stimulation and electrolytic lesion production. In: Glasser O, editor. Medical physics, vol. III. Chicago: Yearbook; 1960. p. 102–5.

McCulloch W, Dusser de Barenne JG. Extinction: local stimulatory inactivation within the motor cortex. Am J Physiol. 1935;224:97–8.

Mihailović L, Delgado JMR. Electrical stimulation of monkey brain with various fragments and pulse durations. J Neurosurg. 1956;19:21–36.

Milner B, Branch C, Rasmussen T. Study of short-term memory after intracarotid injection of sodium amytal. Trans Am Neurol Assoc. 1962;87:224–6.

Penfield W. Pitfalls and success in surgical treatment of focal epilepsy. Br Med J. 1958;1:669–72.

Penfield W, Boldrey E. Somatic motor and sensory representation in the cerebral cortex of man as studied by electrical stimulation. Brain. 1937;60:389–443.

Penfield W, Jasper H. Epilepsy and the functional anatomy of the human brain. Boston: Little, Brown and Co; 1954. p. 896.

Penfield W, Rasmussen T. The cerebral cortex of man: a clinical study of localization of function. New York: Hafner Publishing Company; 1968. p. 248.

Rasmussen T, Milner B. Clinical and surgical studies of the cerebral speech areas in man. In: Zulch KJ, Creutzfeldt O, Galbraith GC, editors. Cerebral localization: an Otfrid Foerster symposium. New York: Springer; 1975. p. 238–57.

Stensaas SS, Eddington DK, Dobelle WH. The topography and variability of the primary visual cortex in man. J Neurosurg. 1974;40:747–55.

Urban H. Zur Physiologie der Occipital region des Menschen. Z Ges Neurol Psychiatr. 1937;158:257–61.

Wada J. A new method for the determination of the side of cerebral speech dominance: a preliminary report on the intracarotid injection of sodium amytal in man. Med Biol. 1949;14:221–2. Japanese.

Wada JA. Epilepsy surgery revisited: conceptual reassessment of generalized seizure. Folia Psychiatr Neurol Jpn. 1982;36:233–5.

Wada J, Rasmussen T. Intracarotid injection of sodium amytal for the lateralization of cerebral speech dominance: experimental and clinical observations. J Neurosurg. 1960;17:266–82.

Walker AE. Electrocorticography in epilepsy. EEG Clin Neurophysiol. 1949a;2(Suppl):30–7.

Walker AE. Post-traumatic epilepsy. Springfield: Charles Thomas; 1949b. p. 86.

Walker AE, Johnson HC, Kollros JJ. Penicillin convulsions: the convulsive effect of penicillin applied to the cerebral cortex of monkey and man. Surg Gynecol Obstet. 1945;81:692–701.

5 Corticectomy

5.1 Introduction

The basic operation in epilepsy surgery is the simple removal of a section of the cortex, e.g., the "corticectomy." The use of subpial resection forms the basis of the technical removal of the section of the cortex. Thus, the periphery, or edges, of the resected area of the cortex is where the attributes of subpial dissection are most important, i.e., precluding, or reducing, the potential injury to the surrounding cortex, which will remain as the intact functioning cortex. However, in addition to the quality of the subpial surgical technique, the operation of corticectomy requires the recognition of other surgical aspects, many of which depend upon the site of the resection. These include: (1) the necessity of the preservation of some of the vessels overlying the cortex to be removed, (2) the lack of the necessity to remove the subcortical white matter underlying the resected cortex, and (3) the mandatory preservation of subcortical white matter in some circumstances.

5.2 Preservation of Overlying Vessels ("Skeletonization")

Some corticectomies, which are at the anatomically peripheral limits of parts of the cerebrum, may be conducted without concern about the preservation of any tissue within the boundaries of the corticectomy. This, for example, would apply to most corticectomies involving the poles of the hemisphere, e.g., temporal, frontal, and occipital. (If sufficiently large, then they are better designated as polar lobectomies, as opposed to corticectomies.) However, it is rare that the surgeon might be faced with difficulties of preserving *en passage* arterial vessels in those instances, as these more peripheral corticectomies will rarely have overlying arterial vasculature that must be preserved, or underlying white matter that must be preserved. This derives from the fact that the vasculature is "end arterial vasculature"; that is to say, the vasculature in these cases ends in the cortex that is targeted for removal. Thus, there is no reason for its special preservation. The same may be said for the underlying

J.P. Girvin, *Operative Techniques in Epilepsy*,
DOI 10.1007/978-3-319-10921-3_5

white matter, in which all of the subcortical afferent and efferent axons are subservient to the cortex being removed.

In the conduct of a resection of a small portion of the cortex (corticectomy), the onus upon the surgeon is to distinguish between two groups of vessels traversing the cortex. One group consists of those vessels whose only areas of irrigations are confined to those within the cortex to be removed, the "end arterial vasculature" referred to in the foregoing paragraph. The other group consists of those vessels, which are traversing the area of the cortex to be removed but are involved in irrigating the cortex that is not to be removed, but rather to be preserved. Such vessels may also provide as well some irrigation of the parenchyma of the proposed corticectomy. Irrespective of whether they irrigate any part of the proposed corticectomy, any such traversing vessels, which provide significant irrigation of the cortex that is to be preserved, are termed *en passage* vessels. Those vessels on the surface of the gyri, whose areas of irrigation are solely within the cortex to be removed, can usually be visualized without difficulty and their resection is straightforward. The *en passage* vessels, whose end fields of irrigation are outside the corticectomy being conducted, must be preserved and can usually be recognized relatively accurately. The best rule of thumb is that *any* arteries, which may be *en passage* vessels, should be preserved, until, with further dissection, they can be clearly shown to be vessels irrigating only the cortex to be removed. The preservation of such vessels may be easily achieved, especially if they simply pass over a small corner of the corticectomy without contributing to the irrigation of the parenchyma of the corticectomy. However, *en passage* arteries that do contribute to the parenchyma of the proposed corticectomy must be what is called "skeletonized."

Skeletonization literally means "reducing to a skeleton." It has become used in vascular surgery to describe the isolation of a portion of a vessel, usually an artery, by the removal of the tissues adherently associated with it over a part of its course. In the conduct of a corticectomy over which an arterial vessel crosses it to irrigate cerebral parenchyma that is to be preserved, then the vessel, which will be called the "parent" vessel, must also be preserved. Its preservation is achieved by its skeletonization. The adherent tissues that must be removed from the artery over its course across the corticectomy site include leptomeninges and any branches of any size leaving the artery to irrigate *only* the corticectomy parenchyma. This requires the identification of the small branches of the *en passage* artery, which irrigate the parenchyma of the corticectomy. The skeletonization is most easily accomplished by initially carefully incising the leptomeninges throughout the course of the artery crossing over the corticectomy site. When this is completed the arteries confined to irrigating the corticectomy parenchyma are exposed over satisfactory lengths for their coagulations and incisions. For the very small branches, small narrow coagulation bipolar forceps blades and the use of very low coagulating current are most valuable in avoiding injury to the parent artery. Injury results from inadequate low current coagulation and an eventual tearing of the branch at its origin from the parent artery. This can nearly always be avoided by spending a small amount of extra time to isolate a good length of the small branches, e.g., 1–2 mm, in order to have sufficiently exposed vessels that their coagulation and incisions are somewhat remote from the parent vessel. Failure to gain such room in which to isolate them properly will, on occasion, lead to the branch vessel being ruptured at its exit from the parent vessel, which can then be a nuisance to stop, and may even end up with obstruction of the parent vessel. This unpleasant complication usually only requires a single occurrence before the described method of securing a satisfactory length of the vessel with which to work, before coagulating and incising it, is *always* followed! Once the small vessels irrigating the corticectomy parenchyma have been incised and the *en passage* vessel is separated from its leptomeningeal investment, it is truly "skeletonized" and the cortex beneath can be removed without injuring the vessel. When an *en passage* vessel is large, or delicate, or there is more than one, the cortex may have to be removed piece meal.

Figure 5.1a is an illustration of an *en passage* branch of the middle cerebral artery ("epMCA"), emerging from the Sylvian fissure, overlying a right posterior temporo-occipital corticectomy, supplying not only the parenchyma of the proposed corticectomy but in addition some occipital cortex near the pole, which is outside of the proposed periphery of the corticectomy. The pebbled linear outlines depict the periphery (A2) of the corticectomy on the occipital cortex and the subcortical depth (A1) of the corticectomy. Figure 5.1b illustrates the "skeletonization" of the *en passage* vessel. This includes incisions in the juxtaposed leptomeningeal investment (B2) of the corticectomy parenchyma and coagulation and incision of those arterial branches irrigating the cortex being removed ("*"). Figure 5.1c illustrates the resection bed of the corticectomy and the preserved *en passage* artery.

While the recognition of the groups of surface vessels, as noted in the foregoing, is usually relatively straightforward, there is also the possible presence of deep, sulcal, arteries, which may not be managed quite so easily. These intrasulcal vessels are smaller in general, more delicate, and less visible, and their fields of irrigation frequently cannot be easily determined. Further, they do not have a leptomeningeal investment, but rather only a *pial* meningeal investment. It is tantamount that the surgeon uses all the gentleness of suction and low current coagulation strength, which have been emphasized previously, in order to not penetrate the pial membrane. There is always some very minor bleeding from the penetration of the pia by these small branches of the intrasulcal vessels, during the subpial dissection, but some simple gentle pressure for a few minutes from an inserted cottonoid patty can nearly always easily stop this bleeding. Again, the potential fragility of the intrasulcal vasculature cannot be over emphasized. Many of the intrasulcal vessels are sufficiently delicate that minimally applied traction to them may cause the rupture of their branches, or even of them. This is where the technique of applying countertraction (see Sect. 2.2.3) on the pia is so important. That is to say, the countertraction must be enough such that the pull of the suction does not disturb the normal position of the pial membrane. If the latter is achieved, then the tributaries of these vessels

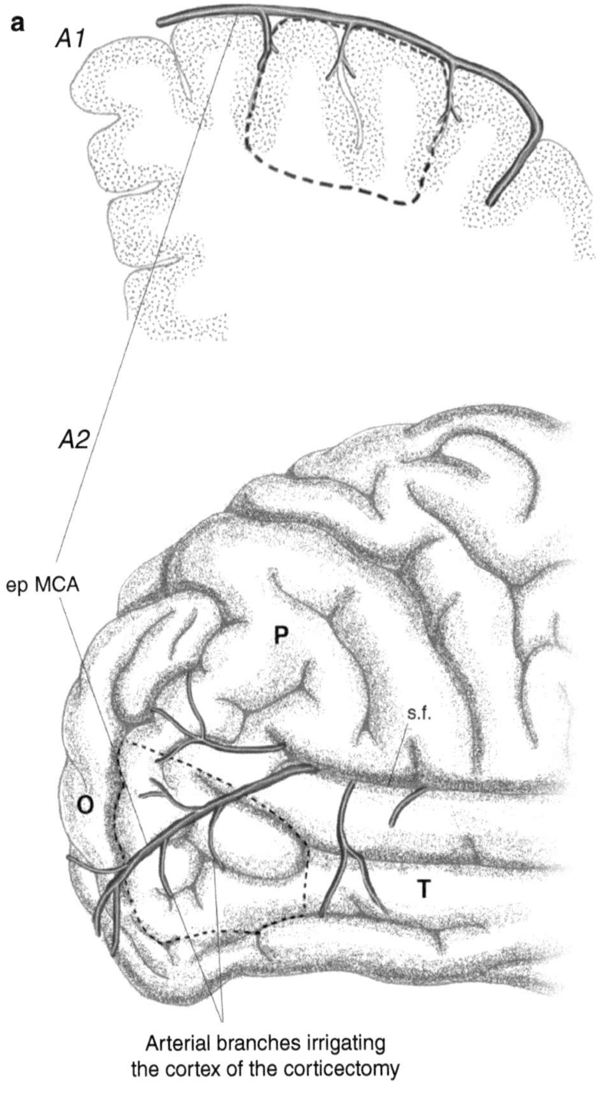

Fig. 5.1 Illustrations of "skeletonizing" *en passage* vessels. An illustration of the steps in the "skeletonization" of an "en passage" artery, a branch of the middle cerebral artery (epMCA), which emerges from the posterior aspect of the Sylvian fissure and courses over the surface of a proposed posterior (*right*) temporo-occipital corticectomy. (**a**) is a diagrammatic representation of the cross section (*A1*) and dorsolateral surface (*A2*) of a potential temporo-occipital corticectomy. *B1* and *B2* depict the achievement of skeletonizing the en passage vessel by coagulating and incising those arteries irrigating *only* the parenchyma of the corticectomy (*), i.e., confined to the corticectomy tissue, in coronal and dorsolateral illustrations, respectively.

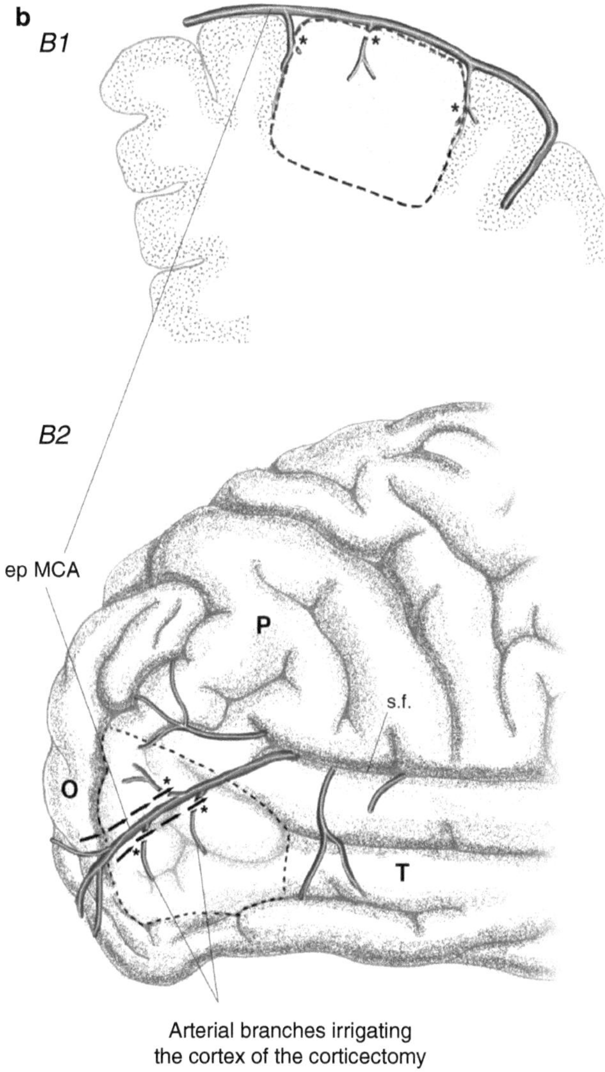

Fig. 5.1 (continued) (**b**) exhibits those arterial vessels (*) that are irrigating *only* parenchyma of the corticectomy and thus require being removed with the corticectomy removal; *B1* depicts three such vessels, the middle one which is over the gyral surface of the corticectomy, arising from the parent vessel, while the other two are secondary branches in that they arise from vessels of the parent artery, irrigating sulcal parenchyma of the corticectomy; *B2* depicts three branches, all of which arise from the parent vessel, irrigating corticectomy parenchyma from the cortex. These branches, outlined in the forgoing, are coagulated and incised, thus leaving the en passage vessels, from which they arose, skeletonized. (**c**) Diagrams of the final resection bed in cross section (*C1*) and on the dorsolateral surface view (*C2*). *epMCA* en passage branch of the middle cerebral artery, *O* occipital lobe, *P* parietal lobe, *S.f.* Sylvian fissure, *T* temporal lobe, * coagulated and incised small branches of the epMCA

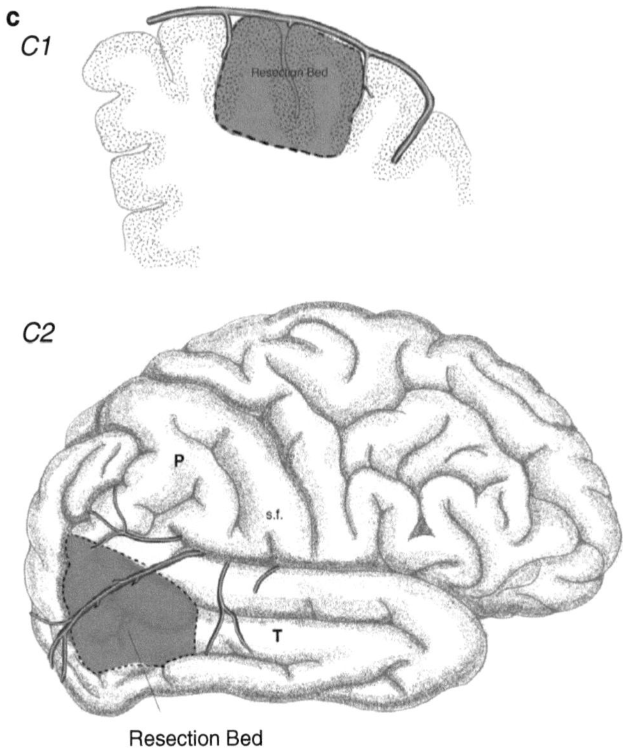

Fig. 5.1 (continued)

will not be compromised. Having said the foregoing, I must confess that very few *en passage* vessels of any significance travel in the depths of the sulci.

There are also specific operative procedures in which relatively predictable preservations of blood supplies are integral parts of the operative procedures, e.g., the peri-callosal and calloso-marginal arteries in frontal lobe resections (see Sects. 7.2.4, 7.2.5, 7.3, and 7.4), the middle cerebral arterial (MCA) branches and posteriorly coursing arteries in an anterior temporal lobectomy (see Sects. 6.2.4 and 6.2.6), the MCA branches irrigating superior dorsolateral Rolandic cortex in an inferior Rolandic corticectomy (see Sect. 8.4), and the arterial branches to the eloquent cortex and white matter in extensive posterior hemisphere corticectomies. These will be considered more completely in later chapters.

5.3 The Subcortical White Matter

The biology of neurons teaches us that their metabolic centers are located in their bodies, or somata, not in their axonal and dendritic branches. Thus, the removal of these somata leads to the death of the neurons. This same consideration applies to the neurons constituting an epileptic focus. The focus resides in the somata of the neuronal population, or network, giving rise to the seizures, i.e., the "gray matter" of the focus. Thus, the surgical treatment of epilepsy is primarily concerned with the removal of the somata of the neurons, or the cortical gray matter. In conducting a corticectomy it is indeed only the gray matter that must be removed. Thus, the removal of any focus can be achieved by the removal of only the gray matter of the focus. Taken to its logical conclusion, therefore, a corticectomy could consist of simply removing only the gray matter of the gyri involved.

The purpose of the foregoing preamble was simply to emphasize that there is no necessity of removing subcortical white matter. In actual fact there is nearly always a significant removal of some white matter in a corticectomy for a number of reasons. First, usually the function of the immediately underlying white matter is entirely associated with the cortex being removed. Under these circumstances its removal has no secondary complications, e.g., such as the involvement of a postoperative neurological deficit. Its vascular counterpart is the removal of only the branches of an *en passage* vessel feeding the corticectomy parenchyma, leaving the parent artery that irrigates healthy parenchyma being left intact. Second, it precludes the possibility of leaving behind some gray matter (e.g., deeper layers of the cortex). It is not always easy to recognize exactly the junction of the deeper layer of gray matter with the superficial subcortical white matter. Thus, in these cases it is safer to remove some of the underlying white matter in order to ensure that all of the cortical gray matter, i.e., the neuronal somata, has been removed. Third, the inclusion of some white matter with the cortical gray mantle often facilitates the actual surgical removal of the cortex. Fourth, a better quality specimen of the cortex, harboring the epileptic focus, is achieved from which to obtain satisfactory morphology.

The maintenance of normal connectivity of the remaining marginal cortex is very difficult about which to be certain. It is most likely never truly achieved completely. However, the surgeon must be at least cognizant that the dissection may significantly alter the neuronal connections and may bring about deafferentation and/or deefferentation of neurons that are being left behind in as normal health as possible. Deafferentation of neurons was considered by Ward to be a significant contributor to the epileptogenicity of epileptic foci (1969). There are specific corticectomies where one is aware of the necessity to take particular caution in preserving the deep white matter and these will be pointed out in later chapters.

The greater the normal connectivity can be preserved, the greater will be the physiological integrity of that cortex that remains behind. As indicated in the foregoing, this is probably never ideally achieved. However, once the cortical neurons of the epileptic focus are removed, then as much of the immediate subcortical white mater as readily possible should probably be preserved.

The reader should now appreciate that there is no reason to be concerned about the removal of small amounts of subcortical white matter, while at the same time there is no necessity to remove large amounts of white matter, or for that matter any white matter! One can usually count on a safe corticectomy consisting of the coincident removal of subcortical white matter that is superficial to the depths of the

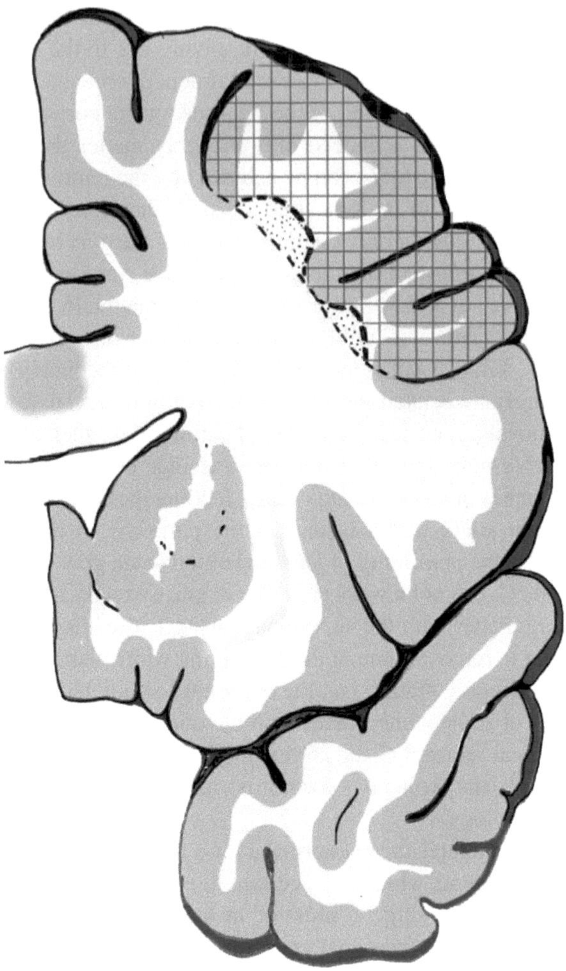

Fig. 5.2 Subcortical resection line of a corticectomy. Illustration of the depth of a (midfrontal) corticectomy, below which there is no reason to resect any deeper white matter. The final resection specimen is outlined in the crosshatching. The *bold* interrupted line outlines the actual deep resection line, i.e., curvilinear, with the deepest points being those beneath the cortex in the depths of the sulci in the specimen. In this manner as much of the subcortical white matter as possible has been saved and thus left intact. The *stippled area* represents subcortical white matter, which may or may not have been part of the resection (See text)

sulci of the cortex being removed. That is to say, so long as the resection is taken only to the bottom of the sulci, then usually the white matter being removed is that which is most likely to be neurophysiologically associated only with the cortex of the corticectomy, e.g., the U-fibers and afferent and efferent fibers to and from the cortical mantle. Once the bottom of a sulcus is reached, the deeper white matter is quite likely to include bundles of axonal fibers whose connectivity is not related to the cortex being removed but may involve tracts that should be preserved. Therefore, the depth of the corticectomy should be no deeper than the cortices at the depth of the sulci of the corticectomy, as demonstrated in Fig. 5.2. Accomplishing the latter requires the surgeon, *during* the conduct of the corticectomy, to initially err on the side of being too superficial after the depth of the gray matter of each sulcus is reached and removed. Therefore, after passing beneath the sulcal gray matter, the line of incision is taken superficially until the next sulcal gray matter is encountered, at which point the incision is taken more deeply to reach a depth just below the deepest extent of the sulcus. When there are a number of sulci involved in the corticectomy, the resection consists of a number of elevations and depressions in the achievement of the deep resection incision line. This is depicted in Fig. 5.2 as the bold interrupted line. It illustrates the fact that after resecting the gray matter of a given sulcus, the direction of the ensuing resection is taken more superficially until the next sulcus in encountered, when once again the relatively pure cortical resection will be taken beneath it. This then constitutes the rather typical curvilinear deep resection line of a corticectomy that involves a number of gyri. In the final analysis the ideal surgical specimen will consist of the surface cortex plus a layer of underlying white matter that is approximately the thickness of the depth of the sulci.

5.4 Mandatory Preservation of Subcortical White Matter

The foregoing statements regarding removal of subcortical white matter during the conduct of corticectomies are generalizations that are important to be remembered. Also very important to be remembered are those instances where there is definitely or very likely knowledge that the subcortical white matter harbors axonal tracts that must *not* be encroached upon; in these cases the deep resection line must be as superficial as possible. In this case its removal may indeed cause an unwanted neurological deficit. These instances will be covered in the specific surgical anatomy associated with certain resections later. However, an example will be cited here in order to outline the theoretical reasons for not compromising such white matter.

Perhaps one of the resections for which the rationale of minimal removal of underlying white matter is most easily understood pertains to parietal lobe corticectomies. Medical students for the first three quarters of the twentieth century learned, primarily from references such as MacDonald Critchley's *The Parietal Lobe*, that the parietal lobe cortex posterior to the postcentral sulcus was involved with right-left (body) recognition, normal picture construction, the ability to dress properly, etc. (1953). However, it is now known that it is not the posterior cortex of the parietal lobe whose destruction leads to right-left confusion, constructional apraxia, dressing apraxia, etc., but rather subcortical white matter tracts beneath the parietal lobe cortex (Corkin et al. 1970). Thus, removal of the parietal cortex must be conducted with the minimal removal of the underlying white matter. If the deeper white matter is encroached upon, then there is risk of creating the traditional postoperative "parietal lobe deficit," which historically was attributed to the removal of the parietal cortex, per se. The previous observations, which arrived at different conclusions (Evans 1935; Semmes et al. 1960), were discussed by Corkin et al.

5.5 The Periphery of the Corticectomy

5.5.1 Parallel to Cortical Sulci

There will be peripheral segments to any corticectomy where all the principles of subpial resection can be utilized. This is particularly so when the periphery is parallel to a sulcus or fissure. In this case the cortex is removed down to the depth of the sulcus, as noted in Sect. 2.2.

5.5.2 Crossing Sulci and Gyri

The foregoing section ideal situation will not exist for the full periphery of a corticectomy, however. Other peripheral segments will not be parallel to the sulci, but in fact may be perpendicular to the sulci. Thus, rather than carrying out subpial dissection down one side of a sulcus, the incision line will cross the gyri and sulci. It is in this case where the achievement of a minimally traumatic incision line reaches its greatest importance. The reason for the latter is that it is this line, if made with high current coagulation that may result in a wide line of destruction at least a portion of which will be left behind within the "normal" cortex. A very fine incision line across the summits of the gyri can be achieved with the use of the bipolar coagulation forceps, with the coagulation current as low as possible, as pointed out in Chap. 2. This will result in a good line of coagulated leptomeninges and very little obviously injured cortex left behind, when the corticectomy specimen is removed.

The sulci, which always contain some of the arterial vasculature, are best managed by small incisions in the coagulated juxtaposed summits of the gyri. Suction is then used to remove the underlying cortex, followed by the removal of the cortex down to the bottom of the sulci on both sides. At this point the two pial membranes, lining the sulcus, may be coagulated bloodlessly and incised. By repeating this series of coagulations and incisions, the white matter is cut across and deepened to a depth, which honors the tenets of the foregoing Sect. 5.4, regarding the preservation of the underlying subcortical white matter.

5.5.3 Juxtaposition of the "Eloquent" Cortex

When a margin of a corticectomy is juxtaposed to an eloquent area of the cortex, there are some extra strategies required. The removal of the cortex that is *immediately* juxtaposed to the eloquent cortex is often associated with a transient deficit from dysfunction of that eloquent cortex. This is particularly striking when the cortex being removed is situated on one side of a sulcus, juxtaposed to the "eloquent" cortex on the other side of the sulcus. The closer the resection incision is to the clinically functional cortex, the more quickly does the transient dysfunction appear. In the case noted in the foregoing, its appearance may be perceived as quickly as a few minutes, but certainly within 15–20 min.

Given the foregoing, the surgeon must *not* allow this time to lapse between the initial juxtaposed surgical resection and any further required surgical resection that could influence the appearance of a deficit or an increased deficit, before completing this particular part of the resection. If the deficit becomes complete before the last part of the resection in the immediate vicinity of the eloquent cortex, then one has lost the whole advantage of carrying out the procedure under local anesthesia. Why is this so? If the function is lost, then further surgery that might produce or enhance the deficit cannot be assessed by the usual continual clinical examination accompanying the progress of the surgery and which helps define the extent of surgery.

What is the surgery that defines the "completion" of the resection in the immediate vicinity of the eloquent cortex? The resection of the epileptogenic cortex, per se, will have been carried out, under the guidance of ongoing clinical examination of the patient's pertinent neurological function. Once this has become completed, employing all the tenets of good-quality subpial dissection and resection, the only other concern resides in the continuum of the next part of the incision and whether it could influence the connectivity of the eloquent cortex to the point of creating or increasing a clinical deficit. It is the surgeon's responsibility to make absolutely certain that in the event of clinical monitoring, which suggests the onset of a neurological deficit during the surgery, to proceed as quickly as possible in completing this phase of the surgery before a "loss" of the function becomes complete. This is best achieved after the incision through the cortex, in carrying out the following subcortical incision promptly. This incision is angled away from the area of the eloquent cortex, as superficially as possible. A subcortical incision of only a centimeter or two is necessary to discharge this hurried obligation. This is illustrated in two diagrams in Fig. 5.3 (see also Sects. 2.2.3.1, 2.2.3.2 and 2.2.3.3). In Fig. 5.3a the junction between eloquent and epileptogenic cortices is at the base of a sulcus (as was the case in Fig. 2.8), and in Fig. 5.3b the junction is on the surface of a gyrus.

In Fig. 5.3 there are three gyri in each of the "a" figures (Aa and Ba). The cross-hatched cortex represents the epileptogenic cortex that is to be removed, while the stippled cortex is the normal eloquent cortex that is to be preserved. The vertical bar indicates the (resection) margin at the junction of the two cortices; in figure A this is at the bottom of a sulcus, while in figure B it is at the top of a gyrus. The thin arrows in figure A exhibit the initiation of the resection of the gyrus, all the cortex of which is epileptogenic. The broad (thick) arrows represent in both figures A and B the point at which the time required for the completion of the remainder of the resections should be minimized, as outlined in the previous paragraph. The "b" figures (Ab and Bb) illustrate the parenchyma of the peripheries of the corticectomy that remain intact following the resections. Note in particular that as much subcortical white matter as possible is left intact, as the greater the remaining white matter the greater is the likelihood that the health of the normal neuronal connectivity of the remaining peripheral cortex will be preserved.

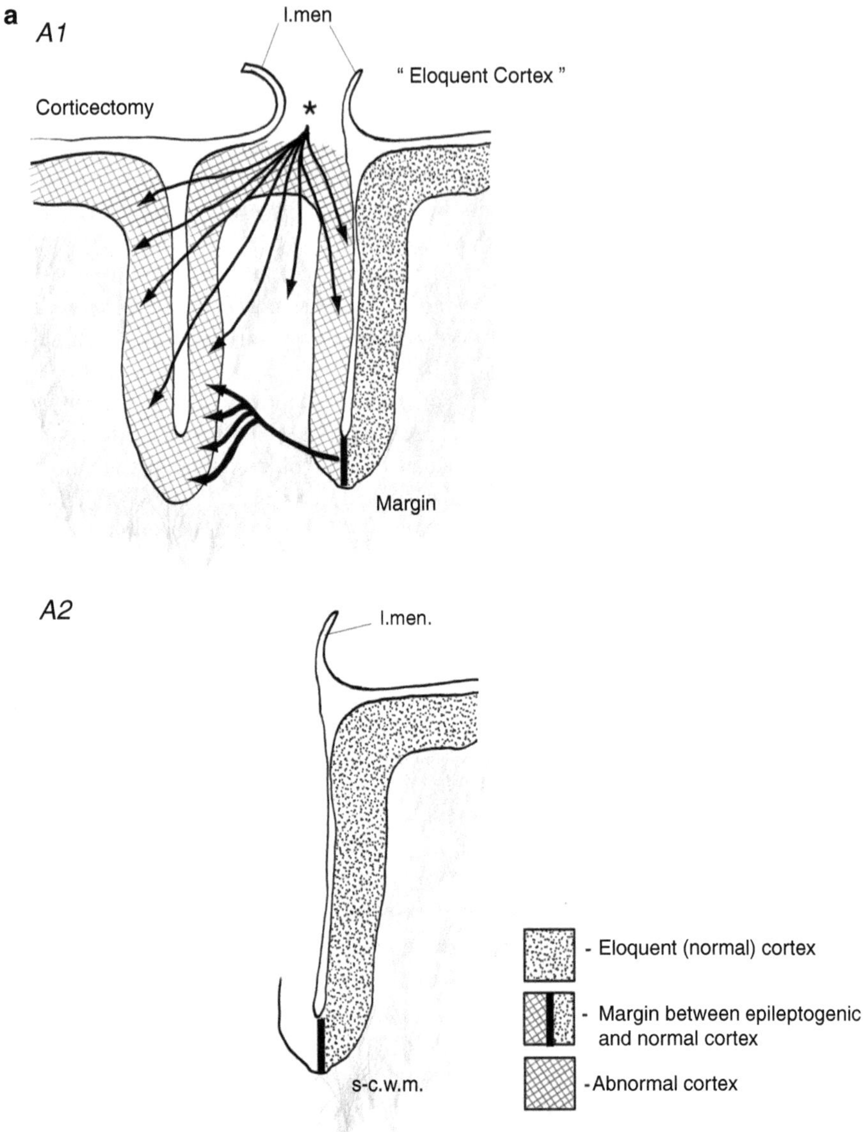

Fig. 5.3 Periphery of a corticectomy, when juxtaposed to the "eloquent" cortex. Illustrations of margins of a resection immediately juxtaposed to "eloquent" cortex, and the associated subcortical incisions, which should promptly follow the cortical incision. (**A1**) An example of the junction between epileptogenic and normal eloquent cortices in the depth of a sulcus; (**A2**) an example of the case where the junction between the two cortices is in the summit of a gyrus. (**B1**) and (**B2**) show the subcortical white matter left intact after the removal of the epileptogenic cortex, per se (see text). *l.men* leptomeninges; *s-c.w.m.* subcortical white matter, ✶ the incision in the leptomeninges, at the starting point of the resection; **I** juncture between epileptogenic and normal (eloquent) cortices; → the (*thin*) *arrows* initiating the subpial resection in **A**; → the (*broad*) *arrows* representing that phase in the operation where the time taken for the resection should be minimized so that the resection is completed before any neurological deficit might emerge

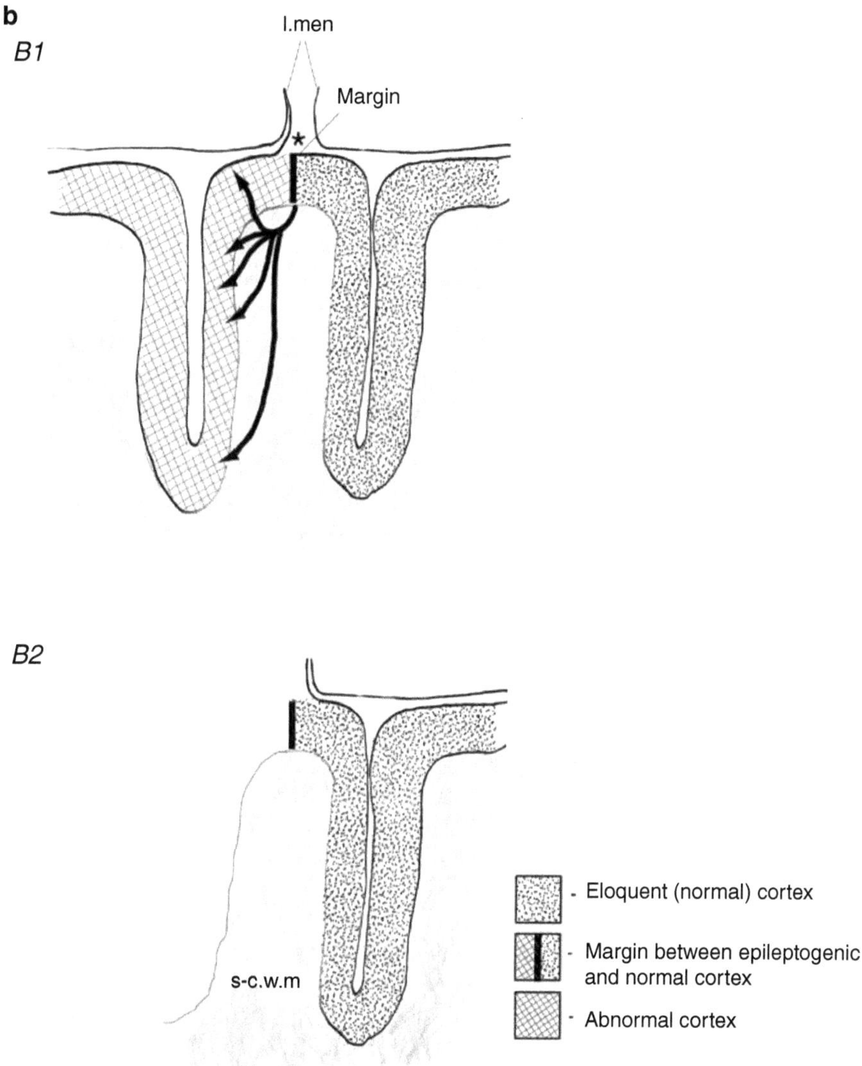

Fig. 5.3 (continued)

5.6 The Determination of the Dimensions and Size of the Corticectomy

The peripheral extent of some resections is perfectly straightforward. For example, there are clear-cut foci of epileptic discharge, determined by preoperative EEG and/or subdural ECoG recordings. This is particularly the case when the corticectomy pertains to one or two surfaces of the poles of a lobe, e.g., frontal and temporal. The latter would include also the occipital pole in those cases where a preoperative hemianopia would preclude a concern of removal of the lobe and leaving the patient with an unwanted visual field defect.

In other cases the peripheral dimensions would be determined intraoperatively through "tailoring" of the resection. That is to say, certain intraoperative findings would influence the size and configuration of the resection. These findings include the definition of the focus by intraoperative ECoG, the mapping of the nearby functional cortex, and the anatomy of the cortical topography.

As in most cases of resection, there is always the question of how much cortex should be removed. The initial philosophy of the Montreal school was similar to what has emerged in the current day practices in most branches of surgery, i.e., a minimally invasive philosophy. In other words, the surgery should involve a minimally potentially injurious surgical pathway to the site of surgery and as minimal a removal as possible, which was considered necessary to achieve the surgical objective. This was the initial philosophy of the Montreal school, and therefore in the early years, the surgery was primarily directed at the removal of only that which was considered to be primary epileptic focus. However, over the years many such resections were followed with second operations, extending the previous resection, amounting to what initially might have been considered a greater-than-minimal resection. The practice of making larger resections emerged as a more satisfactory philosophy and hence the earlier, rather restricted, resections being replaced with larger resections (Penfield and Flanigin 1950; Penfield and Paine 1955; Rasmussen and Jasper 1958; Rasmussen and Branch 1962; Rasmussen 1963).

Dr. Rasmussen, in his 1963 paper on the surgery of frontal lobe epilepsy, noted that in the Montreal school there had been "changes in our concepts of the nature of the focal epileptogenic mechanism" in patients with focal epilepsy in whom "discrete and restricted epileptogenic foci seem to be rare and most patients exhibit larger epileptogenic areas …." And finally he noted "Thus, removals of an atrophic gyrus or two of the temporal lobe carried out in the early years of our experience gave way to removal of the cortex of the entire anterior half or two thirds of the temporal lobe, with the subsequent addition of removal of the medial temporal structures, amygdala and hippocampus, with progressive improvement in the clinical results." He clearly delineated the philosophy of the benefit of conducting larger anatomical resections of the cortex, rather than smaller.

On an occasion in the early 1970s, I called Dr. Rasmussen (1972), as I did not infrequently, and part of our conversation had to do with the size of cortical resections. I asked him (words to the effect) "how do you determine how much cortex to remove?" His response was "There have been many times that I have regretted having carried out small resections, but only very, very rarely have I looked back and had concern with large resections" (personal communication, 1972). I must say that I considered from that time onwards that clearly "larger was better than smaller" when it came to surgical resections for the management of intractable epilepsy, so long as the larger resections could be carried out safely. This was apparently the philosophy of Rossi as well (1975). However, there is still no absolutely clear-cut evidence-based answer to this query (Okonma et al. 2011).

It perhaps may be considered that the exception to the foregoing is the use of the amygdalohippocampectomy, as a substitute for the traditional standard anterior temporal lobectomy.

5.7 "Lesionectomy"

I will exercise my prerogative as author of this monograph and indicate that I do not believe that the word "lesionectomy," referring to a lesion as "foreign tissue" by those who talk about "lesionectomy," has any place in the discussion of epileptic surgery! Epilepsy is a symptom, which may result from a number of causes. The increasing quality of medical imaging has reduced tremendously the category of "idiopathic" etiology, as applied to epilepsy, and thus it has exposed many more lesions than would have been achieved before the availability of the increasing quality of magnetic resonance imaging.

Why do I feel that the use of the so-called lesionectomy, as an operative technique in epilepsy, should be dropped? The origin of epileptic seizures is related to an alteration in the normal discharges of populations of neurons. The possible theoretic neurophysiological alterations for this are many and the exact explanation remains unknown. However, what *is* known is that whatever is the neurophysiological basis, it results in a rhythmical, synchronous discharge of neurons, which then gives rise to a pervasive cascade, which recruits increasing numbers of neurons until a self-sustained, variously transient or self-limited by exhaustion, electrographic seizure occurs. That is to say, unchecked, this electrographic seizure will spread by continual recruitment of neurons until a critical amount of the brain, or all of the brain, is involved, at which point a clinical counterpart to the electrographic seizure will become apparent. The seizures can only arise from excitable cells whose alterations give rise to spontaneous, self-sustained abnormal discharge.

How would a lesion produce such an event? There is possibly a reasonable argument that lesions of various types can lead to seizures. However, nonneuronal lesional tissue, per se, very, very rarely, if ever, is the cellular source of focal epileptic discharge. Rather it is its ability to cause dysfunctional alterations in a critical mass of neurons that give rise to a seizure focus. The way that different lesions might cause such alterations is controversial, but certainly there is little likelihood that lesions in general cause some type of similar uniform abnormality in the surrounding neuronal parenchyma. For the purposes of considering the basis of the understanding of a "lesionectomy," the causes are probably immaterial. By literal understanding a lesionectomy is a removal of a lesion, per se. If one accepts this, then the corollary is that the understanding also includes the view that the cells of the lesion are those giving rise to the electrographic abnormality, e.g., the discharges which give rise to the epilepsy. This, of course, is not the case. Rather, the lesion produces the epileptic focus in some population of neurons outside its own population of cells. From clinical ECoG recordings the altered population of neurons usually resides in the immediate vicinity of the lesion, i.e., outside the lesion in the cerebral parenchyma. However, it is important to be aware of the fact that it may be more remotely located.

I feel, personally, that even a consideration of those tumors and tissues, which are composed of both nonneuronal tissue, usually glial, plus neuronal tissue is also unlikely to be totally responsible for focal epileptic discharge and thereby intractable epilepsy. These examples include such lesions as hamartomas, glioneuronal tumors, and the cortical dysplasias. There have been suggestions, but I don't believe the suggestions have been the product of clear-cut evidence that these lesions may, per se, cause the epilepsy. However, the argument with the greatest likelihood of being the case is certainly that of the cortical dysplasias. Ferrier et al. have provided very good data regarding intraoperative electrocorticography and glioneuronal tumors and cortical dysplasia (2006). However, they did not take the step of indicating that the focal epileptogenic activity emerged purely from the lesional tissue as opposed to the associated surrounding cortex. Further, some of the glioneuronal tumors, primarily the gangliogliomas, were in the white matter alone (see also Blümcke and Wiestler 2002). (If it was demonstrated that the neuronal elements of such tumors were connected to neurons of the cerebral parenchyma, my argument would be more controversial!)

As a result of the foregoing, my personal view is that a so-called lesionectomy is a misnomer and as such primarily provides the name of a morphological entity, the confined removal of which should not be construed as a definitive surgical epilepsy operation! The use of the word detracts from the importance of the removal of the associated parenchyma, which must be removed as well in order to effectively remove the epileptic focus caused by the lesion. That is, it is this part of the operative removal of a so-called lesionectomy, which gives rise to the satisfactory outcome of the operation. I believe that most, if not all, "lesionectomies" that result in satisfactory seizure outcomes are related to the associated resection of surrounding epileptogenic cerebral parenchyma. Spencer provided suggestive evidence of this, even though the evidence certainly did not involve randomization of surgeries of pure lesion tissue resections versus the combination of lesion and cerebral parenchyma resections (see Wieser and ILAE 2004, p. 709).

References

Blümcke I, Wiestler OD. Gangliogliomas: an intriguing tumor entity associated with focal epilepsies. J Neuropathol Exp Neurol. 2002;61:575–84.

Corkin S, Milner B, Rasmussen T. Somatosensory thresholds – contrasting effects of post-central gyrus and posterior parietal-lobe excision. Arch Neurol. 1970;23:41–58.

Critchley M. The parietal lobes. London: Edward Arnold; 1953.

Evans JP. A study of the sensory defects resulting from excision of cerebral substance in humans. Pubic Assoc Res Nerv Ment. 1935;15:331–70.

Ferrier CH, Aronica E, Leijten SS, Spliet WGM, van Huffelen AC, van Rijen PC, Binnie CD. Electrocorticographic discharge patterns in glioneuronal tumors and focal cortical dysplasia. Epilepsia. 2006;47:1477–86.

Okonma SV, Blount JP, Gross RE. Planning extent of resection in epilepsy: limited versus large resections. Epilepsy Behav. 2011;20:233–40.

Penfield W, Flanigin H. Surgical therapy of temporal lobe seizures. Arch Neurol Psychiatr. 1950;64:491–500.
Penfield W, Paine K. Results of surgical therapy for focal epileptic seizures. CMAJ. 1955;73: 515–31.
Rasmussen T. Surgical therapy of frontal lobe epilepsy. Epilepsia. 1963;4:181–98.
Rasmussen T, Branch C. Temporal lobe epilepsy: indications for the results of surgical therapy. Postgrad Med. 1962;31:9–14.
Rasmussen T, Jasper H. Temporal lobe epilepsy: indications for operations and surgical technique. In: Baldwin M, Bailey P, editors. Temporal lobe epilepsy. Springfield: Charles C. Thomas; 1958. p. 440–60.
Rossi GFD. Considerations on the principles of surgical treatment of partial epilepsies. Brain Res. 1975;95:395–402.
Semmes J, Weinstein S, Ghent L, Teuber HL. Somatosensory changes after penetrating brain wounds in man. Cambridge, MA: Harvard University Press; 1960.
Ward AA. The epileptic neuron: chronic foci in animals and man. In: Jasper HH, Ward AA, Pope A, editors. Basic mechanisms of the epilepsies. Boston: Little, Brown & Co; 1969. p. 263–88.
Wieser HG, ILAE. Mesial temporal lobe epilepsy with hippocampal sclerosis. Epilepsia. 2004;45:695–714.

Temporal Lobe Surgery

6

6.1 Introduction

A discussion of "temporal lobectomy," which is more accurately referred to as "anterior temporal lobectomy" (aTLY), for the surgical management of intractable temporal lobe (TL) epilepsy requires two somewhat different strategies, depending upon whether the seizures are considered to be arising in the limbic (anteroinferomesial) structures or in the neocortex. However, the objective of nearly all of the so-called aTLYs, including the more restrictive amygdalohippocampectomy, is the removal of the former, e.g., the antero-infero-mesial limbic cortex, as the majority of intractable temporal lobe seizures arise in this cortex. There is some controversy with respect to the choice of utilizing an aTLY on the one hand, consisting of the removal of some anterior neocortex, as well as the amygdala and hippocampus, or on the other hand an amygdalohippocampectomy, consisting of the restricted removal of the amygdala and hippocampus. There have been earlier papers in the literature outlining some of the surgical aspects of a temporal lobectomy, which are briefly described (Bailey and Gibbs 1951; Penfield and Baldwin 1952; Rasmussen and Jasper 1958; Penfield et al. 1961; Walker 1967; Olivier 1997).

Even in the case of the aTLY, there is controversy as to the choice of a so-called "standard" or "tailored" removal. While both procedures involve removal of the limbic cortex to roughly the same extent, the primary difference between the two procedures is in the amount of neocortex removed. The standard aTLY consists of the simple predetermined extent of removal of neocortex, usually something of the order of 2–4 cm, while the tailored aTLY is one that is influenced by the presence of any preoperatively identified neocortex in which epileptogenicity is considered to be present, either by preoperative electroencephalography (EEG) or subdural electrocorticography (ECoG) or intraoperative ECoG. If such is felt to be present, then if possible, it is removed as part of the neocortical removal. (In essence this author believes that there is really little difference between the two procedures, with respect to neocortical removal!)

J.P. Girvin, *Operative Techniques in Epilepsy*,
DOI 10.1007/978-3-319-10921-3_6

In those cases of pure neocortical seizures, then the removal will be much the same as described in Chap. 5 on corticectomy. That is to say, it is simply a variant of the procedure of corticectomy, with all the considerations of such.

Since the majority of intractable seizure disorders consist of TL seizures and since most TL seizures originate within the limbic cortex of the temporal lobe, the primary thrust of this chapter will be the description of the equivalent of a standard aTLY. Nearly all of the aTLYs that I have conducted were done under local anesthesia. Some aspects of the latter will be mentioned, but the major aspects of the use of local anesthesia have been covered in Chap. 3, pertaining to the preparation of the patient (Sect. 3.2) and the preoperative anesthetic blockade of scalp nerves (Sect. 3.3).

Before leaving this introduction, a brief note should be made with respect to how much hippocampus might be removed in the aTLY. This might have been considered a somewhat controversial feature in the middle of the twentieth century, but it certainly became more controversial during the latter part of the century. The initial view of the Montreal school was that the greater the amount of hippocampus removed, the better is the seizure outcome postoperatively. This controversy, during the latter part of the century, was perhaps expanded somewhat as a result of the back-to-back articles in which 100 cases of aTLY each were reviewed by Rasmussen (Rasmussen and Feindel 1991) that involved a "major hippocampectomy" and by Feindel (Feindel and Rasmussen 1991) that involved a "minimal hippocampal resection," in which there was no significant difference between the two reviews! Wyler and colleagues undertook a randomized prospective study of "total" (back to the colliculi of the midbrain, ~5.5 cm posterior to the temporal pole) versus "partial" (back to the anterior midbrain, ~3.5 cm posterior to the temporal pole) hippocampectomies, which disclosed 69 % versus 38 % seizure-free outcomes, respectively (1995). There have been some concerns regarding some of Wyler's methodological aspects, but in general it has been accepted as indicating the greater the hippocampal resections, the greater is the likelihood of better outcomes. (I have always used, simply by habit, the 5–6 cm hippocampal resection.)

6.2 Anterior Temporal Lobectomy (aTLY)

6.2.1 Introduction

The general technique of aTLY has been noted elsewhere (Girvin 1992). With some modifications, it will be similarly repeated here. The modifications will include some alterations of surgical anatomy, through both the text and figures.

6.2.2 The Scalp Incision

There are a number of different scalp flaps used for access to the temporal lobe. I will only note that which I believe to be the best. It is the one that I learned at the Montreal Neurological Institute and is demonstrated in Fig. 6.1. It is certainly the

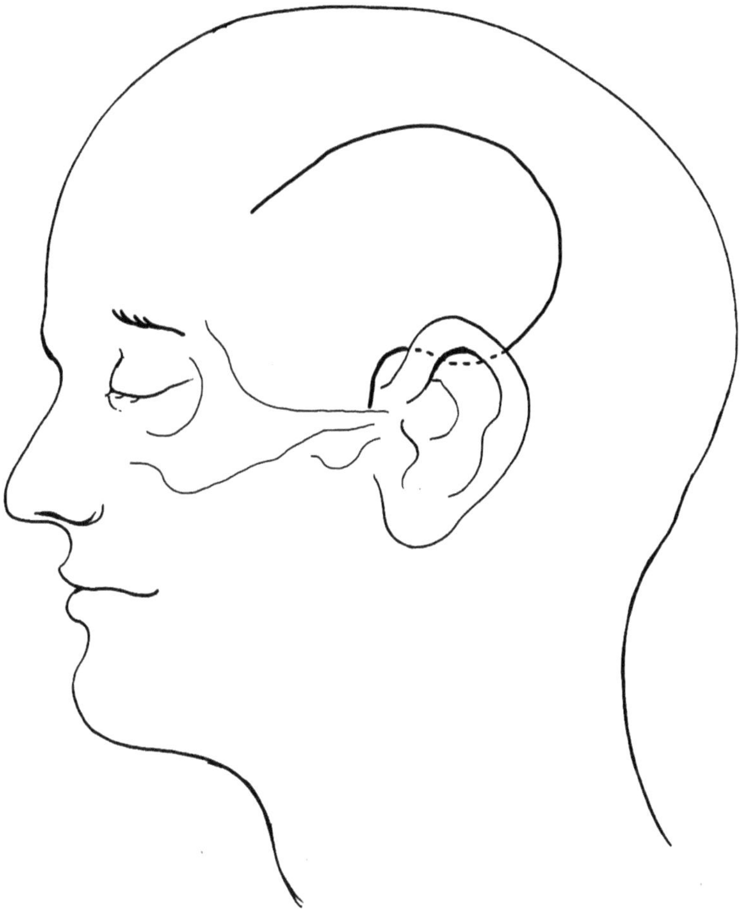

Fig. 6.1 Scalp incision for an aTLY (anterior temporal lobectomy). Scalp flap, which typically begins just in front of the tragus of the ear at the zygoma. It then is taken vertically for 1–2 cm and turned posteriorly just above the ear lobe to whatever amount of lateral cortex is required to be exposed. (Note: just in front of the ear is ~5 cm, and at the back of the ear ~8 cm, behind the anterior pole of the temporal lobe.) At the posterior extent of the proposed incision, it is simply curved superiorly and then anteriorly approximately halfway between the ear and the midline, to end just behind the hairline above the eye

best flap from the cosmetic point of view and thus it has significant advantages, particularly in the case of young women. It lacks having to cut through the temporalis muscle, which is required to some extent in any T-shaped incision. It also precludes in the latter the potential of a vertical anterior arm of the flap coursing just inside the hairline anteriorly. Thus, I do feel that the described flap provides a better cosmetic result. In addition, I believe that the larger single flap is easier to retract and to close at the termination of the operative procedure.

To reiterate, the proposed scalp incision is injected with 0.33 % bupivacaine hydrochloride (Sect. 3.3.4). When the incision is made, bleeding arteries can be coagulated and the use of peroxide gauze, with rare exception, is all that is needed for the remainder of hemostasis if the initial scalp injection has been satisfactory (see Sect. 3.6.3). (If the surgery is to be done under local anesthesia, see Sects. 3.3.2, 3.3.4, and 3.6.2.)

6.2.3 Craniotomy

The craniotomy, using local anesthesia and neuroleptanalgesia, has been outlined earlier (Sect. 3.6). The sphenoid wing of the temporal bone creates a special difference between the routine craniotomy on the one hand and the ideal craniotomy for the removal of an anterior temporal lobe. I had initially performed the craniotomy in what I believed was the usual fashion, placing a burr hole on either side of the sphenoid wing and then simply running the Gigli saw, or craniotome, between the two holes. When the bone flap was removed the final part of the craniotomy was composed of a large removal of the outer portion of the sphenoid wing and the inferior temporal bone with rongeurs. This was a perfectly reasonable method for such a craniotomy. However, I came to be very often disappointed in the final cosmetic appearance of the characteristic depression in the skin over the anterior temporal region. In the case of young girls, my disappointment was the greatest and it soon became associated with embarrassment. I eventfully considered that this should not have to be the case!

Given the fact that I performed nearly all the temporal craniotomies under local anesthesia and the fact that under the latter the inferior dura is the most important dura to be anesthetized for the relief of discomfort, I began using the air drill for making the inferior bony incision. The normal burr holes are placed inferiorly and in the so-called "key hole" area above the base of the sphenoid wing. Using the medium-sized diamond burr in the air powered drill and small rongeurs, the inferior bony incision line is achieved in a series of steps, involving the intermittent injection of local anesthetic between the leaflets of the dura. As noted earlier (Sect. 3.6.7), it is very advantageous to initiate the craniotomy inferiorly in order to anesthetize the inferior dura in a temporal craniotomy, as this usually is nearly all the dural anesthesia that is required for the craniotomy. (If the craniotomy is initiated in the superior part, then local anesthesia will be required two times, e.g., superiorly and then later in the inferior part.) The line is taken anteroinferiorly *through* whatever part of the sphenoid wing that needs removing; a large part of the sphenoid wing is included in the bone flap (The resulting craniotomy, from this simple small linear incision through the sphenoid wing, *never* results in *any* unwanted cosmetic suggestion postoperatively of an individual having had a craniotomy.).

One other feature that I have found to save significant time of operation, if using sutures for closing the bone, is to, just prior to raising the bone flap, mark the holes for the sutures and drill them after raising the flap, something that takes no more than about 30 s. (It is one of the reasons that allow a satisfactory closure in ~30 min.)

I open the dura in a simple X shape, with the bases of the X being in the corners of the craniotomy, fold them, and use rubber bands for retraction. I have used other openings, but I have found this to provide the easiest satisfactory closure for me.

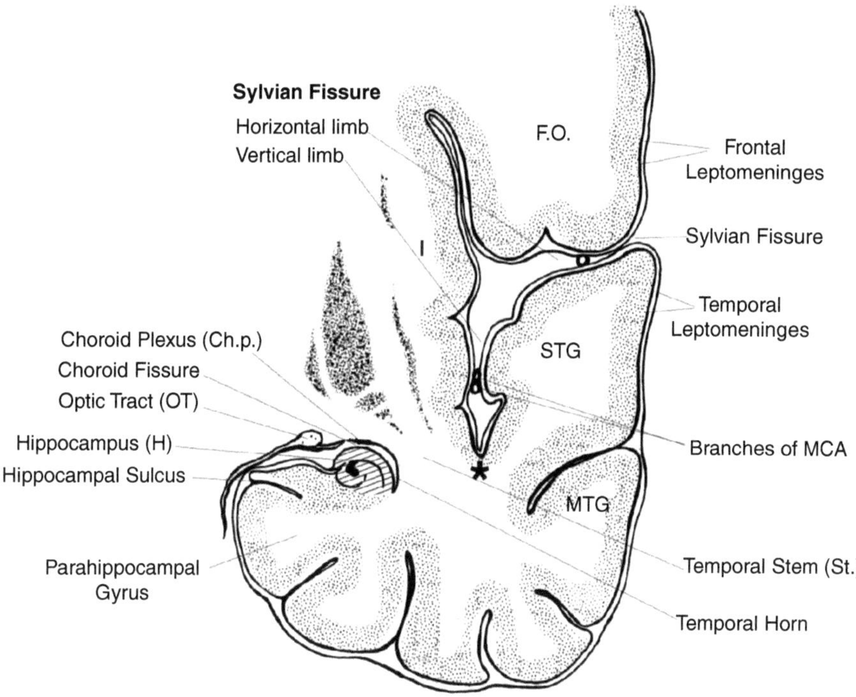

Fig. 6.2 Pertinent anatomy of the TL in the conduction of an aTLY. Coronal section (~3–4 cm behind the tip of the temporal pole) through the temporal lobe. *F.O.* frontal operculum, *I* insula, *MTG* middle temporal gyrus, *STG* superior temporal gyrus, ✱ the inferior edge of the leptomeningeal investment of the medial surface of the temporal lobe (also the bottom of the vertical limb of the Sylvian fissure)

6.2.4 The Initiation of the aTLY

Walker (1967) advocated making the initial incision through the middle temporal gyrus (MTG), thus preserving the superior temporal gyrus (STG), but gave no reason for doing so. Some have adopted this, often giving the reason as that of "safety," e.g., decreasing the likelihood of injuring the underlying middle cerebral artery vasculature (MCA). I have seen exactly the opposite on more than one occasion, when the middle temporal gyral path had been utilized, in order to save the STG! In two or three of these instances, the incision was taken too inferiorly, as it was directed medially, and ended up below the lower edge of the leptomeningeal investment of the medial surface of the superior temporal lobe, in among the insular cortex, external capsule, and on one occasion the internal capsule. The ease of this eventuality can be appreciated from viewing Fig. 6.2, an illustration of a coronal view through the middle of the temporal lobe; a perpendicular incision through the MTG could quite easily end up inferior to the bottom of the vertical limb of the Sylvian fissure. Quite apart from the fact that I believe this to be a dangerous approach, especially in the hands of a less experienced surgeon, it also leaves tissue (primarily the STG) that is at least partially denervated, i.e., de-afferented and/or de-efferented—a potential for the origin of epileptogenicity and thus a contraindication to the principles of good epilepsy surgery. There is *no* good reason for saving the STG! Thus, I dogmatically believe that the initiation should be through the STG for reasons discussed in the following, especially now with the current practice of only very rarely extending the posterior resection line in the STG beyond ~4 cm posterior to the temporal pole.

Using an initial incision through the STG allows the surgeon to expose the leptomeninges not only over the lateral surface but also over the superior and medial surfaces, i.e., the horizontal and vertical limbs, respectively, of the Sylvian fissure, right from the beginning of the procedure. Therefore, the surgeon can take full advantage of the anatomy and the protective value of the leptomeningeal barrier by remaining within the confines of the leptomeninges of the horizontal and vertical parts of the Sylvian fissure. Through the leptomeninges the underlying anatomical structures, e.g., MCA branches and insula, can always be visualized. Further, it also provides ready visualization of the boundaries of leptomeningeal investment of the Sylvian fissure with the progression of surgery.

Often the superficial middle cerebral vein is large, follows the Sylvian fissure, and empties into the sphenoparietal sinus anteriorly or into draining veins posteriorly, such as the vein of Labbe. It important to be aware that it may also veer off the Sylvian fissure, particularly more posteriorly, and lead to misinterpretation of its course in conducting an aTLY or inferior Rolandic corticectomy, i.e., some of the superior temporal gyrus may appear above the vein or a part of the frontoparietal operculum below the vein! The best accurate strategy under this circumstance is to follow the leptomeningeal barrier, which has been incised more anteriorly, as it defines the Sylvian fissure, irrespective of the course of the superficial middle cerebral vein.

The leptomeningeal investment of the lateral aspect of the STG is coagulated in an anteroposterior direction about 3–5 mm below the Sylvian fissure, within the proposed AP extent of removal (Fig. 6.3). Small incisions are then made in the coagulated leptomeninges *in between* the MCA branches, which emerge out of the Sylvian fissure over the STG and which supply a part of the temporal lobe parenchyma being removed. There are usually three or four such vessels. Through these incisions the subpial dissection of the underlying STG is initiated. Removal of parenchyma from beneath the arterial branches overlying the STG isolates them, and 3–5 mm provides adequate length for their being safely picked up with their overlying leptomeninges, coagulated, and incised. The incision throughout the extent of proposed STG removal is now relatively complete. This now provides a clear, unimpeded path for the advancement of the subpial dissection.

Using the barrier provided by the leptomeninges, the subpial dissection initially is taken over the superior surface, thus separating the STG from the horizontal limb of the Sylvian fissure and the frontal operculum (and the anterior parietal operculum in more radical aTLYs, e.g., posterior to the Rolandic fissure). The continuation of dissection then separates the medial surface of the STG from the leptomeninges of the vertical limb of the fissure, thus separating the medial aspect of the STG from the underlying insula and the MCA vessels. In the whole of this resection, the double layer of leptomeninges is usually easily preserved. This layer, which had covered the STG, serves to provide a sturdy protective covering of the MCA vessels and

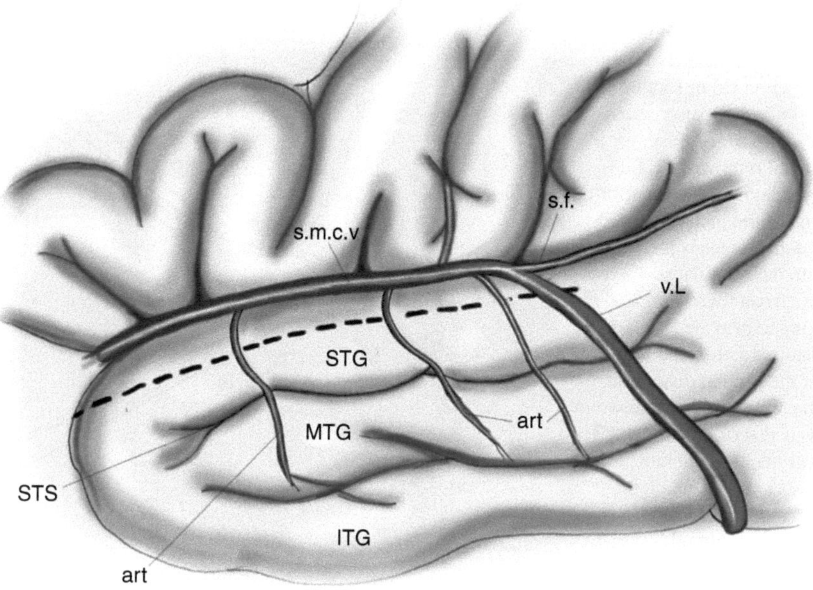

Fig. 6.3 The initial parenchymal incision in an aTLY. Illustration of the exposure of the lateral surface of a left temporal lobe. In the AP direction, ~3–5 mm below the Sylvian fissure, the leptomeningeal investment of the superior temporal gyrus (*STG*) is coagulated. The latter is incised between the arterial vessels emerging from the Sylvian fissure over the STG and each of these incisions is utilized to remove the STG parenchyma subpially from the frontal operculum. Once this is achieved the arteries can be picked up with the coagulation forceps, coagulated, and incised (see text). *art.* arteries emerging from the Sylvian fissure, *ITG* inferior temporal gyrus, *MTG* middle temporal gyrus, *S.f.* Sylvian fissure, *s.m.c.v.* superficial middle cerebral vein, *STG* superior temporal gyrus, *STS* superior temporal sulcus, *v.L.* vein of Labbe

the insula. As noted in Sect. 2.2.3, this may be achieved by blunt dissection or by suction or perhaps most commonly by a combination of both. This is illustrated in Fig. 6.4, which is very similar to the illustration used earlier in Fig. 2.6. The subpial dissection, removing first the superior and then the medial STG cortex, is carried inferiorly until the symbol ✱ is reached, which is illustrated in cross sections in Figs. 6.2 and 6.4. This point represents three important anatomical features: (1) the inferior aspect of the leptomeningeal investment of the medial temporal (STG) cortex, (2) the bottom of the vertical limb of the Sylvian fissure, and (3) the superior aspect of the temporal stem. Interestingly, this point is nearly always only 1 mm or so below a large, primarily anteroposteriorly oriented, MCA vessel within the Sylvian fissure. During the dissection this point is easily recognized by the fact that there ceases to be evidence of the leptomeningeal barrier combined with the uncovered appearance of the very white temporal stem (see also Fig. 6.5b), which is composed of the connecting fibers of the anterior part of the temporal lobe to the interior of the hemisphere, e.g., orbitofrontal cortex, hypothalamus, anterior commissure, inferior occipitofrontal and longitudinal fasciculi, etc. Also, at this juncture there is often some very minor venous bleeding, which can be simply packed for a minute

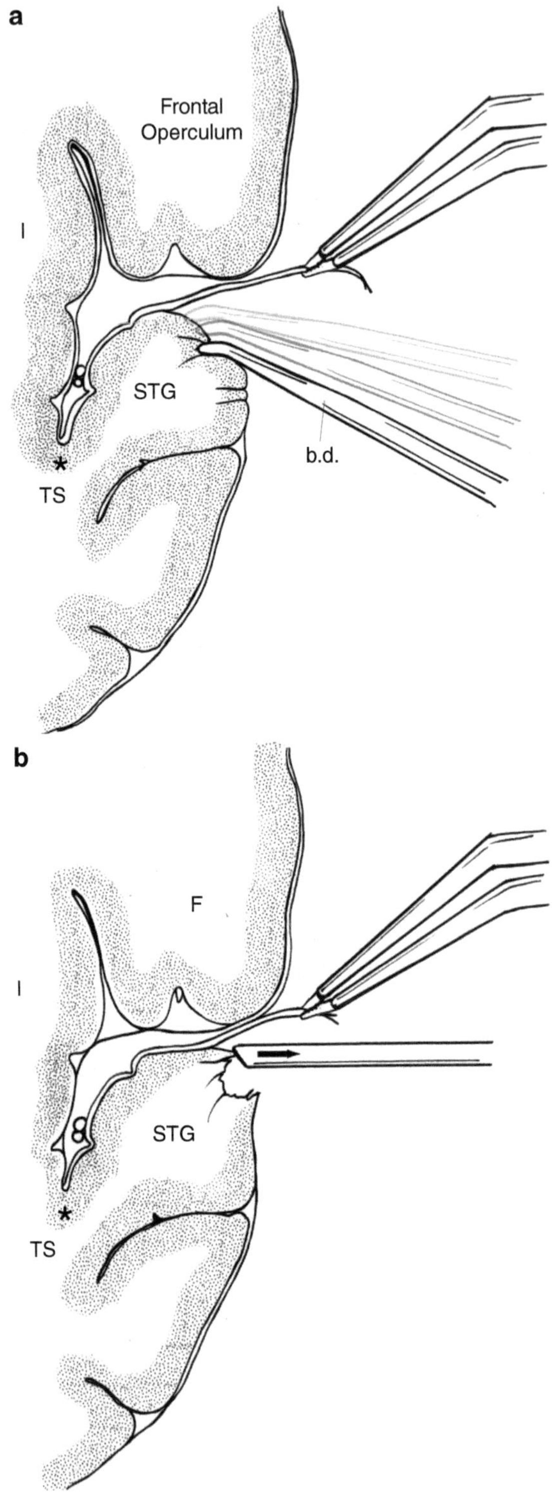

Fig. 6.4 Subpial removal of STG (superior temporal gyrus). Coronal sections, illustrating the use of blunt dissection (**a**) or suction (**b**), as similarly demonstrated earlier in Fig. 2.6a, c, for the subpial removal of STG parenchyma. The superior limb of the incised leptomeninges is picked up with the coagulation forceps, which can then be moved along to provide countertraction and stability for the subpial dissection. The blunt dissector shown in (**a**) is that of a Penfield # 2 instrument. *b.d.* blunt dissector, *F* frontal lobe (operculum), *I* insula, *STG* superior temporal gyrus, *TS* temporal stem, ✱ a designation of the bottom of the vertical limb of the Sylvian fissure (as also shown in Fig. 6.2), the inferior edge of the leptomeningeal investment of the medial surface of the TL, and the superior aspect of the temporal stem (Redrawn, with permission, from Girvin (1992))

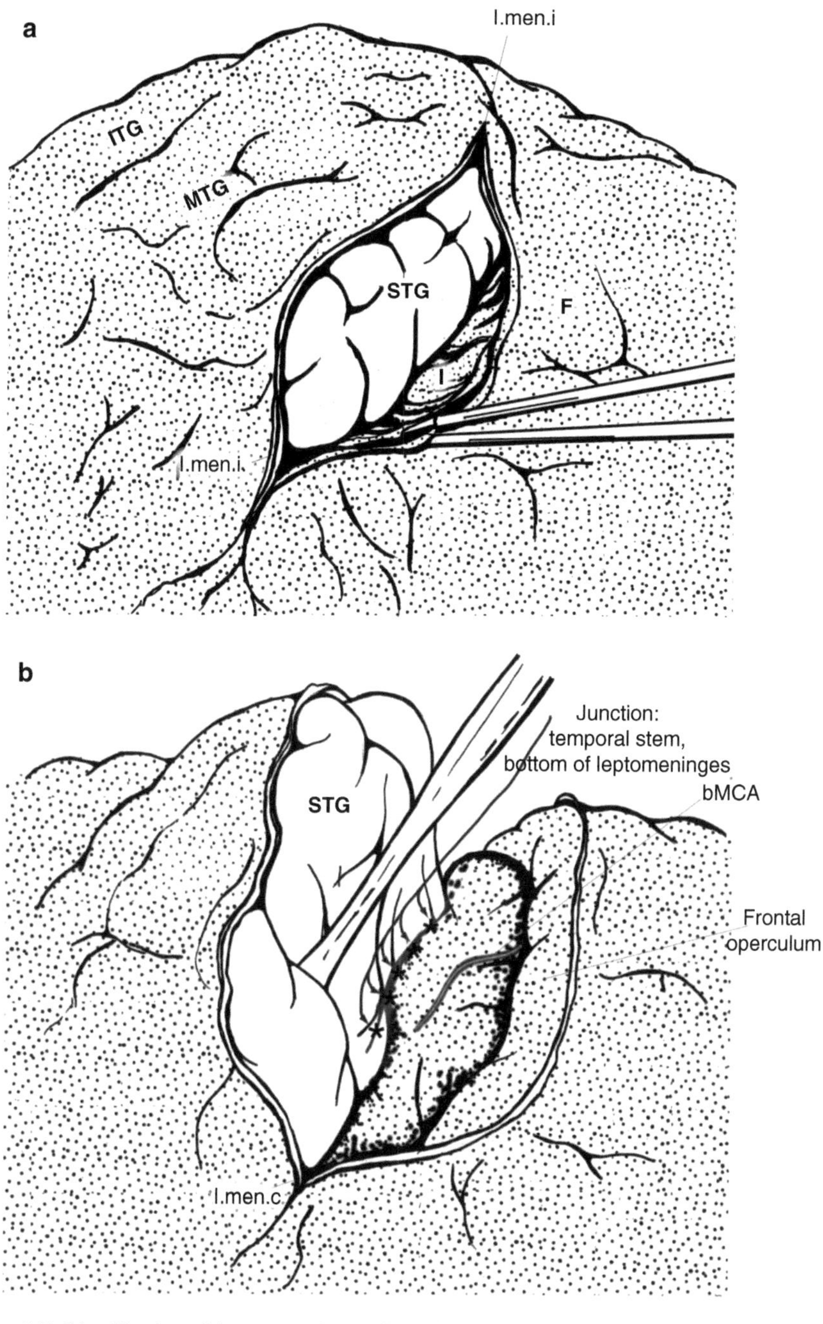

Fig. 6.5 Identification of the temporal stem. Dorsolateral illustrations of (**a**) the beginning of the subpial dissection of the STG, after the completion of the lateral anteroposterior incision of its leptomeninges. (**b**) With further dissection the bottom of the leptomeninges of the Sylvian fissure is reached and the temporal stem comes into view. *F* frontal lobe (operculum), *I* insula, *ITG* inferior temporal gyrus, *l.men.i* leptomeningeal incision over the STG, *MTG* middle temporal gyrus, *STG* superior temporal gyrus, *bMCA* branch of the middle cerebral artery in the Sylvian fissure, * the junction of the inferior edge of the medial temporal leptomeningeal barrier and the temporal stem (Redrawn, with permission, from Girvin (1992))

or so with a cottonoid patty; rarely is coagulation necessary. However, since this is also the line along which the temporal stem will be incised further on, it is often advantageous to simply coagulate a shallow (~1–2 mm) incision through the stem at this point, along the bottom of the leptomeninges. The best direction for deepening this incision can be better estimated later in the resection.

6.2.5 The Isolation of the Anterior Neocortex

Once the vessels overlying the STG are coagulated and incised a large majority of the blood supply to the anterior TL will have been interrupted. In order to isolate and devascularize the majority of the remaining part of the most anterior temporal lobe, the leptomeningeal incision of the STG is now carried anteriorly by subpial dissection associated with coagulation of vessels over it. Providing that the leptomeninges are incised as far as the dissection has progressed, then at this point inferolateral retraction of the anterior aspect of the lobe from beneath the sphenoid wing facilitates better exposure of the operative field. With the continual anterior extension of the subpial resection of the STG along the underside of the sphenoid wing, a point is reached where there is no longer any juxtaposed frontal operculum on the other side of the leptomeninges, but rather simply the anteromedial bony wall of the anterior middle fossa, covered with the dura mater. Continuing further, eventually the floor of the middle fossa is reached. At this point the free (isolated) leptomeningeal membrane can now be gradually incised coincident with the progression of the subpial resection. (If the patient is under local anesthesia and coagulation is required, the membrane must be lifted away from the dura for the coagulation, or the dura anesthetized, so that it does not result in discomfort.) Eventually, with this progression, the dissection will extend anteriorly, then leave the Sylvian fissure inferiorly around the anterior part of the temporal stem, and finally move somewhat posteriorly. This is illustrated in Fig. 6.6a, the point at which the part of the TL anterior to the temporal stem is partially freed as a result of the subpial dissection and incision of its leptomeningeal investment medially. With retraction of the anterior TL at this point, not only can the superolateral aspect of the temporal stem be seen at the bottom of the anterior Sylvian fissure, which was initially seen when the STG was being resected (Figs. 6.4 and 6.5), but now its anterior extent can be visualized. Thus, the subpial resection can be taken around the anterior extent of the temporal stem, which actually occurs between Fig. 6.6a, b. Continuation of the dissection will now progress posteriorly, under the stem, back along the underside of the inferomedial surface of the TL.

At this juncture, approximately 2 cm behind the temporal pole, the subpial dissection will be continued posteriorly over the inferomesial aspect of the temporal lobe separating the parenchyma from its leptomeningeal investment. Continued posterior dissection at this point is over the bony floor of the middle fossa and eventually the anteromedial tentorium cerebelli. This provides some increased exposure along the deep inferomedial surface of the anterior temporal lobe—one of the most important parts of the surgery of the aTLY, but the surgeon cannot easily visualize the inferomesial structures being stripped of their leptomeningeal investments. Taken about as far as the dissection can be carried out at this point, the vicinity of the uncus will have been reached. It is difficult to continue the dissection further posteriorly because of the bulk of the temporal stem (see also Fig. 6.6b).

If the aTLY is being carried out under local anesthesia, nearly always once there is retraction required on the anterior part of the lobe, when rounding the anterior end of the Sylvian fissure, or carrying out the subpial dissection of the inferomedial side of the lobe, the patient will begin to experience discomfort. It is at this point

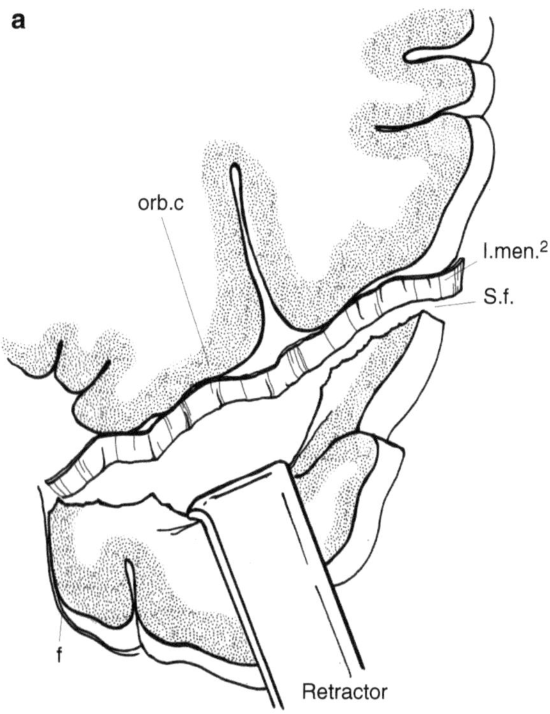

Fig. 6.6 Subpial resection anteriorly around the temporal stem. Illustrations of the gradual progressive subpial dissection around the anterior end of the temporal stem of a left TL. (**a**) A coronal section immediately anterior to the temporal stem, displaying the incision of the leptomeningeal investment of the very posterior part of the temporal pole, e.g., just anterior to the temporal stem (under the S.f), probably ~15–20 mm behind the temporal pole. (**b**) A cross section through the amygdala, posterior to the anterior aspect of the temporal stem and anterior to the tip of the ventricle, ~ 25–30 mm behind the temporal pole. (**c**) Cross section through the posterior extent of the amygdala; the anterior part of the hippocampus, e.g., the pes hippocampus; and the anterior aspect of the temporal horn, ~30–35 mm behind the temporal pole. *f.* floor of the middle fossa; *I* insula; *l.mem.* leptomeninges (single layer); *l.men*^{2} leptomeninges (double leptomeningeal layers); *orb.c.* the posterior part of the orbitofrontal cortex; *S.f.* Sylvian fissure; *TS* temporal stem; *V* temporal horn (ventricle); the junction of the bottom of the Sylvian fissure, the inferior aspect of the medial leptomeningeal investment of the TL, and the temporal stem; ••••• a potential line of incision through the temporal stem (Redrawn, with permission, from Girvin (1992))

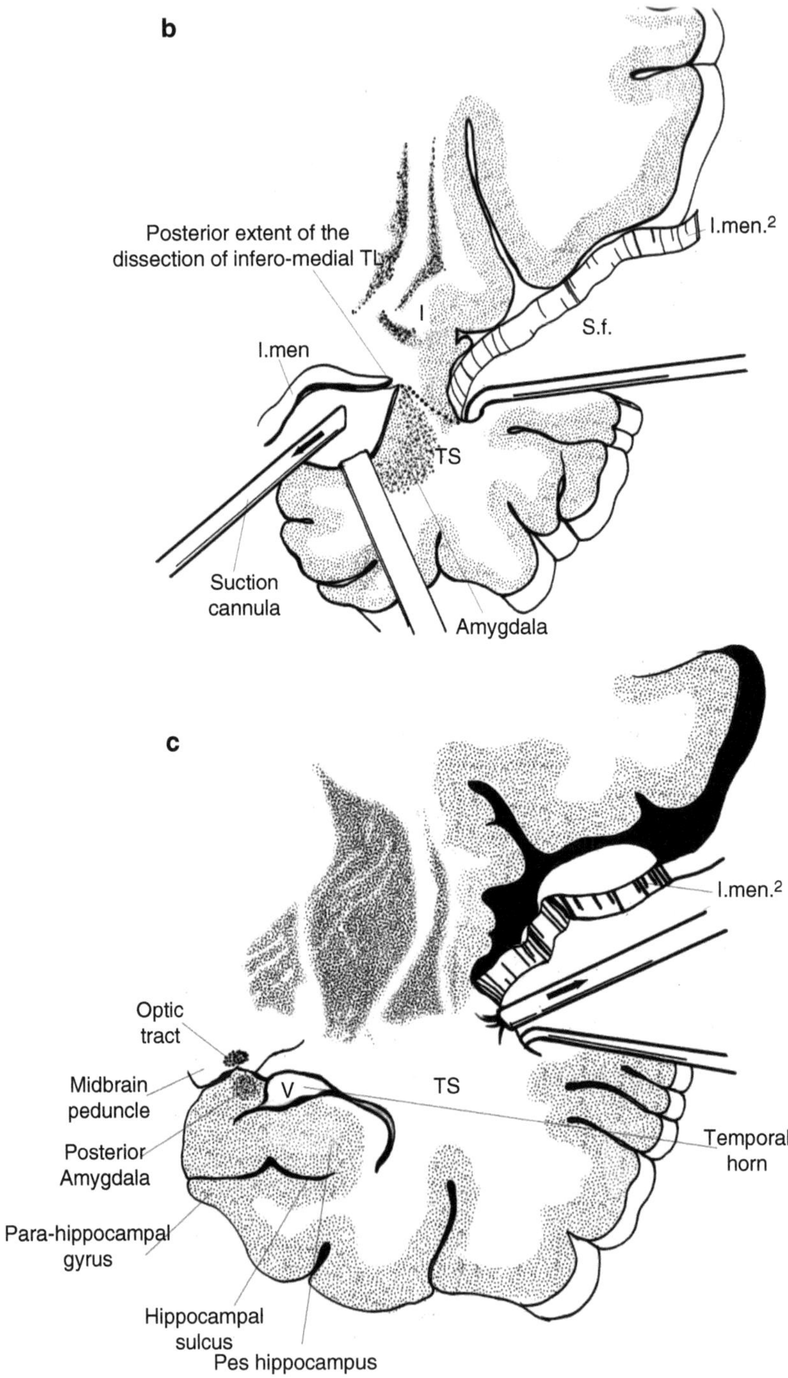

Fig. 6.6 (continued)

that the injection of some local anesthesia into the anterior part of the tentorium, lateral to the third nerve (which can be seen through the leptomeninges), into the area of the trigeminal nerve will be somewhat painful, but it is usually the last requirement for the use of local anesthesia in the operation of an aTLY. This is shown in Fig. 6.7, which illustrates the cranial base. The very slow injection of

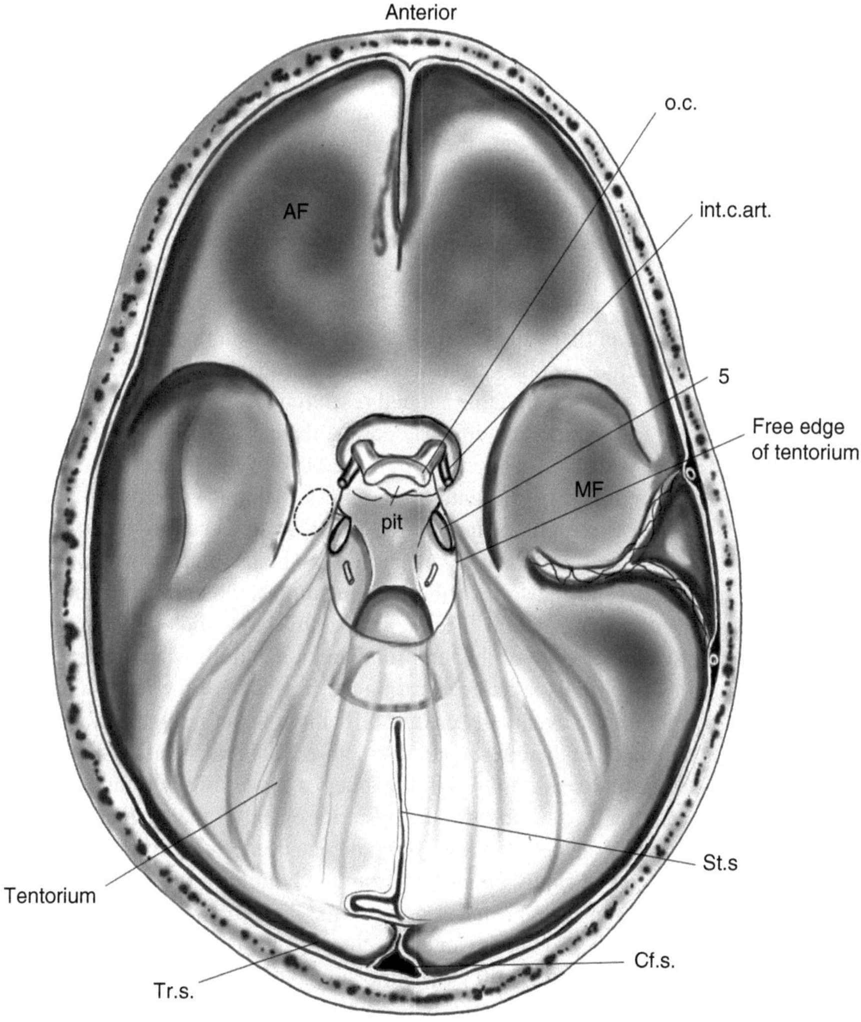

Fig. 6.7 The site of injection of local anesthetic in the basal dura for analgesia. A postmortem diagram of the floor of the anterior and middle cranial fossae. The *dotted circle* illustrates the site of injection within the dura mater and/or just below the dura mater of local anesthesia, which is most effective in reducing potential discomfort associated with dissection in the anteromedial temporal lobe. *5* cranial nerve, *AF* anterior fossa, *Cf.s.* confluence of the dural venous sinuses, *MF* middle fossa, *int.c.art.* internal carotid artery, *o.c.* optic chiasm, *pit.* pituitary gland, *St.s.* straight sinus, *Tr.s.* transverse sinus; the broken line circle depicts the region of the injection of local anesthetic for abolishing pain in patients operated upon under local anesthesia (see text)

0.5–1.0 ml of anesthetic can be administered through the use of a long #25 needle into the region, between the leaflets of the dura, within the dashed circle of the figure. This is very close to the underlying branches of the ophthalmic division of the trigeminal nerve, emerging in this area, that give rise to the most important innervation of the tentorium, as shown in Fig. 3.4. As outlined by Feindel and his colleagues it "forms a major contribution to innervation of intracranial structures" (1960, p. 563). It is likely the fact that the needle is inserted into this bundle of nerves, within the dura leaflets, which is usually somewhat painful. Because of the likely discomfort of the injection, I always warn the patient at the time of this likelihood. However, the benefit of the injection far outweighs the very brief discomfort, as it nearly always abolishes not only the immediate discomfort of the patient but is often sufficient to abolish *any* residual discomfort associated with the finishing of the operation. Infrequently there will be a partial anesthesia of the trigeminal, oculomotor, or trochlear cranial nerves, which are in the very near area of the injection, which may last for a few hours.

At this juncture the anterior aspect of the free edge of tentorium, probably the third cranial nerve and perhaps the internal carotid artery, can be seen through the partially translucent leptomeninges from which the cortical parenchyma has been removed. The farther posterior that this subpial resection is able to be conducted on this (deep) underside of the medial temporal cortex, the easier will be the later part of the aTLY dealing with the incision through the bulk of the temporal stem and then eventually the removal of the anteroinferomesial (limbic) parenchyma. The ease of visualizing these structures and the reduction in the necessity of excessive retraction of the most anterior part of the neocortex can be facilitated by an ongoing associated coagulation and incision of the leptomeninges, which have been freed and isolated by the subpial resection. The incision at this point should be conducted roughly parallel to the free edge of the tentorium and a few millimeters lateral to it, i.e., thus leaving its free (incised) edge covering the free edge of the tentorium.

The intact temporal stem eventually creates difficulty of continuing further posteriorly along the underside of the inferomedial structures. This can be at least partially rectified by initiating the incision through the anterior aspect of the temporal stem and gradually extending it posteriorly to the posterior extent of the subpial incision, ending in the vicinity of the pebbled line (•••••) depicted in Fig. 6.6b; that is to say, the TS incision line can be safely conducted from the bottom of the Sylvian fissure through the stem to the furthest posterior point of the dissection over the inferomedial surface. This incision through the anterior stem will form the initial incision the completion of which (vide infra) will isolate the amygdala from the anterior temporal lobe. The surgeon will not be aware of the presence of the amygdala at this point, but in fact it is juxtaposed to the anterior part of the uncus and actually accounts for part of the medial protuberance of the uncus. However, the fact of the amygdala at this time is not something that can be appreciated by the surgeon. After the incision the uncus/amygdala will have been separated from its medial leptomeningeal investment. Its final isolation at its base will be achieved after the removal of the neocortex (vide infra). Thus, while the incision of the anterior stem and subcortical white matter must be "tight" to the superficial (above) and deep (below) leptomeningeal barriers, respectively, yet it must not encroach on the surrounding parenchyma. At this point, an alternative to continuing the dissection more posteriorly along the inferomedial surface, one may choose to put a cottonoid patty in the resection bed of the incision in the anterior stem and return to the posterior resection extent of the STG and proceed to establish the posterior resection line (PRL).

In my view the preferred alternative is to continue with the more posterior dissection along the deep part of the medial surface, *only* if it can be conducted satisfactorily. If this alternative is chosen, then the adequacy of progressively viewing this dissection is not only facilitated by, but also dependent upon, the coincident continuation of the incision through some of the temporal stem subcortical white matter between the two boundaries noted in the foregoing paragraph. With very little more posterior dissection, the choroidal point will be reached, which is just outside the medial aspect of the ventricle at the posterior part of the amygdala. This is illustrated in Fig. 6.6c. Although perhaps the surgeon will be unaware, a coronal section at this point would reveal that the incision is posterior to the protrusion of the amygdala into the lateral wall of the ventricle and posterior to the anterior part of the pes (head) hippocampus. Further, at this point the lateral surface of the brain stem (midbrain) may be visualized through the double layer of partially translucent leptomeningeal barriers, e.g., that adherent to the lateral side of the midbrain peduncle and that which has been separated from the medial side of the TL. (This is also a location where the optic tract, coursing anteroposteriorly from the optic chiasm to the lateral geniculate body, is less than a millimeter away!) If the incision through the temporal stem and basal amygdala is sufficiently posterior, the "mantle" of the ventricle at this point is less than 1 mm in thickness, as seen in Fig. 6.6c. The "mantle" here is the last tissue that needs to be incised (into the ventricle) in order to complete the deep anteroposterior separation of amygdala and uncus from its overlying leptomeningeal investment. The entry of the ventricle through this thin mantle now wholly isolates the anterior temporal lobe anteriorly. Its only neuronal connectivity is that now coursing through its posterior parenchyma. At this point, the most difficult part of the aTLY has been achieved!

A consideration of this part of the resection would not be complete without declaring that if at any point after turning posteriorly along the medial temporal cortex there is a concern about the surgical anatomy, then further dissection should be ceased and the continued surgery should be directed at defining the PRL and removal of the neocortex.

6.2.6 The Posterior Resection Line (PRL)

The location of the posterior resection line (PRL) at this point may have already been determined or, if not, will be determined now. It is determined by a number of factors. As noted earlier, in the majority of aTLYs, it is the limbic cortex (amygdala and hippocampus) that is the source of seizures. It is this fact which has given rise to the prominence of the operation of amygdalohippocampectomy in which there is little or no removal of associated neocortex (see Sect. 6.4). The description here will be based upon the usual or "standard" aTLY. In this case the amount of neocortex removed will be simply that which facilitates a satisfactory visualization and the safe proposed removal of the hippocampus. There is no reason to go further back than about 4 cm behind the temporal pole in the STG in which to provide the pathway from a satisfactory removal of the hippocampus. While much more of the STG may be removed in the nondominant hemisphere, nevertheless there is little reason to remove more than 4–5 cm of the STG.

In the choice of exactly where in the STG the initiation of the PRL should be, it is worth examining the topographical anatomy of the lateral surface of the lobe. If a vertical (e.g., perpendicular to the Sylvian fissure) sulcus is in the vicinity of the proposed resection line, then it should be used, as good subpial dissection technique will leave a clean, minimally traumatized PRL through the STG. This is the principle utilized in the planning of all resection lines, e.g., the use of natural sulci wherever possible, so that any potential epileptogenicity from the surgical trauma will be minimized. Large arterial vessels that occur in the proximity of the STG PRL, which obviously irrigate cortex in the STG and/or the middle temporal gyrus (MTG) posterior to the proposed resection line, must be preserved. This may determine the posterior extent of the STG resection line or if the very unusual circumstance exists that such a large vessel is significantly anterior to the proposed PRL, then it should be "skeletonized" and thus preserved, as outlined in Sect. 5.2. Large veins sometimes require preservation as well. Some such veins, even veins of Labbe, which drain, or primarily drain, only portions of the temporal lobe that are being removed may be sacrificed, so long as they are noted to have connections to other good anastomotic draining veins, such as the superficial middle cerebral vein. However, veins which are large and which obviously drain portions of the temporal lobe that will be left behind or which do not possess obviously patent collateral (venous) drainage should be preserved (again, see Sect. 5.2).

The PRL will normally cross all of the temporal gyri at some angle, often perpendicular (i.e., 90°). In this case the use of subpial resection, in the ordinary sense, is not the primary resective surgical methodology. Rather, in this case the surgeon is "crossing" the sulci and gyri, and the methodology, which is described in Sect. 5.5.2, is quite different. Starting at the posterior end of the chosen resection line in the STG, the PRL is then angled inferiorly and posteriorly such that it meets the junction of the lateral and inferior surfaces approximately 6 ± 1 cm behind the temporal pole (Fig. 6.8a). The PRL in the MTG should not be further posterior than about 5 cm behind the temporal pole, especially in the dominant temporal lobe. The depth of the PRL in its upper part will be similar to that described in the foregoing (Sect. 6.2.4), with respect to the initiation of the removal of the STG. That is to say, the PRL incision of the STG follows the subpial removal of cortex and white matter from its leptomeningeal investment over the frontal operculum, MCA branches, and insula down to the leptomeningeal investment of the depth of the Sylvian fissure. Once this is reached the remainder of the MTG is incised to a depth of its sulci, similar to what was outlined in the peripheral incision in a corticectomy (see Sect. 5.5.2). This will leave the subcortical white matter overlying the lateral aspect of the temporal horn.

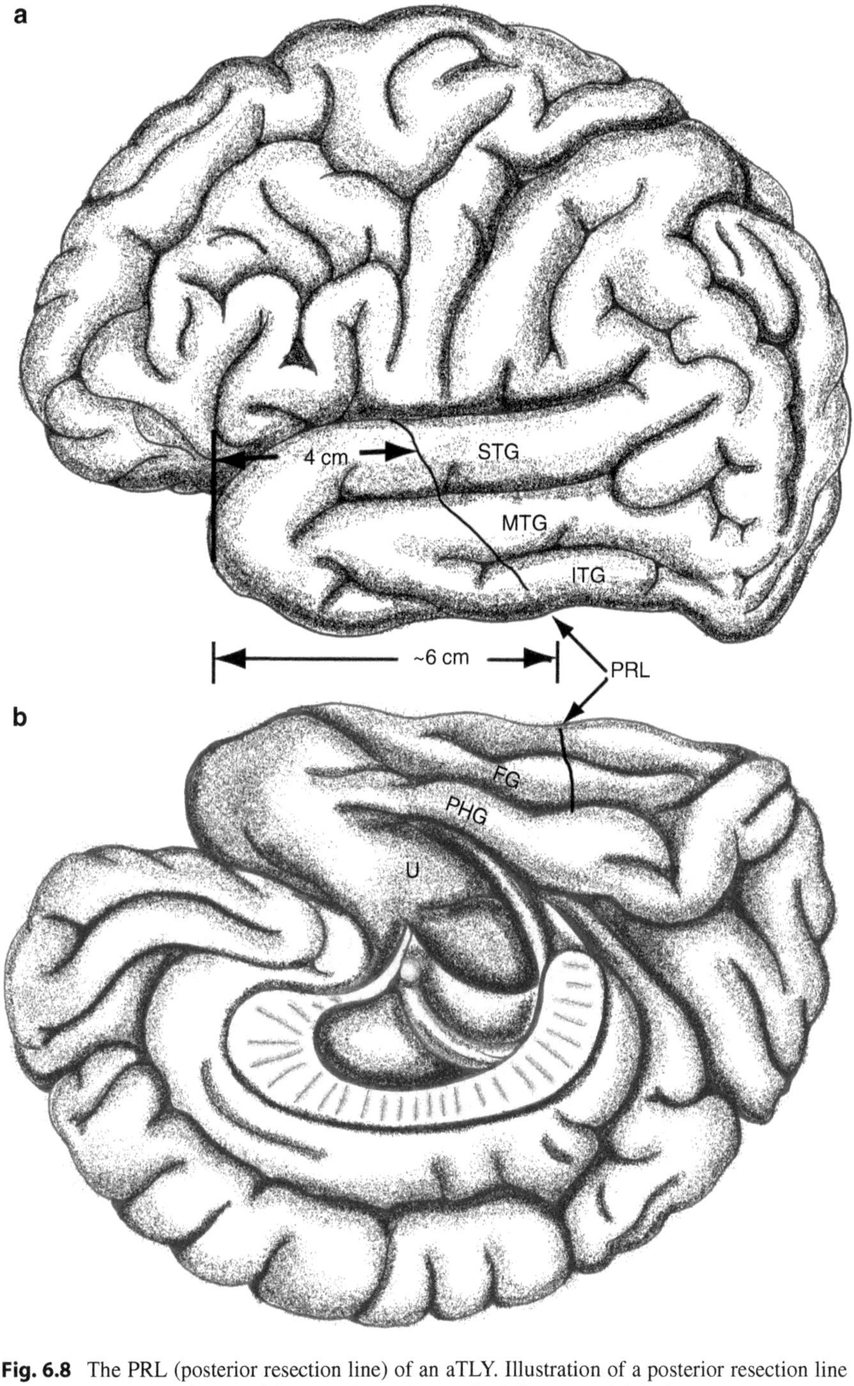

Fig. 6.8 The PRL (posterior resection line) of an aTLY. Illustration of a posterior resection line (PRL) over the lateral (**a**) and inferior (**b**) surfaces of a left temporal lobe in a typical standard aTLY. *FG* fusiform (occipitotemporal) gyrus, *ITG* inferior temporal gyrus, *MTG* middle temporal gyrus, *PHG* parahippocampal gyrus, *STG* superior temporal gyrus, *U* uncus

There are really no restrictions with respect to the posterior extent of the PRL through the inferior temporal gyrus (ITG). For example, in some cases of posteriorly located tumours in the inferior part of the temporal lobe the ITG incision may be at the very back of the TL (~9 cm behind the temporal pole), or even into the occipital lobe, order to achieve a safe pathway to the tumour. Similarly, those rare cases which require a standard aTLY along with significant removal of posterior ITG epileptogenic neocortex can be conducted without any real post-operative concerns.

On the inferior temporal surface, the PRL is further angled somewhat more posteriorly as it is carried medially across the inferior surface of the inferior temporal gyrus (ITG) and occipitotemporal (fusiform) gyrus towards the parahippocampal gyrus (Fig. 6.8b). There is not an absolute necessity to angle this part of the PRL, but there is nothing lost in doing so, and more importantly it provides easier achievement of a very posterior PRL through the hippocampus, as it decreases the requirement of forceful retraction of the remaining posterior temporal lobe in doing so.

6.2.7 Identification of the Temporal Horn of the Lateral Ventricle

There are a number of ways of finding the ventricle. The most important considerations are those that are the safest in avoiding "getting lost" in attempting to identify its location. The approach may be from above in the superior part of the PRL or inferiorly through the inferior temporal gyrus (ITG) or the undersurface of the lobe. Superiorly, the initial attempt to find the ventricle can usually be made by deepening the superior part of the PRL within the temporal stem, by about 5–10 mm below the inferior aspect of the (vertical) Sylvian fissure leptomeninges (Fig. 6.9a). With respect to the latter, it may be remembered that the last the last sentences of Sect. 6.2.4, regarding this superior area of the temporal stem, were "However, since this is also the line along which the temporal stem will be incised, it is often advantageous to simply coagulate a shallow (~1–2 mm) incision through the stem at this point, along the bottom of the leptomeninges. The best direction for deepening this incision can be better estimated later in the resection." This is the point of "later in the resection!" If this deepening of 5–10 mm does not reach (i.e., "find") the ventricle, then another of two potential strategies for reaching it is safer.

The first strategy is the recognition that there is a choice of various directions of the 5–10 mm exploratory incisions for reaching the ventricle. In Fig. 6.9b I have used the two extremes (#s 1 and 3) and the ideal (# 2). One can appreciate that using # 1 is very likely to encroach upon the optic tract or, if the PRL is more posteriorly located, the lateral geniculate body and/or the internal capsule, with the consequence of producing a neurological deficit. It is this risk that leads me to the fact that no more than 5–10 mms should be used, if the ventricle is not reached. The # 3 incision looks safe and indeed it is. However, while it is safe, it is also lateral enough that the bulk of the temporal stem medially will nearly always preclude easy visualization of the medial part of the ventricle, without significant retraction, which must exist for eventually removing the hippocampus. The # 2 exploratory incision is ideal

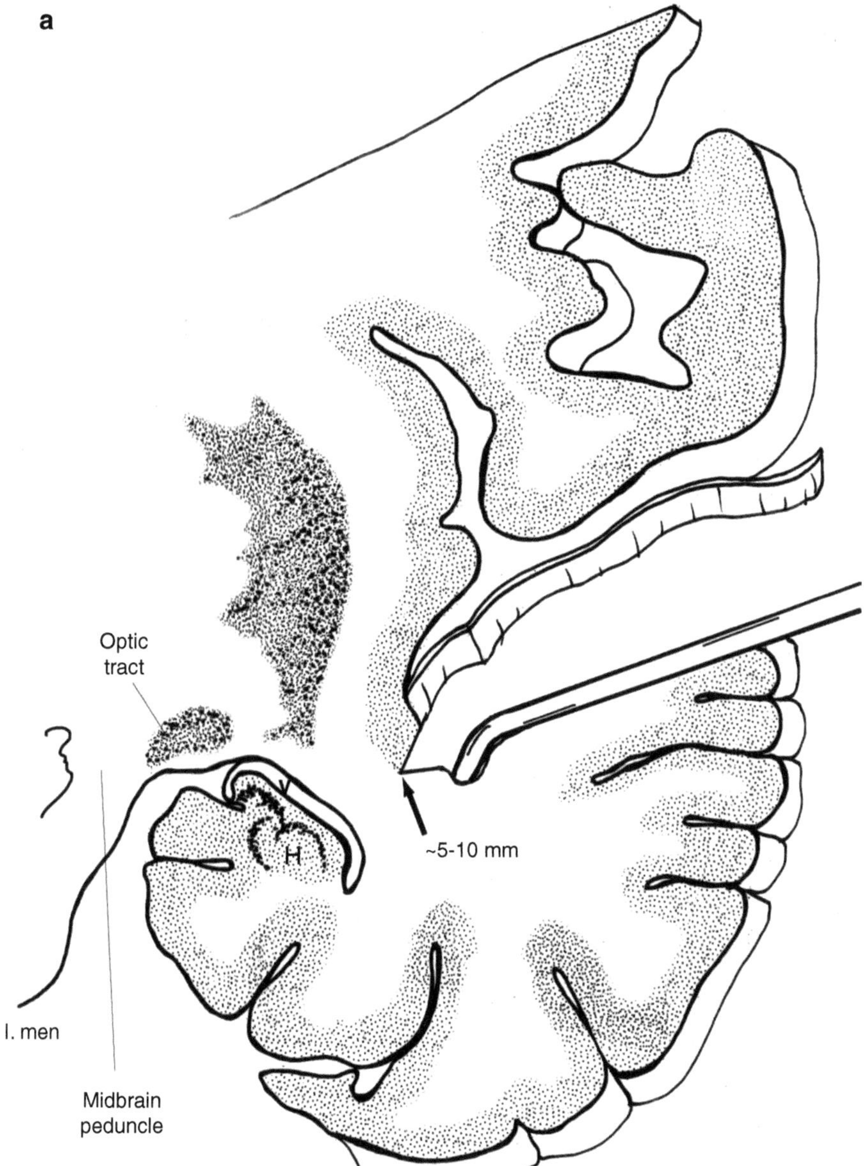

Fig. 6.9 The identification of the temporal horn of the lateral ventricle. An illustration of a coronal section through the posterior resection line (PRL) of an aTLY. (**a**) A point in the PRL about 5–10 mm below the bottom of the Sylvian fissure leptomeningeal fold, from which the ventricle may be approached. (**b**) Illustrates three potential lines of incision through the temporal stem in order to identify the temporal horn of the lateral ventricle. There are individual advantages and disadvantages associated with incision lines # 1 and # 3 (see text). *H* hippocampus, *l.men.* leptomeninges, *v* temporal horn of the lateral ventricle (Redrawn, with permission, from Girvin (1992))

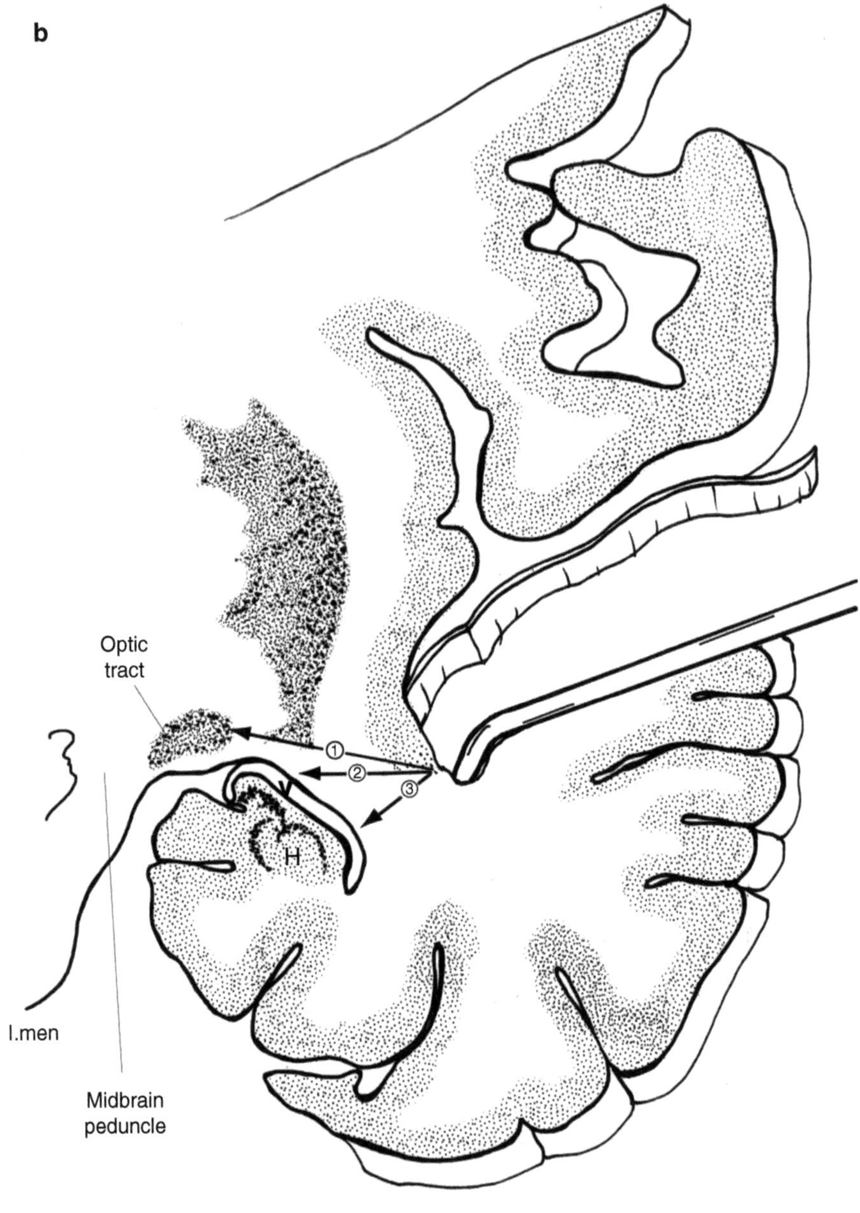

Fig. 6.9 (continued)

because it is not associated with a risk of producing a neurological deficit, nor does it require removing further bulk of the temporal stem after the ventricle is reached. In summary, the # 1 must not be used. Numbers 2 and 3 can be used safely, but with the latter further white matter (temporal stem) must be removed until it is roughly the same as # 2. From the foregoing, the reader will appreciate that the best initial attempt at safely and satisfactorily finding the ventricle should be initiated more laterally than medially!

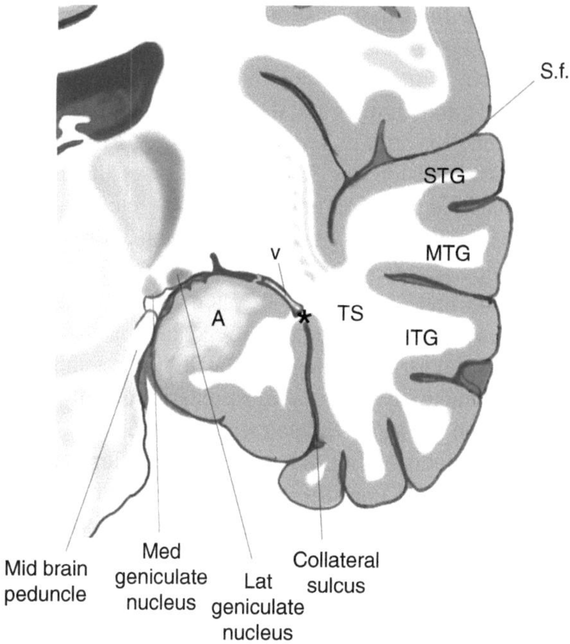

Fig. 6.10 A coronal section, illustrating the distance between the depth of the collateral sulcus and the temporal horn. Illustration of the very small distance between the bottom of a sulcus (in this case, the collateral sulcus) of the underside (inferior surface) of the temporal lobe and the temporal horn of the lateral ventricle. *A* amygdala, *ITG* inferior temporal gyrus, *MTG* middle temporal gyrus, *S.f* Sylvian fissure, *STG* superior temporal gyrus, *TS* temporal stem, *v* temporal horn of the lateral ventricle, ✱ the middle of the small distance between the depth of the collateral sulcus and the temporal horn

If the foregoing is not satisfactory in safely reaching the ventricle, then there is yet another approach. "Getting lost" can always be avoided by completing the PRL over both the lateral and inferior surfaces as far as the depths of the sulci. If the ventricle is not found at this point then the surgeon should consider that now "getting lost" is a risk, particularly if the choice of the ensuing strategy is that of simply deepening the lateral incision (PRL) further, which certainly can lead to disappointing postoperative neurological deficits! Under these circumstances, the better choice is to use the approach from the inferior surface.

The inferior surface exploratory approach to the ventricle simply involves largely what was suggested in the foregoing paragraph and much as if it was to be the periphery of a corticectomy (Sect. 5.5.2), i.e., it should be deepened initially only to the bottom of the sulci. The distance between the depths of the medially located sulci on the inferior temporal surface and the ventricle usually are no more than 1–2 mm. This is illustrated in Fig. 6.10. By deepening the incision at the bottom of the sulci of the medial area of the *inferior* surface, e.g., the inferior temporal and/or collateral sulci, the ventricle is usually safely and relatively easily found.

The exposure of the ventricle is easily appreciated by the drainage of CSF (abundance of clear colorless fluid), the appearance of the bulging choroid plexus, or the appearance of the strikingly pure white glistening surface of the hippocampus. The placement of a cottonoid patty in the ventricular incision will decrease the likelihood of blood entering the ventricle, but more importantly it remains as a landmark by which to continually localize the ventricle. With the ventricle now identified, the temporal stem can now be incised, beginning at the PRL, with the bipolar coagulation forceps one blade of which is placed inside the ventricle and the other along the bottom of the Sylvian fissure. The forceps blade in the bottom of the Sylvian fissure will follow the small incision that was made in the Sylvian fissure (see the end of Sect. 6.2.4), as mentioned earlier in this section. The line of coagulation should be conducted, as medial as possible, and superficially it will be at the junction of the Sylvian leptomeninges and the temporal stem. If the 1–2 mm incision was initiated in this junction after its original exposure, then this incision will form the superficial part of the incision line. The coagulation of the incision (in the stem) is conducted in an anterior direction until it meets the incision line, which had been carried out earlier in order to better visualize the subpial dissection of the deep anteroinferomedial temporal cortex, referred to in Sect. 6.2.5.

As the incision through the stem is completed, the ventricle (temporal horn) becomes more visible and the amygdala is easily recognized as a protrusion into the inferomedial aspect of the anterior tip of the temporal horn. If the incision is taken "tightly" medially, then the most anterior extent will be at the anterior or posterior base of the uncus/amygdala (see Figs. 6.6b and 6.11a). Irrespective of which, the end of this incision line is best carried anterior to the amygdala, as illustrated in the anterior stippled line in Fig. 6.11a; at this point the temporal stem is completely incised and the anterior part of the neocortex has been separated from the inferomedial temporal lobe that contains the limbic structures. This allows the preservation of a good, intact amygdala for histological examination. If it is easily visualized, the amygdala can be removed now (see Sect. 6.2.8, vide infra); often, it is more easily removed later (see Sects. 6.2.8 and 6.2.9).

Gloor lamented the paucity of articles in the literature dealing with the postoperative histological examination of the amygdala, especially in contrast to the attention paid to the hippocampus from the same operations (1997). He also provided reasons for this in his indications that "for technical reasons, comparable samples of amygdala have not become available, because it cannot safely be removed en bloc" (p. 692) or that it "is often damaged at surgery because of its location and anatomical formation" (p. 709). This perhaps was reflecting the views of the surgical group at the Montreal Neurological Institute in the very early days; in the article of Penfield et al. in 1961, Rasmussen outlined his technique of an aTLY (pp. 773–6) in which my interpretation of the technique is that the amygdala was removed with piecemeal suction. It is a contention with which I certainly cannot agree currently. My own teaching of residents and fellows is that clear recognitions, and en bloc resections, of both the hippocampus and the amygdala is mandatory, as part of the surgical anatomy of an aTLY, and should accompany that of the anterior neocortex as the three specimens made available for histological study in *every* aTLY! Further, in my view, I think that without any doubt they can be removed safely!

If the superior incision, composed of the joined anterior and posterior incisions, has been completed, and the PRL has been taken medially to the collateral sulcus of the inferior surface, then the anterior neocortex, now ready to be removed, will have been largely devascularized. Its remaining attachment will consist of the cortex and white matter of the gyri of the inferior surface, e.g., inferior temporal and/or fusiform gyri, and their leptomeningeal investments, a few small arterial vessels, and the amygdala and hippocampus. The small arterial vessels will be minimal if the subpial resection beneath the anterior end of the Sylvian fissure has been taken

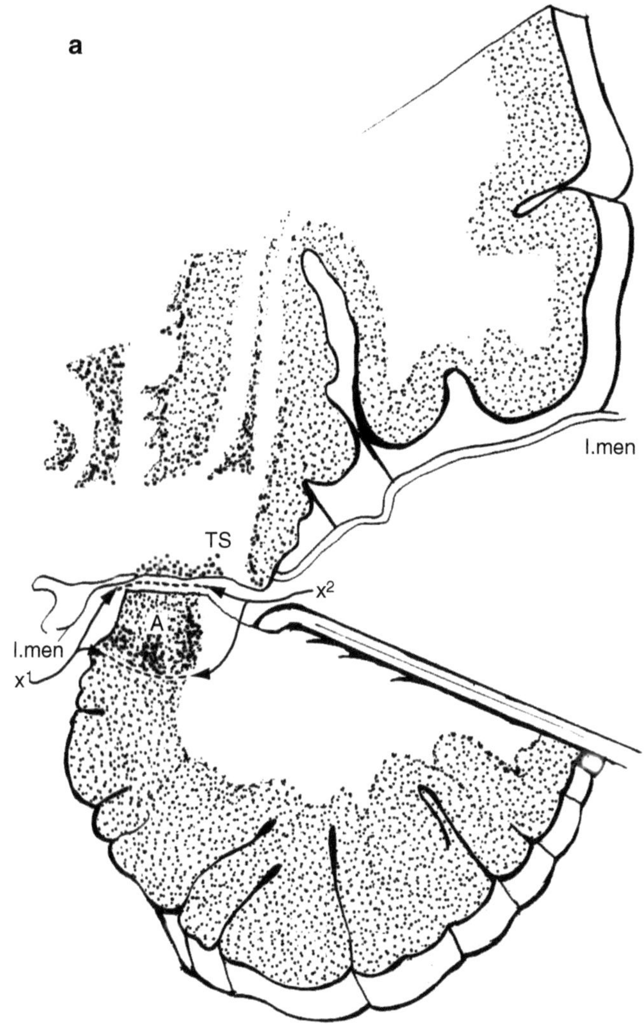

Fig. 6.11 Isolation of the anterior temporal neocortex in an aTLY. It illustrates the incisions that disconnect the anterior temporal neocortex of a left TL for its isolation. (**a**) Coronal section. ~30–35 mm behind the pole of the TL, illustrating the anterior coronal incision, from inside the ventricle, near the posteromedial base of the amygdala, thus separating the anterior part of the TL from the more posterior inferomedial hippocampus (see text). (**b**) Coronal section, ~40–45 mm behind the TL pole, illustrating the hippocampus, now separated from the amygdala, remaining connected to the isolated temporal neocortex (see text). (**c**) Coronal section, ~ 50–60 mm behind the TL pole, illustrating the final incision (*dotted line*) that provides the separation of the inferomedial cortex from the now isolated anterior temporal neocortex (see text). *A* amygdala, *H* hippocampus, *l.men* leptomeninges, *ph.g* parahippocampal gyrus, *S.f* Sylvian fissure, *TS* temporal stem, *U* uncus, $\mathbf{x}^1$ the furthest posterior point (outside the uncus/amygdala, i.e., "extrinsic") reached by the subpial resection around the temporal stem in the undersurface of the medial TL (see Fig. 6.9b), $\mathbf{x}^2$ the point of an internal (e.g., "intrinsic," i.e., within either the TS of the anterior TL or the ventricle) location (Redrawn, with permission, from Girvin (1992))

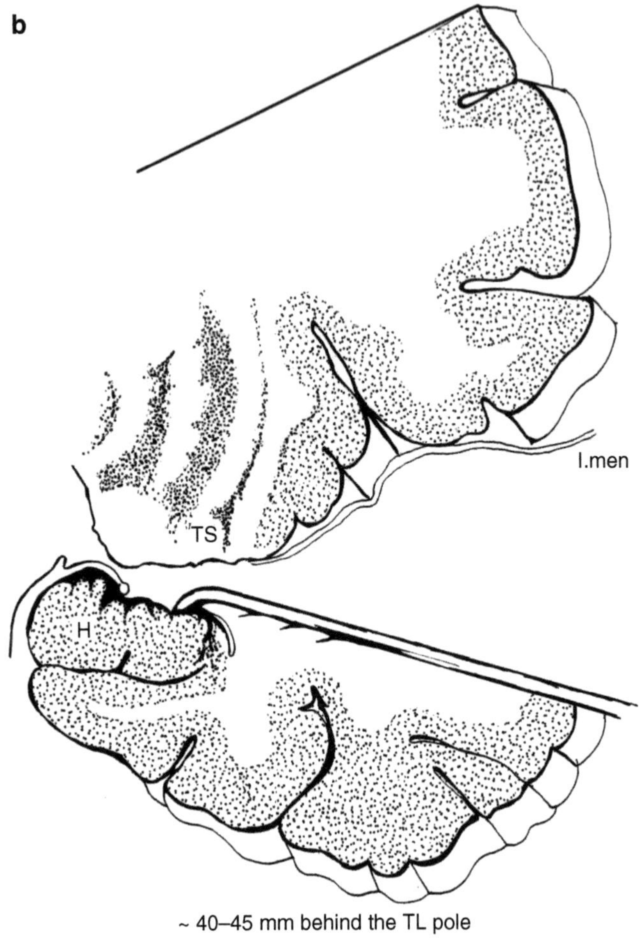

Fig. 6.11 (continued)

c

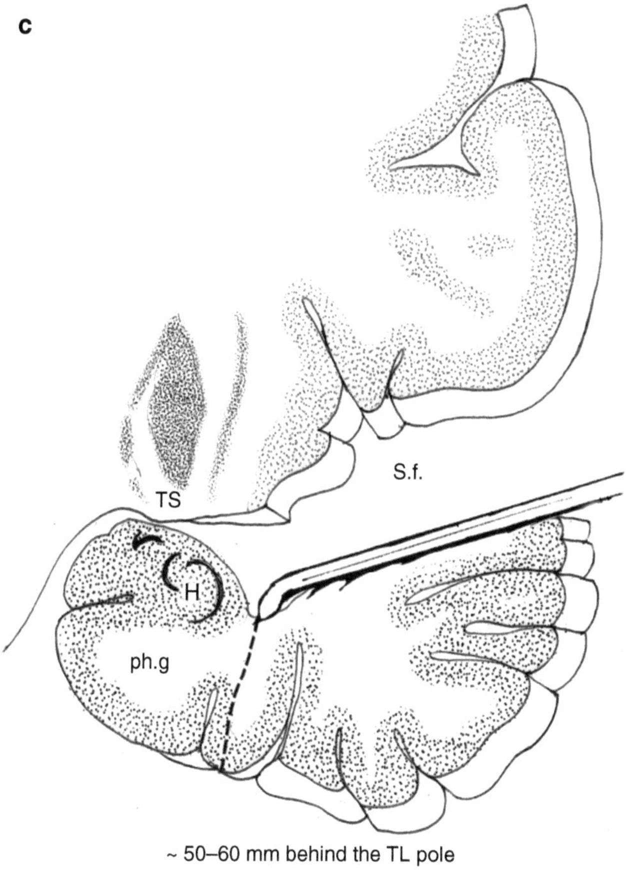

Fig. 6.11 (continued)

as far posteriorly as possible on the undersurface of the inferomedial cortex (see end of Sect. 6.2.5 and Fig. 6.6b).

6.2.8 Removal of the Neocortex

The ease and completeness of the eventual, final removal of the hippocampus is greatly facilitated by the absence of the overlying neocortex. At this point the ventricle is fully open for visualization, the PRL of the neocortex is completed medially to roughly the area of the fusiform gyrus or the collateral sulcus, and the neocortex to be removed has been largely devascularized. As noted in the foregoing, now the only connectivity of the partially isolated anterior neocortex is to the inferior surface and the anteroinferomedial limbic structures, e.g., amygdala and hippocampus.

Figure 6.11 is a series of coronal sections, extending between ~3 and 6 cm behind the tip of the temporal lobe pole, illustrating the final incisions leading to isolation of the temporal neocortex. Figure 6.11a depicts a section approximately 30–35 mm behind the temporal pole. In that figure $\mathbf{x}^1$ represents the furthest posterior point that was achieved from the subpial dissection that was initiated in the Sylvian fissure and then continued around the anterior extent of the temporal stem and then finally posteriorly on the undersurface of the inferomedial TL. Its posterior extent was aided by the initiation of the incision of the anterior temporal stem (see Sect. 6.2.5 and Fig. 6.6b). In figure A it is outside (extrinsic to) the vicinity of the uncus/amygdala; however, it could be at any part of the amygdala or even in front of, or behind, the amygdala, depending upon where the subpial dissection had been terminated. It could have ended anywhere from before to behind the amygdala near the anterior hippocampus. As noted earlier, when the temporal horn was opened fully, the inner (intrinsic) side of the amygdala is easily recognized as a bulge in the inferomedial wall of the anterior tip of the temporal horn (see Sect. 6.2.7).

If the amygdala has not already been removed (see Sect. 6.2.7), then it can be removed now. The designated $\mathbf{x}^2$ can be defined as the intrinsic end point of an incision line in which the extrinsic point $\mathbf{x}^1$ is the other end. In Fig. 6.11a $\mathbf{x}^2$ is in the parenchyma of the anterior TL, but more often it would be somewhat further posterior and thus would be in the wall of the ventricle. An incision between $\mathbf{x}^1$ and $\mathbf{x}^2$, as illustrated by the dotted line in Fig. 6.11a, would not only be one of the incisions involved in removing the amygdala, but it would also contribute to the isolation of the anterior TL as a result of removing its connectivity with the inferomedial hippocampus.

Figure 6.11b is a coronal section ~40–45 mm behind the TL pole and is simply a reminder that the hippocampus remains connected to the neocortex throughout its extent by the gyri of the inferior surface. The more lateral part of the neocortex can now also be relatively devascularized by coagulating the inferior surface and underlying white matter moving either from this point or the PRL along an anteroposterior line parallel to one of its anatomical structures, e.g., collateral sulcus, fusiform gyrus, and/or inferior temporal gyrus. The latter can be done from within the ventricle in which case it is parallel, and a few millimeters lateral, to the hippocampus. Figure 6.11c is a coronal section about 50–60 mm behind the TL pole, which is at the back of the midbrain and within a centimeter or so of what will be the PRL of the hippocampus. It demonstrates by the stippled line the anteroposterior incision through the fusiform gyrus, leaving the parahippocampal gyrus and the hippocampus intact. The leptomeningeal investment is coagulated and incised, leaving the neocortex isolated. If the anteroposterior incision was conducted from within the ventricle, the neocortex should be removed only after gently raising the specimen and verifying that there is no connecting vein to its undersurface that might be ruptured at its exit.

It is sometimes difficult to join the anterior and posterior incisions through the anterior neocortex because of the bulk of the lobe, which requires retraction to do so. Thus, once the incisions have been carried as close as possible to one another the majority of the vasculature to the lobe has been removed and the cortex can be removed. I have always simply used a pair of curved Mayo scissors to cut through the remaining mantle at its base, along an approximate incision in the ITG/fusiform gyrus, in order to remove the neocortex. In doing this the scissors must be oriented inferolaterally, so as to avoid encroaching on the hippocampus. There are usually a few vessels coming into it medially, which will be cut across in the maneuver, but these can easily be identified with the use of a cottonoid patty, suction, and some saline irrigation and then coagulated. For those who feel that this is too wildly barbaric (!), bipolar coagulating forceps may be used to achieve stepwise the same appropriate incision.

6.2.9 Removal of Anteroinferomesial (Limbic) Cortex

Once the neocortex has been removed, at least 2–4 cm of the hippocampus is clearly seen. If the amygdala happens to still be present (see Sects. 6.2.7 and 6.2.8), which is likely, it can at this juncture be very easily removed with a pair of small curved scissors and submitted as a separate specimen. At this point there are no anterior connections to the hippocampus. That is to say, whatever connections remain at this point are located posteriorly, through primarily the hippocampal crura and commissure.

Using a small cup curette such as the curette end of the Penfield # 1, the anterior end of the hippocampus can be gently separated from the underlying leptomeninges by slipping it in between them. This is facilitated by countertraction through the use of a sucker on a cottonoid patty applied to the leptomeninges that have been disclosed by removal of the anterior temporal lobe in front of the anterior end of the hippocampus. As this separation is conducted, it will eventually become difficult because of the intact posterior hippocampus. However, it is worthwhile immobilizing as much of the anterior hippocampus as possible at this juncture and the coagulation and incision of any small arterial vessels that bridge the plane of separation. A cottonoid patty is then wedged gently into the plane, as far posteriorly as possible.

At this point, attention is turned to the completion of the PRL through the hippocampus. An appropriately placed retractor, containing an angled end, in the ventricle, can be utilized to retract the temporal lobe posteriorly and laterally, well posterior to the lateral temporal PRL. The hippocampal PRL should be as posterior as can be achieved, usually at least 6–7 cm behind what was the tip of the temporal pole and which will be roughly 10–15 mm behind a coronal plane of the posterior surface of the midbrain. The incision can be made by progressing mediolaterally or lateromedially in any combination. (It might be mentioned here that Spencer et al. 1984 have an article setting out a clear manner in which this may be achieved, after removing 4.5 and 3 cm of the nondominant and dominant temporal lobe neocortex, respectively.) In the former, the choroidal fissure is identified, usually after the medial retraction of the choroid plexus—best achieved by covering it with a cottonoid patty and using a separate small retractor. Retraction of it medially allows easy identification of the fimbria. The latter can be raised up and separated from the underlying leptomeningeal investment with a small blunt dissector (the Penfield # 4 dissector or a "blunt hook" are both ideal instruments) and coagulated. The blunt dissector is used for stripping as much of the hippocampus of its leptomeningeal investment, starting with the fimbria, which can be achieved satisfactorily.

Combining the achievements of the blunt dissector and the retraction, the surgeon can then choose the location of the PRL as posteriorly as possible. It is initiated in typical subpial fashion, using the suction cannula and bipolar coagulating forceps. Figure 6.12 illustrates the directions in which the PRL can be conducted. Figure 6.12a1–3 starts medially through the fimbria and then the body of the

Fig. 6.12 The *PRL* (posterior resection line) through the hippocampus. It illustrates the two directions by which the completion of the posterior resection line (PRL) through the hippocampus can be executed. It may be accomplished by working (**a**) medial to lateral within the proposed PRL or (**b**) lateral to medial (see text). *b.d.* blunt dissector, *c.s.* collateral sulcus, *fim.* fimbria of the hippocampus, *H* hippocampus, *h.g* hippocampal gyrus, *h.s.* hippocampal sulcus, *IC* internal capsule, *ph.g.* parahippocampal gyrus, *re* retractor, *MP* midbrain peduncle, *OT* optic tract (Redrawn, with permission, from Girvin (1992))

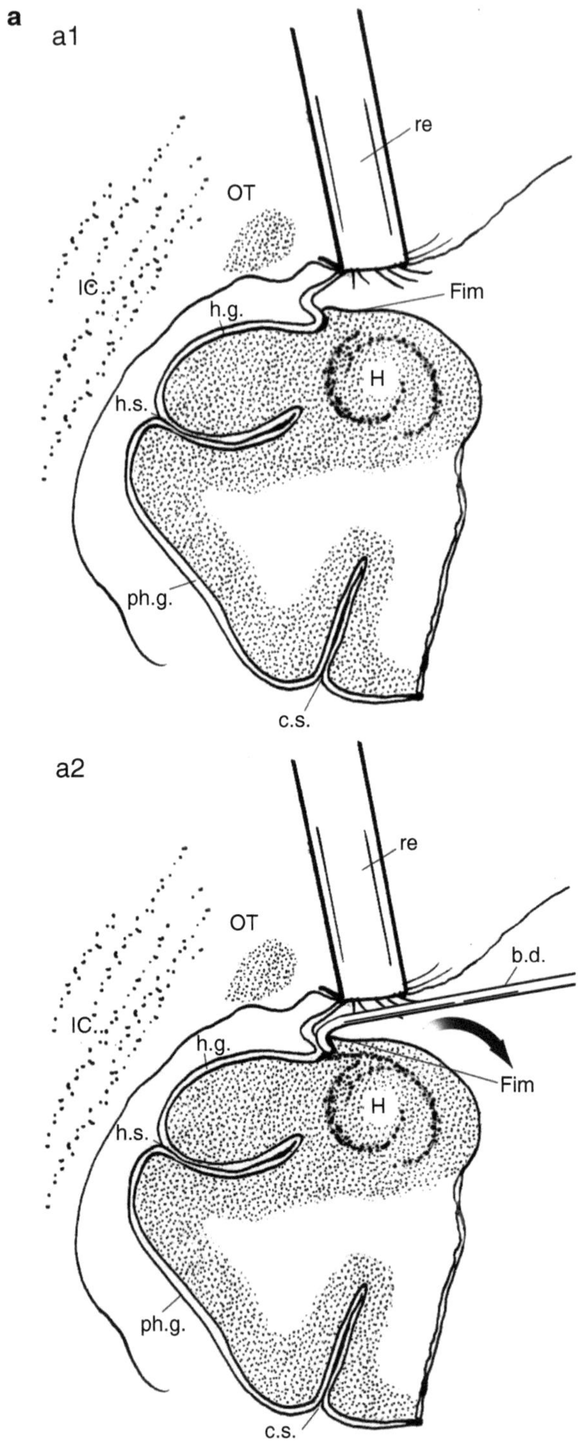

Fig. 6.12 (continued)

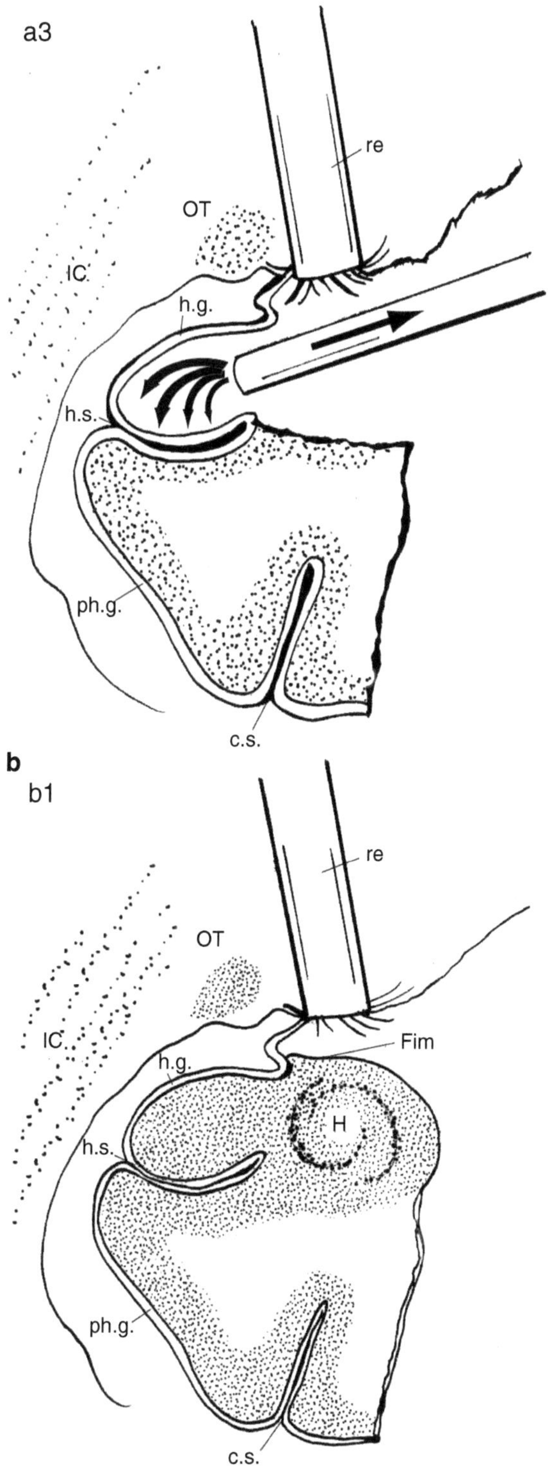

Fig. 6.12 (continued)

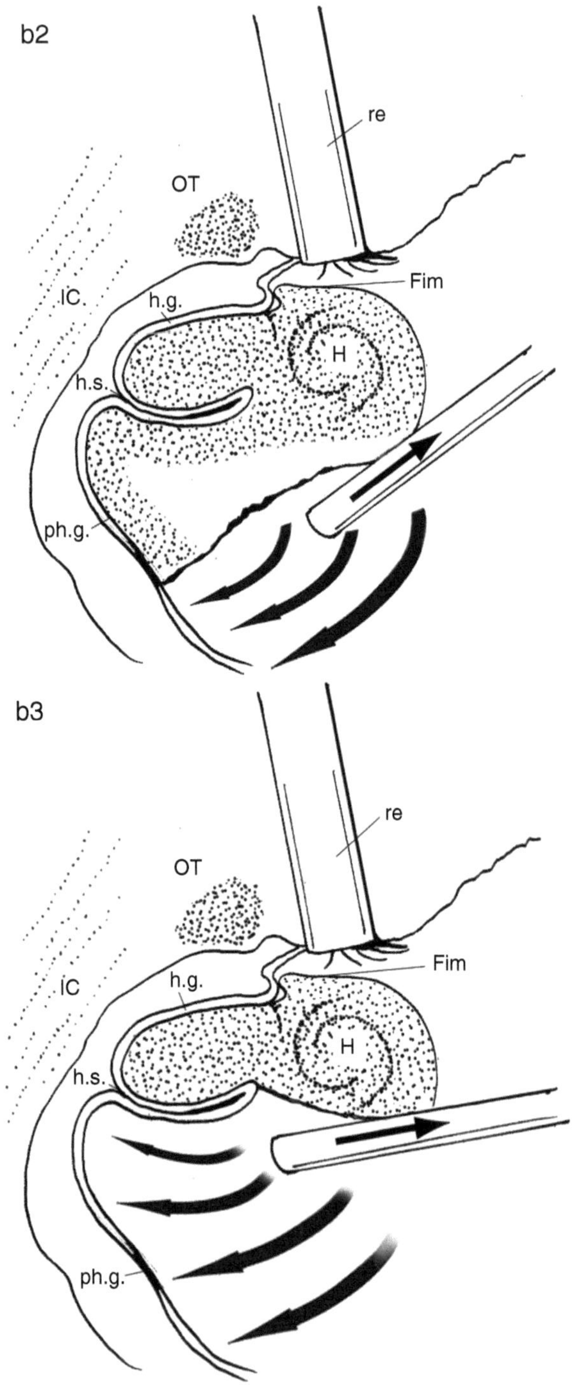

hippocampus down to the upper side of the hippocampal sulcus. Figure 6.12b1–3 is the reverse of Fig. 6.12a, starting laterally from the incision that freed the neocortex (see Sect. 6.2.8 and Fig. 6.11c) then proceeding laterally towards the undersurface of the hippocampal sulcus. In both of these the incision can be continually deepened, until the leptomeningeal barrier is reached. At the same time it is well worth while widening the incision lines posteriorly by ~2–3 mm; by doing so, this removes more of the hippocampal cells, if they are still present beyond the PRL, and the wider incision is very helpful in the final separation of the body of the hippocampus from the leptomeninges. The use of cottonoid patties with the forceps aids in retraction of the resection incisions. Very little coagulation is necessary and thus most of the resection is conducted by suction alone. Irrespective of whether the resection is conducted mediolaterally or lateromedially, once the hippocampal sulcus is encountered, the remaining resection line can usually be more easily achieved by now turning to the opposite approach. As these incisions are advanced, the retraction becomes much easier. If there is a significant amount of the occipitotemporal (fusiform) and parahippocampal gyri remaining at the time of initiating the hippocampal PRL, then there is an advantage of starting on the lateral side, thereby reducing the bulk of the inferomedial neocortex early on and thus making the retraction required to complete the remaining hippocampal PRL easier.

Once the PRL is completed, then once again the curette end of a blunt dissector—my choice is the Penfield # 1—can be employed to gently separate the hippocampus from its leptomeningeal investment, working both posteroanteriorly and anteroposteriorly. As one proceeds with the separation, there will usually be two or three very small vessels (from the anterior choroidal and/or posterior cerebral arteries), which can be coagulated and incised easily, finally freeing the hippocampal specimen.

If the aTLY has been carried out gently in following the foregoing described procedure, there should be no bleeding whatsoever. Thus, at this point the resection bed should be irrigated freely with saline. If there is some minor bleeding, then packing with some cottonoid patties for a few minutes should be sufficient to deal with it. If insufficient, a small piece of fibrin foam or, often, low current coagulation will suffice.

6.2.10 Anatomy of Resection Bed Following aTLY

If a good quality aTLY has been carried out, then the resection bed should *always* reveal, through the partially translucent leptomeninges, the insula with the overlying MCA vessels, the free edge of the tentorium, the oculomotor nerve, the internal carotid artery, and the lateral side of the midbrain. It *usually* reveals the anterior choroidal artery, the posterior communicating artery, the posterior cerebral artery, and the basal vein of Rosenthal. It *rarely* reveals the optic tract, the superior cerebellar artery, or the trochlear nerve.

6.3 Neocortical aTLY

The only real variation between the pure neocortical aTLY and the standard aTLY is how much subcortical white matter is left behind. From the foregoing the isolation and removal of the neocortical anterior temporal lobe in the standard aTLY is as outlined in the foregoing sections (Sects. 6.2.1, 6.2.2, 6.2.3, 6.2.4, 6.2.5, 6.2.6, 6.2.7, and 6.2.8). I would also include the amygdala, as outlined in Sects. 6.2.7, 6.2.8, or 6.2.9.

If one wishes to not enter the ventricle, for whatever reason, then Sects. 6.2.1, 6.2.2, 6.2.3, 6.2.4, 6.2.5, and 6.2.6 can be followed after which the lateral temporal neocortex quite easily can be removed in a similar fashion to a corticectomy, following the steps noted in Chap. 5. The inferior surface is somewhat more difficult to achieve without entering the ventricle, but can be done with care not to carry the resection in the inferior sulci deeper than the deepest gray matter in their depths. Less difficult is making certain that the medial extent of the inferior surface corticectomy is the collateral sulcus. Thus, the parahippocampal gyrus will be left completely intact.

The usual reason for the preservation of ventricular integrity is to preclude the presence of blood entering the ventricular system in cases in which the amygdala and hippocampus are left intact. If that is truly the reason, then I would point out that if the neocortical aTLY is carried out properly, the paucity of blood remaining in the ventricle is never a reason for concern. Thus, I would encourage one to not engage in this much longer procedure, which may give rise to blood having seeped into the ventricle unknowingly through an unidentified rent in the ventricle wall.

6.4 Amygdalohippocampectomy (AHPy)

The amygdalohippocampectomy (AHPy) was introduced by Niemeyer in 1958. His original surgical approach was through a small (2 cm) incision in the MTG into the temporal horn of the lateral ventricle. It was really popularized as an epilepsy operation by Wieser and Yasargil in the 1980s (Weiser and Yasargil 1982a, b; Yasargil et al. 1985, 1993; Weiser 1986, 1988, 1991). Their surgical approach to the temporal horn of the lateral ventricle is through the anteroinferior Sylvian fissure and the temporal stem. Other approaches have been reported through the superior temporal sulcus (Olivier 1987, 1997, 2000) and the STG (Rougier et al. 1992) or subtemporally (Hori et al. 1993).

In most of these operations, the surgical pathway into the amygdala and hippocampus has been heralded as "minimally invasive." If the cortical incision is small, then usually the passage way is limited, the visualization is somewhat restricted and the achievement of an en bloc resection of the removed tissue is much more difficult. If the cortical incision is enlarged to provide very good visualization, then the procedure is much less minimally invasive from the point of view of one of the tenets of epilepsy surgery in that there is more injured cortex left behind. The approach of Yasargil invades very little cortex and can be enlarged through increasing the incision in the temporal stem. It has been considered by some as being more difficult and particularly more risky by virtue of the fact that the pathway of the surgical dissection is through the MCA vasculature in the Sylvian fissure. A very good review of this approach has been provided by Comair (2001).

The very increased popularity of use of the AHPy toward the end of the twentieth century occurred as a result of its adherence to the minimalist philosophy at the time, as it relates to the amount of surgery and the intuitive view that there might be a better postoperative neuropsychological assessment after it, in contrast to the larger standard aTLY. As it turns out there is apparently little or no evidence to support this intuitive notion.

6.5 Obligations for Tissue Histopathology

Just as the recognition of certain anatomical features of the resection bed following an aTLY is usually an accompaniment of a satisfactory resection, the specimens submitted to the pathologist for histopathology are similarly reflective of an adequately achieved resection. There should be specimens of "anterior temporal lobe neocortex," "amygdala," and "hippocampus." My feeling is that the submissions of these specimens are an obligation of the surgeon, from the points of view of the ability to correlate histopathology with the potential cause of the epilepsy, the resulting improved academic understanding of the pathophysiology of the epilepsy that accrues from such correlations, the increased understanding of the surgical anatomy, and finally the training of young surgeons.

It is obvious from the foregoing that this author favors as much "en bloc" resection as possible, rather than piecemeal resection. One of the disadvantages of the use of an ultrasonic aspirator is the difficulty in obtaining a good en bloc resection. The latter provides better morphological specimens, makes the neuropathologist much happier, and provides one of the important bases for better understanding of the pathophysiology of epileptic entities. There is nothing wrong with the use of the aspirator in my view. However, also in my view, there is no advantage in its use!

6.6 Safe Limits of Resection

Historically, when greater amounts of lateral cortex were being removed, a removal of 5–5.5 cm on the dominant side and 6.5 cm on the nondominant side were accepted as the posterior limits of resection behind the temporal pole in order to preclude significant deficits of speech or visual field, respectively. Penfield and Rasmussen (1968, p. 188) wrote that removal of more than 5 cm of the cortex and subcortical white matter resulted in a homonymous hemianopia. In my experience one can go a centimeter or so beyond the 5 cm mark and not necessarily suffer a hemianopia, but rather commonly only a contralateral upper quadrantanopsia. However, as noted in the foregoing, since the advent of the recognition of the importance of the limbic TL, as opposed to temporal neocortex, most aTLYs do not require a removal of

Table 6.1 MRI measurements of the distance from the temporal pole to more posteriorly related anatomy of the lobe

Anatomical structure	Distance behind temporal pole (cm)	Range
Anterior end of temporal stem	2	1.7–2.3
Center of amygdala	2.6	2.1–3.0
Tip of temporal horn of the lateral ventricle	3	2.2–3.7
Anterior aspect of midbrain (peduncle)	3.5	3.2–4.0
Posterior edge of midbrain (quadrigeminal plate)	5.9	5.6–6.5

Table 6.2 Intraoperative measurements of the distance of speech areas and the Rolandic fissure from the temporal pole (measured with a red rubber catheter)

Anatomical designation	Distance behind temporal pole (cm)	n	Range
Rolandic fissure	6.1	89	4.3–7.5
Temporal speech area	7.4	63	6.0–9.4
Broca's area	4.0	47	2.3–5.8

more than 3.5–4.5 cm, and this removal is primarily to facilitate the easy visualization of the limbic cortex and its removal en bloc.

The surgical anatomy of the aTLY is easier to understand when there is an awareness of the relationship of its intrinsic structures to the tip of the temporal pole. Table 6.1 shows the measurements ($n = 20$) of some of the anatomical landmarks of the anterior temporal lobe in relation to the tip of the temporal pole. These were derived from medical imaging, primarily MRIs (see also Fig. 7.8 and Tables 6.2 and 7.1).

I would be remiss in not acknowledging some measurements made by others and more particularly surgeons of the Montreal Neurological Institute. Dr. Feindel noted that "the amygdala lies between 3 and 4 cm from the tip [of the temporal pole] while the hippocampus extends from 3.5 cm to about 7 cm from the tip." I am uncertain as to how many observations led to these measurements, but the one picture shown (Fig. 111) was a sagittal section that was obviously a postmortem example (Feindel 1964).

It is clear that the inferior temporal gyrus is *never* involved in speech in the dominant hemisphere. Thus, this gyrus can be removed for purposes of removing epileptic cortex or can be entered and/or removed for purposes of the provision of a surgical pathway to deeper structures.

Penfield noted in a lecture in 1957, "Removals of the superior convolution on either side is followed by no defect of vestibular function …." I am not quite sure what he meant by this, but since the paper was primarily associated with the localization of auditory and vestibular function, I have interpreted the "removals" as only involving the STG as far behind the temporal pole as the posterior extent of the auditory cortex, e.g., 6–6.5 cm.

Table 6.2 outlines the distances behind the tip of the temporal pole where the Rolandic fissure, temporal speech area, and Broca's area are found. These

Table 6.3 Outlines of the safe (and unsafe) limits of the temporal lobe cortical resections

	Resection safe?			Postoperative course		
				Deficit		
Temporal resection	Yes	No	?	Transient	Permanent	Uneventful
Speech area	–	√		–	Aphasia	–
Routine unilateral aTLY	√	–		Contralateral upper quadrantanopsia	Partial contralateral upper quadrantanopsia	√
Radical aTLY (9 cm)	–	–	√	? Transient contralateral hemianopia	Contralateral superior quadrantanopsia or hemianopia	–
Bilateral polar (<3 cm) corticectomies	√	–		–	–	√
Bilateral conservative aTLY (<5 cm)	–	√		–	At least some impairment of anterograde memory	–
Bilateral hippocampal removal	–	√		–	Anterograde amnesia	–

measurements were made intraoperatively (initially with a Penfield #2 dissector + 5 mm), as outlined in Chap. 2 (Sect. 2.3).

Table 6.3 summarizes the potential clinical results, which may be the postoperative accompaniments of the variety of resections that might be carried out in the management of temporal lobe epilepsy.

6.7 Complications

6.7.1 Dysphasia

Operations that suggest that significant amounts of lateral neocortex require a consideration of removal should be conducted under local anesthesia. If the operations are to be carried out under general anesthesia, then the foregoing Tables can be utilized to help avoid complications, but they are *never* as predictably accurate under general anesthesia as stimulation and clinical monitoring are in patients under local anesthesia! Pilcher and Rusyniak have provided a very extensive and intensive report of the complications of epilepsy surgery, not only those related to the actual surgical techniques but also those that occur in the various preoperative investigative strategies that accompany the potential surgical procedures (1993).

Most temporal lobe operations that require removals within a cm or so of the speech area will almost always experience a transient dysphasia, often with the characteristics, interestingly enough, of a Broca's dysphasia. This often starts within 24–48 h and disappears by the end of a week or so. Further, if while operating under local anesthesia there is no suggestion of a neurological deficit at the completion of the resection, then any emergence of a deficit afterwards will only very, very, very rarely be permanent. This is certainly in keeping with the statement of Penfield and Paine, specifically related to dysphasia, that "When no aphasia appeared while the patient was on the operating table, its subsequent appearance proved to be of little moment." (1955). Lüders et al. observed that stimulation of the dominant fusiform gyrus of a 38-year-old patient, 3.5–5.5 cm posterior to tip of the temporal lobe, gave rise to both receptive and expressive aphasia (1986). Whether this might be the cause of the transient dysphasia following aTLYs is unknown so far as I know.

Some evidence of aphasia after the conduct of an aTLY of the dominant hemisphere is not uncommonly observed. It is nearly always transient, gradually disappearing over the postoperative course of a few days or weeks and only very infrequently over the course of a few months. This is always the case, as noted in the foregoing, in cases conducted under local anesthesia when speech is normal after the surgical resection. However, even the presence of some dysphasia after a standard aTLY conducted under general anesthesia is very likely to follow the same course.

6.7.2 Hemiparesis/Hemiplegia

The term "manipulation hemiplegia" occurred in 5 % of the temporal lobectomies carried out by Penfield and colleagues from 1948 to 1955, of which half were permanent (Penfield et al. 1961; see also 1958). In the eight cases in which this occurred, it was during the removal of "very deep" scars, and six of which the dissections were "near the middle cerebral artery." In none was there any hemorrhage nor suggestion of the ligation of a significant sized artery. However, interestingly most were associated with homonymous hemianopia. Penfield considered that the lesion was probably in the vicinity of the internal capsule and that it "was probably related to manipulation of arteries," more particularly the "slender arteries" supplying the internal capsule.

I do not consider that the cause of the hemiplegia was "manipulation" and I would guess that this would have been Dr. Rasmussen's view as well, as he indicated that no such complication had occurred in the use of a newer technique, as more recently he had performed over 110 cases of aTLY without the complication (Penfield et al. 1961, p. 761). The technique was outlined in the latter part of the paper (pp. 773–6), as well as earlier in the articles of Penfield and Baldwin (1952) and Rasmussen and Jasper (1958).

6.7.3 Visual

In 1952 Penfield and Baldwin indicated that resections reaching to greater than 5.5 cm behind the temporal pole resulted in permanent contralateral upper quadrantic field defects. Two years later Penfield noted that such defects occurred when the resection was greater than 6 cm from the tip of the pole (1952). Further, at that time he indicated that removals of greater than 8 cm or more would likely give rise to a contralateral homonymous hemifield defect! It is not uncommon to find a contralateral superior quadrantanopsia in the immediate postoperative period; however, these nearly always gradually decrease in size and frequently they disappear all together. The upper quadrantic visual defects that become permanent nearly never cause a significant clinical impairment. Interestingly, the only two patients I have had who did have impairments upper quadrantanopsia were two sportsmen. One was a golfer who had intermittent difficulty in always seeing where his drives fell in the distance. The other was a tennis player who had opponents who learned that if they hit a high ball into the side of the visual defect he would often have some delayed trouble in dealing with it!

6.7.4 Cognitive Impairment

Brenda Milner thoroughly investigated patients before and after aTLY and remotely postoperatively throughout the majority of the last half of the twentieth century—a period of remarkable growth of the discipline of neuropsychology. Her contribution in 1958 is a very early discussion of the neuropsychological alterations that can be found in patients following aTLYs. Over the lateral part of the twentieth century, there has been increasing evidence that the dominant aTLYs may be associated with some cognitive impairment (Ojemann and Dodrill 1985, 1987; Invik et al. 1987). Further, the better the dominant temporal lobe function is preoperatively, the greater is the chance of such a postoperative cognitive alteration. Recent reviews agree fully with these observations. It should also be noted that Ojemann and Dodrill have provided evidence of some memory function in temporal neocortex.

Helmstaedter et al. in longitudinal studies looked at memory decline in a cohort of patients with chronic temporal lobe epilepsy, 147 of whom were operated upon and 102 of whom were treated medically (2003). They disclosed a number of very interesting observations, but the one most pertinent to this discussion was in the group of patients who had dominant temporal lobe surgery and continued to have seizures postoperatively. There was memory decline in the whole cohort, but it was greatest in this group. This was in striking contrast to the group of patients whose seizures were abolished by surgery who had the least decline in memory. Further, as was suggested in the foregoing, the decline was steeper in those with the better baseline performances. Interestingly, they also found that those with "tailored" resections had fewer declines in memory than those with a "standard two-thirds anterior lobectomy."

Sherman et al. reported a very recent meta-analysis of neuropsychological outcomes, using the increasingly more accepted techniques of RCI (reliable change index) and SRB (standardized regression-based) for measuring cognitive changes after surgery for epilepsy (2011). The estimated risk to verbal memory with left aTLYs was 44 %, in contrast to 20 % for right aTLYs. There was a 27 % gain in verbal fluency in the left aTLY group.

There is some controversy from studies in the literature with respect to the relationships of psychosocial outcomes to the abolition of seizures. Early studies left the epilepsy field with the view that seizure freedom was the primary responsible factor for social improvement following aTLY. In a relatively recent article, Tanriverdi et al. provide a summary of a prospective study outlining the benefit of seizure freedom, but social improvement also occurred in those patients who still had postoperative seizures, and in many of the investigative aspects, the difference between the two groups failed to reach statistical significance (2008).

References

Bailey P, Gibbs FA. The surgical treatment of psychomotor epilepsy. JAMA. 1951;145:365–70.

Comair YG. The transsylvian functional hemispherectomy: patient selection and results. In: Lüders HO, Comair YG, editors. Epilepsy surgery. 2nd ed. Philadelphia: Lippincott Williams & Wilkins; 2001. pp. 702–3.

Feindel W. Memory and speech function in the temporal lobe in man. In: Brazier MA, editor. Brain function, vol. 2, RNA and brain function; memory and learning. Berkeley-Los Angeles: University California Press; 1964. pp. 277–98.

Feindel W, Rasmussen T. Temporal lobectomy with amygdalectomy and minimal hippocampal resection: review of 100 cases. Can J Neurol Sci. 1991;18:603–5.

Feindel W, Penfield W, McNaughton F. The tentorial nerves and localization of intracranial pain in man. Neurology. 1960;10:555–63.

Girvin JP. Temporal lobectomy. Chapter 11. In: Apuzzo MLJ, editor. Neurosurgical aspects of epilepsy. Park Ridge: American Association of Neurological Surgeons; 1992. p. 157–70.

Gloor P. The temporal lobe and limbic system. Oxford: Oxford University Press; 1997. 865 pp.

Helmstaedter C, Kurthen M, Lux S, Reuber M, Elger CE. Chronic epilepsy and cognition: a longitudinal study in temporal lobe epilepsy. Ann Neurol. 2003;54:425–32.

Hori T, Tabuchi S, Kurosaki M, Kondo S, Takenobu A, Watanabe T. Subtemporal amygdalohippocampectomy for treating medically intractable temporal lobe epilepsy. Neurosurgery. 1993;33:50–7.

Invik RJ, Sharbrough FW, Laws ER. Effects of anterior temporal lobectomy on cognitive function. J Clin Psychol. 1987;43:128–37.

Lüders H, Lesser RP, Hahn J, Dinner DS, Morris H, Resor S, Harrison M. Basal temporal language area demonstrated by electrical stimulation. Neurology. 1986;36:505–10.

Niemeyer P. The transventricular amygdala-hippocampectomy in temporal lobe epilepsy. In: Baldwin M, Bailery P, editors. The temporal lobe epilepsy. Springfield: Charles C Thomas; 1958. p. 461–82.

Ojemann GA, Dodrill CB. Verbal memory deficits after left temporal lobectomy for epilepsy. Mechanism and intraoperative prediction. J Neurosurg. 1985;62:101–7.

Ojemann GA, Dodrill C. Intraoperative techniques for reducing language and memory deficits with left temporal lobectomy. Adv Epileptology. 1987;16:327–30.

Olivier A. Cortical resections (commentary). In: Engel J, editor. Surgical treatment of epilepsy. New York: Raven Press; 1987. p. 405–16.

Olivier A. Surgical techniques in temporal lobe epilepsy. Clin Neurosurg. 1997;44:211–41.

Olivier A. Transcortical selective amygdalohippocampectomy in temporal lobe epilepsy. Can J Neurol Sci. 2000;27 Suppl 1:S68–76; discussion 92–6.

Penfield W. Temporal lobe epilepsy. Br J Surg. 1954;41:337–43.

Penfield W. Pitfalls and success in surgical treatment of focal epilepsy. Br Med J. 1958;1:669–72.

Penfield W, Baldwin M. Temporal lobe seizures and the technique of subtotal temporal lobectomy. Ann Surg. 1952;136:625–34.

Penfield W, Paine K. Results of surgical therapy for focal epileptic seizures. Can Med Assoc J. 1955;73:515–31.

Penfield W, Rasmussen T. The cerebral cortex of man: a clinical study of localization of function. New York: Hafner Publishing Company; 1968. 248 pp.

Penfield W, Lende RA, Rasmussen T. Manipulation hemiplegia. An untoward complication in the surgery of focal epilepsy. J Neurosurg. 1961;28:760–76.

Pilcher WH, Rusyniak WG. Complications of epilepsy surgery. Neurosurg Clin N Am. 1993;4: 311–25.

Rasmussen T, Feindel W. Temporal lobectomy: review of 100 cases with major hippocampectomy. Can J Neurol Sci. 1991;18:601–2.

Rasmussen T, Jasper H. Temporal lobe epilepsy: indications for operations and surgical technique. In: Baldwin M, Bailey P, editors. Temporal lobe epilepsy. Springfield: Charles C. Thomas; 1958. p. 440–60.

Rougier A, Saint-Hillaire J-M, Loiseau P, Bouvier G. Evaluation and surgical treatment of the epilepsies. Neurochirurgie. 1992;38:3–12.

Sherman EMS, Wiebe S, Fay-McClymont B, Tellez-Zenteno J, Metcalfe A, Hernandez-Ronquillo L, et al. Neuropsychological outcomes after epilepsy surgery: systematic review and pooled estimates. Epilepsia. 2011;52:857–69.

Spencer DD, Spencer SS, Mattson RH, Williamson PD, Novelly RA. Access to the posterior medial temporal lobe structures in the surgical treatment of temporal lobe epilepsy. Neurosurgery. 1984;15:667–71.

Tanriverdi T, Poulin N, Olivier O. Psychosocial status before and after temporal lobe epilepsy: a prospective clinical study. Neurosurgery. 2008;62:1071–9.

Walker AE. Temporal lobectomy. J Neurosurg. 1967;26:642–9.

Weiser HG. Selective amygdalohippocampectomy: indications, investigative technique and results. In: Symon L, Brihaye J, Guidetti B, editors. Advances and technical standards in neurosurgery, vol. 13. Vienna: Springer; 1986. p. 39–133 [6.4].

Wieser HG. Selective amygdalo-hippocampectomy for temporal lobe epilepsy. Epilepsia. 1988;29 Suppl 2:100–13.

Wieser HG. Selective amygdalo-hippocampectomy: indications and follow-up. Can J Neurol Sci. 1991;18:617–27.

Wieser HJ, Yasargil MG. Die to "Selektive Amygdala-Hippokampektomie" als chirurgische Behandlungsmethode der mediobasal-limbischen Epilepsie. Neurochirurgia. 1982a;25:39–50.

Wieser HG, Yasargil MG. Selective amygdalohippocampectomy as a surgical treatment of mesiobasal limbic epilepsy. Surg Neurol. 1982b;17:445–57.

Wyler AR, Hermann BP, Somes G. Extent of medial temporal resection on outcome from anterior temporal lobectomy: a randomized prospective study. Neurosurgery. 1995;37:982–91.

Yasargil MG, Teddy PJ, Roth P. Selective amygdalohippocampectomy: operative anatomy and surgical technique. In: Symon L, Brihaye J, Guidetti B, editors. Advances and technical standards in neurosurgery, vol. 12. Vienna: Springer; 1985. p. 93–123.

Yasargil MG, Weiser HG, Valavanis A, von Ammon K, Roth P. Surgery and results of selective amygdala-hippocampectomy in one hundred patients with nonlesional limbic epilepsy. Neurosurg Clin N Am. 1993;4:243–61.

7 Frontal Lobe Surgery

7.1 Introduction

Unlike other cerebral lobes that involve resective surgery for focal epilepsy, the array of frontal resections is much greater. This derives primarily from the fact of its size. The frontal lobe comprises nearly half of a given cerebral hemisphere. Thus, the myriad of different potential resections is striking and serves as surgical management not only of the intractable frontal lobe epilepsies but also resections for the treatment of non-epileptic disorders, more particularly frontal lobe arteriovenous malformations (AVMs) and tumors.

Perhaps the most common frontal lobe operation is simply that of the traditional corticectomy. Corticectomies may involve any of the three surfaces of the frontal lobe – inferior, medial or dorsolateral. In addition to corticectomies lesions, including epileptic foci, may occur in a wide variation of the anterior part of the frontal lobe, which leads to the removal of the frontal pole. These lesions and/or epileptic foci may involve a small part of the polar cortex, per se, or as much as the majority of the whole lobe. Because of this I have arbitrarily named three increasingly sized resections from the frontal pole anteriorly to the posterior cortex anterior to the Rolandic cortex. (Dr. Rasmussen was always of the opinion that the Rolandic cortex was sufficiently functionally different from the frontal and parietal lobes that it should be considered a separate lobe. I have fully accepted that 1)

The arbitrary resections are: (1) fronto-polar lobectomy (F-PL), which includes removal of portions of the initial 5 cms posterior to the tip of the frontal pole; (2) radical anterior frontal lobectomy (radical aFLY), which involves removal of the entire frontal lobe cortex except the eloquent areas of speech and motor representations; and (3) anterior frontal lobectomies (aFLYs), which involve resections of cortex somewhere between the fronto-polar lobectomy and the radical aFLY. These three now-called arbitrary frontal lobe resections are illustrated in Fig. 7.1. The entire Rolandic cortex, both motor and sensory, will be considered as an individual entity in the next chapter.

The craniotomy exposure for any of the aFLYs requires that there is easy access to at least two, and preferably all three, surfaces of the lobe. The dorsolateral

J.P. Girvin, *Operative Techniques in Epilepsy*,
DOI 10.1007/978-3-319-10921-3_7

surface will always be exposed, but if a sufficiently placed bone flap does not achieve an easy pathway of access to at least one of the other two surfaces, preferably the medial surface, then the operative exposure and resection may be very troublesome. If access to the medial and inferior surfaces is covered with significant amounts of bone, then the flexibility of approaching these surfaces is severely compromised. The most obvious disadvantage is that the initiation of the resection

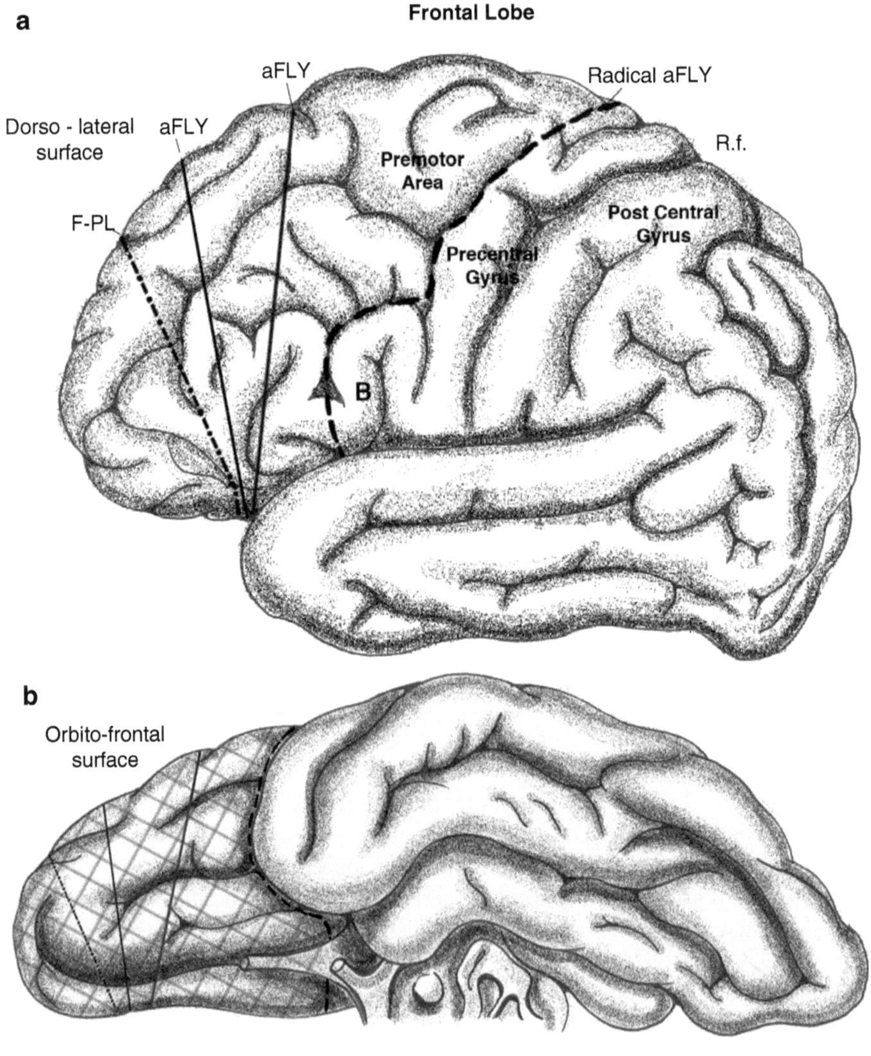

Fig. 7.1 The various surgical resections of the frontal lobe for epilepsy. An illustration of the pure *arbitrary* designations given to the various resections of the frontal lobe. These consist of: – frontopolar lobectomy (F-PL: — • — • —); – anterior frontal lobectomy (aFLY: ———); – radical aFLY (– – –). Figures (**a**–**c**) are the arbitrarily designated resections of the dorsolateral, orbital, and medial surfaces of the frontal lobe. *B* Broca's area, *R.f.* Rolandic (central) fissure, *SMA* supplementary motor area. The *cross-hatched area* depicts the orbitofrontal cortical removal in the radical frontal lobectomy

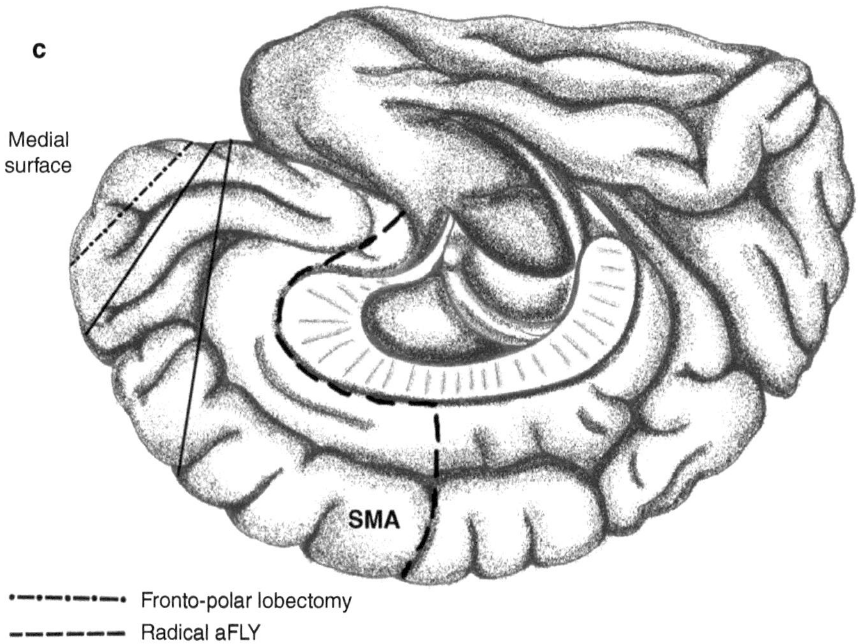

Fig. 7.1 (continued)

usually cannot be undertaken over these surfaces, in large part because the full bulk of the frontal cerebral parenchyma is still intact at this point. Put in another context, if a reasonable amount of the resection has been carried out, it is always associated with somewhat easier access to the other surfaces in spite of the bony overlay. Finally, put into an even further context, the greater the excess of bone overlying the deeper surfaces, the greater must be the extent of the surgical exposure of the dorsolateral resection line, before entering into a contiguous resection of other partially inaccessible surfaces. This is particularly disadvantageous if the medial, or parasagittal, cranial exposure is significantly lateral to the midline. If this eventuality presents itself, it disallows the surgeon from easily inspecting the superior sagittal sinus (SSS) visually, which is terribly disadvantageous if there is a complex arrangement of parasagittal veins. Thus, as a mandatory rule of thumb, the craniotomy should be planned such that access to at least two, and preferably all three, surfaces is straightforward.

The naïve student, introduced to the surgery of frontal lobe epilepsy (FLE), will have been made aware of the general consensus of the relatively poorer outcomes of surgery of FLE than TLE. The paper by Rasmussen, entitled "Characteristics of a Pure Culture of Frontal Lobe Epilepsy," is probably the earliest and perhaps the best paper outlining the clinical characteristics, the pre-incision and post-incision ECoGs, the postoperative EEGs, and the outcomes of patients who were seizure-free immediately postoperatively or within a few years (1983). This article is a treasure for a surgeon who has a concern with respect to how much cortex might or should be removed in a patient with given intractable focal epilepsy of the frontal lobe upon which she/he has been asked to manage surgically. One has to understand the vicissitudes of frontal focal epilepsy, which includes its potential assessment of the focus, the awareness of its spread, and its outcome of potential resection before feeling satisfied with making a decision about management. Wennberg et al., also from the Montreal Neurological Institute, also noted the vagaries of frontal lobe epilepsy, in an article that describes in particular the use of and the importance of the pre-incision and post-excision ECoGs in the surgery of FLE (1998). Perhaps the greatest information in this article is the statistically significant prognoses pertaining to the outcomes of the surgeries that are provided by the pre- and postoperative ECoGs.

7.2 Frontal Corticectomy

7.2.1 Introduction

The corticectomies need very little individual description, outside of the general principles outlined in Chap. 5. That is to say, they include the general technique of subpial dissection/resection, the adherence to sulcal boundaries where possible, the preservation of any blood supply that is *en passage* over the corticectomy designated for resection, the preservation of as much subcortical white matter as possible, and the minimization of the scar left behind.

7.2.2 Dorsolateral

The commonest frontal corticectomies are those of the dorsolateral and orbital surfaces. The former are usually large. If it is remote from the precentral sulcus and Broca's area, then it is not a complex resection and requires only the reiterated summary of the surgical principles, pertaining to corticectomies in general, as outlined previously (Chap. 5).

In those corticectomies encroaching upon the precentral sulcus and/or the sulcus immediately in front of Broca's area, there is emphasis on making certain that there is no associated injury to the gyral surfaces across these sulci that are being left behind and the preservation of their function is mandatory in order to preclude a postoperative neurological deficit. In my view *all* such resections in which the eloquent cortex is involved should be undertaken in the awake state and with continual clinical monitoring of the function of the eloquent cortex that must not be compromised.

As was outlined under the periphery outline of a corticectomy (Sect. 5.5.3) and in the chapter devoted to a description of Rolandic cortical resection (see Chap. 8), the dissection at the bottom of the sulci around the speech and motor areas should be kept as shallow as possible. Thus, when the depth of the sulcus has been reached, then the immediate subcortical white matter should be left as completely intact as possible. This is outlined in Sect. 5.5.3 and is illustrated again here in Fig. 7.2. Figure 7.2a is very similar to previously illustrated examples (see Figs. 2.8 and 5.3a), in which the depths of sulci are junctions between epileptic and eloquent cortices and in which the former is to be removed, while the latter is to be preserved with respect to its integrity and connectivity. In this particular case the sulcus is the precentral sulcus. Figure 7.2b illustrates the very restricted removal of the cortex on the side of the sulcus while leaving the eloquent cortex intact on the other side of the sulcus. Finally, Fig. 7.2c illustrates that once the inferior extent of the gray matter of the cortex in the depth of the sulcus has been reached, then the ensuing incision in the subcortical white matter should not be taken more deeply, but rather should be brought out superficially. This will guarantee optimizing the preservation of the normal neuronal connectivity of those afferent and efferent fibers of the eloquent cortex. In this case the incision will be directed anteriorly, e.g., "away from" the precentral gyrus, as also previously illustrated in Fig. 5.3a2. Further, and most importantly, it should be done immediately after reaching the bottom of the sulcus. Any resection of the abnormal cortex juxtaposed to the eloquent cortex usually will be associated with at least some transient clinical deficit, which reflects the function of the eloquent cortex, as discussed in Sect. 5.5.3. If there is a significant delay

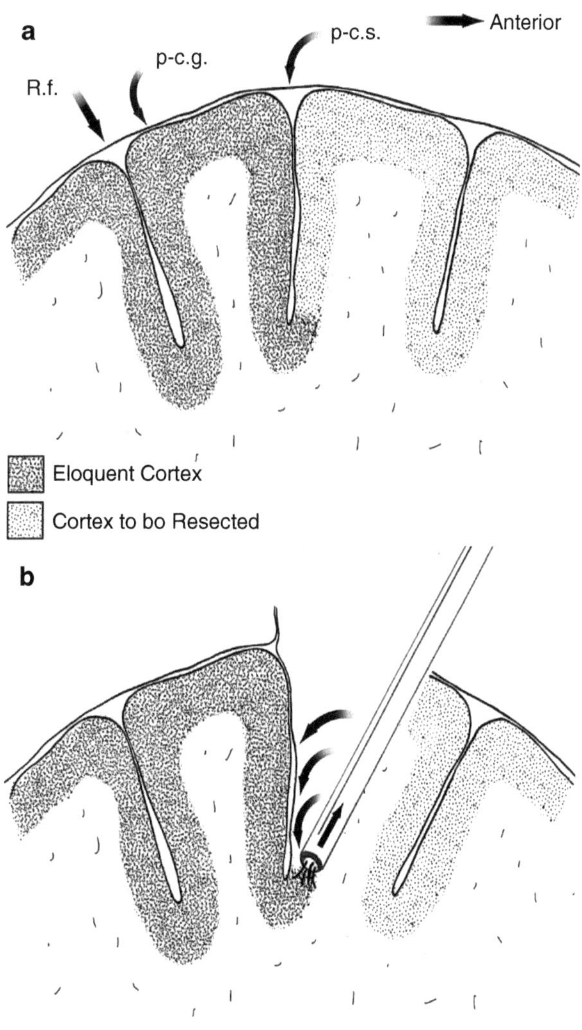

Fig. 7.2 Surgical resection next to juxtaposed "eloquent" cortex. An illustration of a precentral sulcus in which the epileptogenic focus includes the cortex of the anterior part of the sulcus and the gyrus anterior to the sulcus. (**a**) Illustration of the sulcus separating precentral cortex (to be left intact) from the anteriorly juxtaposed cortex, which is to be resected. (**b**) The removal of the cortex on one side of the sulcus, only to the depth of the gray matter at the bottom of the sulcus. (**c**) Depiction of the importance of continuing the dissection in the subcortical white matter in a superficial direction (*solid arrow*) in order to not impinge on potential connectivity of the eloquent cortex beneath the resection. *p-c.g* precentral gyrus, *p-c.s* precentral sulcus, *R.f* Rolandic fissure

Fig. 7.2 (continued)

c

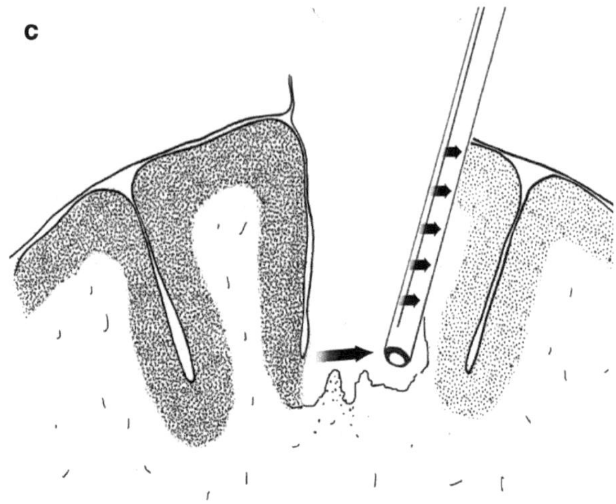

between the removal of the abnormal cortex that initiates a clinical deficit and the termination of the resection of that area of the cortex, there is always a risk that the surgeon may lose the clinical marker by which to judge whether additional surgery in the area is encroaching on parenchyma, the destruction of which may produce a permanent postoperative neurological deficit. Taken to the extreme, if the delay allows a completed deficit of the function of the eloquent cortex, then the safety of any further resection is completely unknown (again this was strongly emphasized in Sect. 5.5.3). Thus, in this circumstance the length of the time to complete this part of the surgery should be minimized as much as possible.

7.2.3 The Potential Adherence of Leptomeninges in Medial Corticectomies

"Pure" medial corticectomies are the least common of the frontal lobe corticectomies. However, all of the resections of the frontal lobe that involve the medial surface, e.g., within the interhemispheric fissure (IHF), may encounter adherence between the leptomeningeal investment of the two hemispheres over those areas in which there is not an intervening dural membrane, e.g., the falx cerebri or crista galli. The latter, if present, precludes any such adherence. If this bihemispheric leptomeningeal adherence is either very patchy or very weak, then it may be relatively easily separated and it is usually an advantage to separate it. However, if the adherence is very strong, e.g., to one another, in which the eventuality of its separation is difficult and thought to possibly be associated with parenchymal damage in the contralateral hemisphere, then it is better to cease trying to separate it and use an alternative strategy.

Under these circumstances the retraction of the leptomeningeal investment along with the underlying parenchyma, in the presence of bilateral adherence of the leptomeninges, is best discontinued in favor of simply utilizing pure subpial dissection over the area of adherence. The adherent leptomeningeal investment is then simply left attached to its contralateral counterpart and is incised around its periphery (of the adherence). In this way the adherence is circumvented and the ipsilateral meningeal investment is simply left intact with its contralateral counterpart. This is illustrated in Fig. 7.3. Figure 7.3a is a diagrammatic representation of the interhemispheric fissure (IHF) between the frontal lobes anterior to the corpus callosum in which there is an area of adherence of the bilateral medial leptomeninges, i.e., bihemispheric leptomeningeal adherence ("bh.l.ad"), above and below which there is lack of adherence. Figure 7.3b discloses the initiation of the right frontal corticectomy

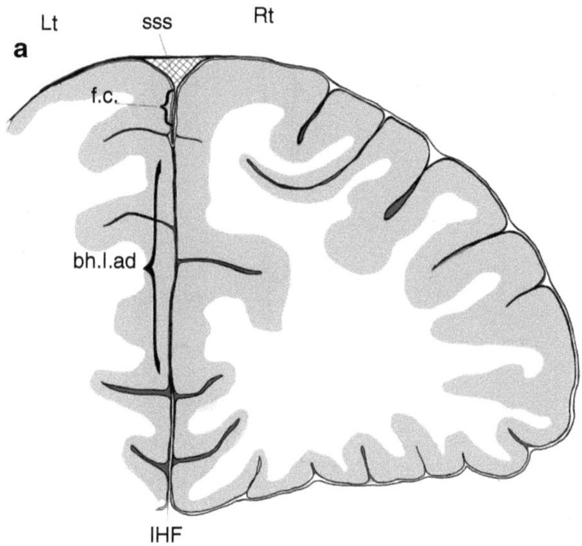

Fig. 7.3 Preserving contralateral medial frontal cortex when adherence between medial leptomeningeal barriers cannot be separated. Illustration of the steps in avoiding injury to the contralateral medial frontal lobe cortex (in this case the left frontal lobe), when resecting the other (*right*) side, in the presence of adherence between the leptomeningeal investments of the medial surfaces of the two frontal lobes. (**a**) Coronal section through the frontal lobe, exhibiting bihemispheric leptomeningeal adherence within the interhemispheric fissure. (**b**) Illustrating the initial isolation of the right frontal medial surface, approaching the area of bilateral leptomeningeal adherence. (**c**) Upon encountering the adherence, the surgical strategy is changed from simple retraction of the leptomeninges of the right side from that on the left and replaced by subpial resection of the parenchyma underlying the adherence, which is achieved by incising the leptomeninges surrounding the area of adherence and leaving the bilateral adherent leptomeninges in place. (**d**) Illustration of the remainder of the removal of the corticectomy inferiorly below the adherence where, as at the beginning superiorly, the two hemispheric leptomeninges can be satisfactorily separated by simple traction (see text). *bh.l.ad.* bihemispheric leptomeningeal adherence, *f.c.* falx cerebri, *IHF* interhemispheric fissure, *l.i.1* leptomeningeal incision, approaching from superiorly, upon transferring from the isolation of the frontal lobe cortex by retraction to that of subpial dissection, at the point of encountering significant bilateral leptomeningeal adherence, *l.i.2* the leptomeningeal incision, when the adherence with the contralateral hemispheric leptomeninges no longer exists, allowing reemergence from the use of subpial dissection to the use of retraction for the separation of the frontal cortices, *SSS* superior sagittal sinus. The *parenthetic symbol* represents the expanse of the adherence

Fig. 7.3 (continued)

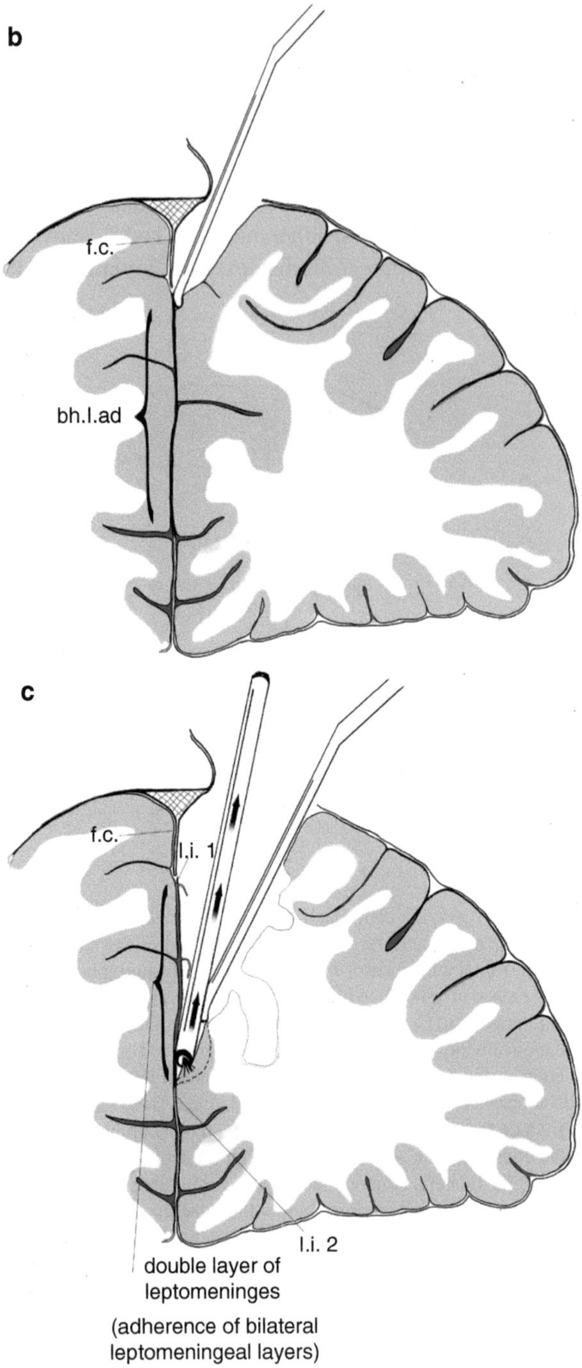

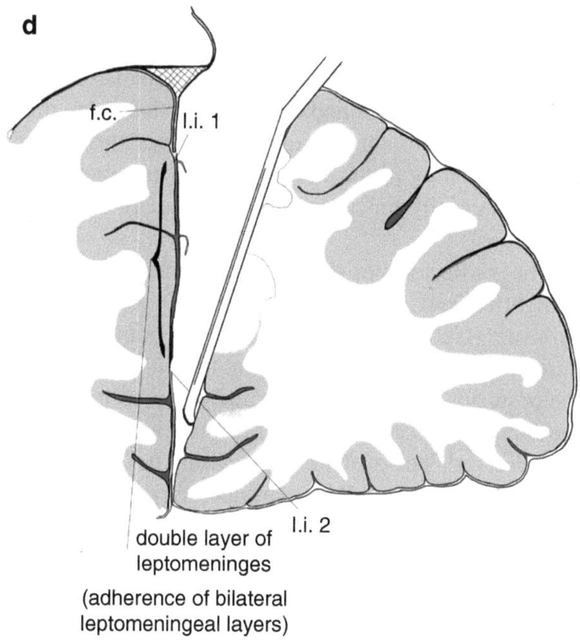

Fig. 7.3 (continued)

with the retraction of the right frontal superomedial cortex inferiorly until the upper part of the area of bilateral leptomeningeal adherence is reached. Prior to reaching this adherence, the isolation of the medial cortex, preparatory to its removal, has been achieved by simply retracting the superior frontal gyrus. However, upon encountering the very adherent middle part the simple retraction is supplanted by an incision in the leptomeninges superior to the adherence ("l.i.1") and then progressing with subpial resection (Fig. 7.3c). The latter is then continued until the inferior aspect of the leptomeningeal adherence is reached after which a further leptomeningeal incision ("l.i.2") is made and carried around the remainder of the periphery of the adherence. Following this, as illustrated in Fig. 7.3d, the adherence has been taken care of and is now followed by the same technique that was used initially at the superior frontal gyrus, i.e., the simple separation of the remaining inferior medial cortex of the corticectomy. The ipsilateral adhering membrane is thus simply left intact with its contralateral counterpart.

7.2.4 Anteromedial Corticectomy

The least common of these medial frontal corticectomies are those that are anterior to the genu of the corpus callosum. Many of these involve also one of the juxtaposed surfaces, i.e., inferior (orbital) or the parasagittal part of the dorsolateral surface. The latter usually involves the parasagittal surface of part of or the entire superior frontal gyrus. Since this parasagittal cortex represents the watershed between the anterior (ACA) and middle cerebral (MCA) arteries, there is less concern about compromising the blood supply of the dorsolateral cortex being left behind. This is true for the anterior boundary of this corticectomy that is nearly always taken to the pole, and it is similarly true of the inferior surface, which, again, is nearly always taken to the floor of the anterior fossa. Thus, these three peripheries of the corticectomy are usually functional watershed areas, forming the equivalent of end arterial irrigations.

The posterior periphery of the anteromedial corticectomy is also usually straightforward. However, if the posterior boundary is at the genu of the corpus callosum (CC) and the callosomarginal branch of the pericallosal artery leaves the parent artery anterior to the genu, then it becomes an *en passage* artery overlying the posterior surface of the corticectomy, as it is usually a major branch irrigating the functional cortex (e.g., paracentral lobule) more posteriorly, and thus it must be preserved. The problem confronting the surgeon at this point is whether indeed it is the important callosomarginal artery or whether it is the frontopolar artery. Usually the distinction between the callosomarginal and frontopolar arteries can be achieved by simply following the course of the artery in question until its primary direction, e.g., anterior or posterior, is clarified. The frontopolar artery proceeds anteriorly and irrigates the medial and parasagittal cortex that is being removed and thus can be sacrificed, while the former proceeds posteriorly, as noted in the foregoing, and requires preservation. Under these circumstances the easiest manner of achieving its preservation is simply by "skeletonizing" it (see Sect. 5.2). Thus, incisions through the covering leptomeningeal investment of the curvilinear portion of the artery allow the removal of underlying parenchyma of the corticectomy and coagulation and incision of any associated branches that are irrigating it.

It should be recorded that it is not uncommon to find the bilateral leptomeningeal adherence between the two frontal lobes, requiring the procedure noted in the last section (Sect. 7.2.3 and Fig. 7.3).

7.2.5 Posteromedial Corticectomy

The posteromedial corticectomy is that which is behind the genu of the corpus callosum. It is more complex by virtue of the fact that it usually involves some part of the supplementary motor cortex (SMA), may involve a posterior resection line (PRL) in the depth of the precentral sulcus, and will nearly always involve the necessity of preserving at least one major branch of the pericallosal artery, i.e., the callosomarginal artery. Often the latter artery or additional arteries will course throughout the anteroposterior extent of the corticectomy and irrigate parenchyma behind the PRL; that is to say, they are *en passage* vessels. These then must be skeletonized and preserved (see Sects. 5.2, 7.2.3, 7.2.4, 7.3, 7.4, and 8.4).

Once again, if the periphery is composed of the precentral sulcus, then the resection in an awake patient is much more satisfactory than one under general anesthesia. There is no doubt that a potential postoperative weakness of the contralateral leg is less alarming than one in the arm, which would be the risk of a similar corticectomy involving the dorsolateral cortex. Nevertheless, I would consider that the ability to clinically monitor the patient for any threat to the motor function of the leg during such surgery makes it mandatory to carry out such operations under local anesthesia. Further, once the resection down to the depth of the precentral sulcus is reached, then the immediately ensuing subcortical incision should be carried superficially in the subcortical white matter, for at least a centimeter or more (see previous Sects. 7.2.2 and 5.5.3).

The surgical preservation of the pericallosal branches in a large posteromedial corticectomy is similar to other resections that require the preservations of significantly sized arteries, e.g., the radical aFLY (*vide infra*), the radical TLY, the inferior Rolandic corticectomy, etc. In both this corticectomy and the radical aFLY, the approach to the posteromedial cortex area will be from above, e.g., superior to the major vascular branching of the pericallosal artery. If the corticectomy involves the dorsolateral aspect of the superior frontal gyrus (SFG), then the lateral resection line will be initiated over that surface, as well as the posterior resection line (PRL) in the SFG, prior to engaging the medial surface. The posterior incision line, including the parenchyma with its overlying investment, will then be continued over the junction of the dorsolateral and medial surfaces down the medial side of the SFG. Assuming that the inferior margin of the corticectomy includes the entire cingulate gyrus, then, as this incision is advanced inferiorly, there must be an ongoing continual visual examination of the incision line for arterial vessels. Those on the surface will be seen easily, but it is the surgeon's responsibility to examine very carefully each (medial) sulcus during the advancing subpial dissection, *before* it is coagulated and incised, in order to be certain that it does not contain a vessel that must be retained. In the absence of a significant vessel in the depth, then the sulcal leptomeninges can be coagulated along with some more inferior medial surface leptomeninges and incised. This forms the first of such steps in the gradual establishment of a medial surface PRL, e.g., coagulation and incision of gyral surface leptomeninges followed by subpial dissection of the next sulcus and in the absence of a significant vessel its coagulation and incision, and so on! This is illustrated diagrammatically in Fig. 7.4. Figure 7.4a shows the callosomarginal artery located in the depth of a medial sulcus in both the coronal section (a1) and in the medial midline sagittal section (a2). Once a vessel is encountered, the onus on the surgeon is to determine its importance, vis-à-vis whether it needs to be saved. In nearly all instances in this very posterior location, any reasonably sized vessel should be saved, as almost certainly its size would primarily be a reflection of a significant field of irrigation posterior to the posterior resection line.

Once a significant vessel is encountered, the incision, which up to this point has included both parenchyma and leptomeningeal investment, will now be one which involves only cortical parenchyma, as the surgical strategy will now involve only subpial resection, per se. It may be conducted by blunt dissection or suction and is similar to the leaving behind of the area of bilateral leptomeningeal adherence outlined in the preceding section (Sect. 7.2.3) and illustrated in Fig. 7.3. That is to say, the remaining part of the incision, down to the corpus callosum, must be conducted subpially, involving therefore only removal of parenchyma and leaving the leptomeningeal investment intact. Figure 7.4b illustrates the gradual deepening of the PRL involving leptomeningeal incision and resection, during which the callosomarginal artery is identified within the cingulate sulcus. In this figure the

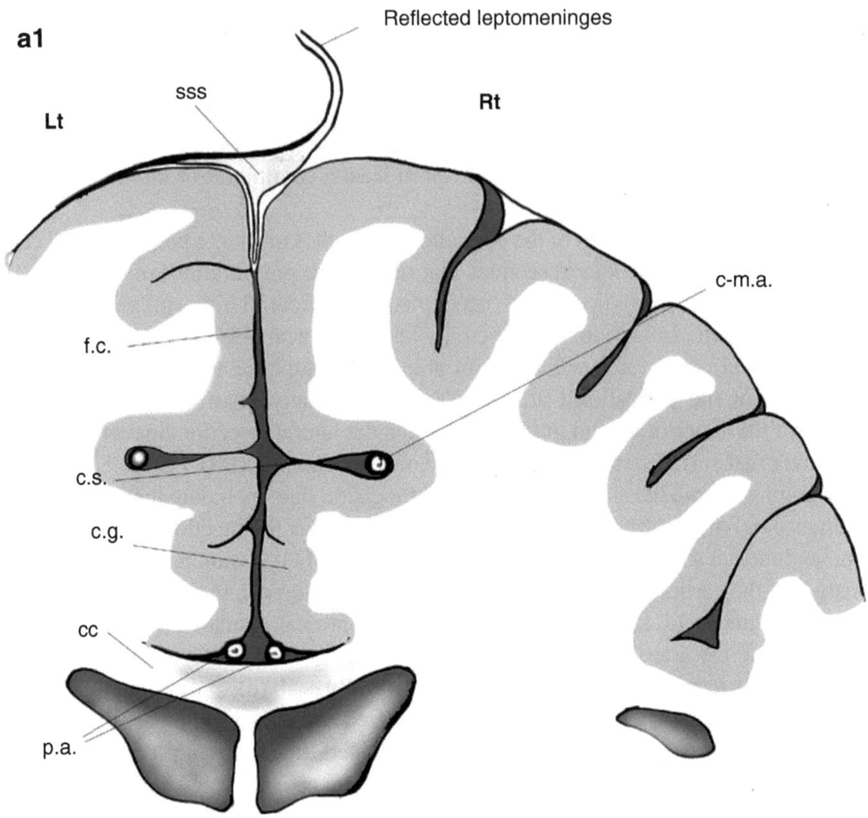

Fig. 7.4 Preserving the callosomarginal artery in a posteromedial frontal resection. Coronal and medial surface illustrations of the subpial dissection/resection of a portion of a posteromedial corticectomy of the right frontal cortex, preserving the callosomarginal artery. (**a1**) A coronal section through the location of the posterior resection line (*PRL*) of the corticectomy, illustrating the location of the callosomarginal artery in the cingulate sulcus; (**a2**) an illustration of the medial surface depicting the posterior-medial part of the resection line and the cingulate sulcus in which the callosomarginal artery resides (the dashed part of the artery represents that which is in the depth of the cingulate sulcus). (**b1**) A coronal section depicting the initiation of the removal of the superior frontal gyrus (SFG) and its associated medial cortex inferiorly to the cingulate sulcus where the callosomarginal artery is isolated and preserved (see text).; (**b2**) the medial surface after the initial part of the posterior resection. (**c**) Illustrations of coronal (**c1**) and midline medial (**c2**) sections just posterior to the anterior boundary of the genu of the corpus callosum (see text). *CC* corpus callosum, *c.g.* cingulate gyrus, *c-m.a.* callosomarginal artery, *c-m.a.** callosomarginal a., on the other (contralateral) side of the preserved leptomeninges, *c.s.* cingulate sulcus, *f.c.* falx cerebri, *f.p.a.* frontopolar artery, *g.* genu of the CC, *g.a.* anterior boundary of the genu of the CC, *l.i.* leptomeningeal incision, *p.a.* pericallosal artery, *p-a.l.i.* the posterior-anterior leptomeningeal incision, parallel to and just superior to the callosomarginal artery, *p.p-c.art.* posterior pericallosal artery, R^n superior-lateral retraction of the superior part of the partially separated frontal cortex, *PRL* proposed posterior resection line, *SSS* superior sagittal sinus

a2

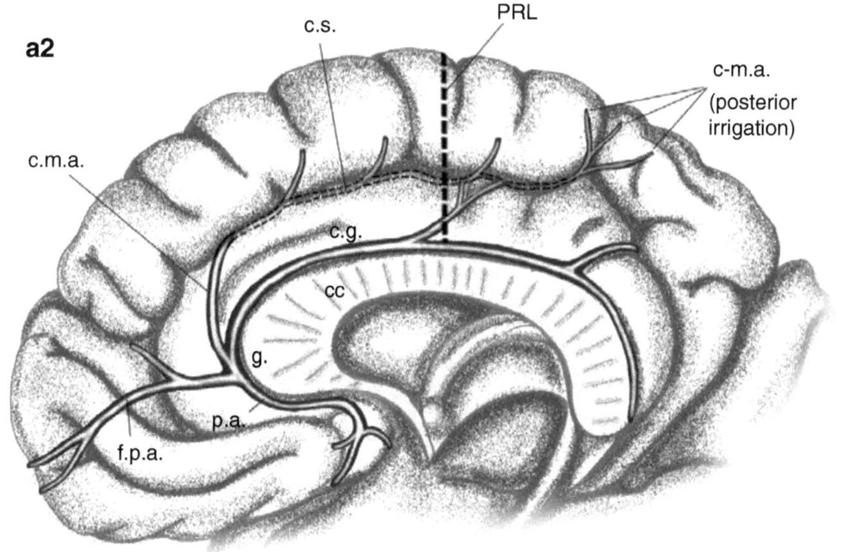

b1

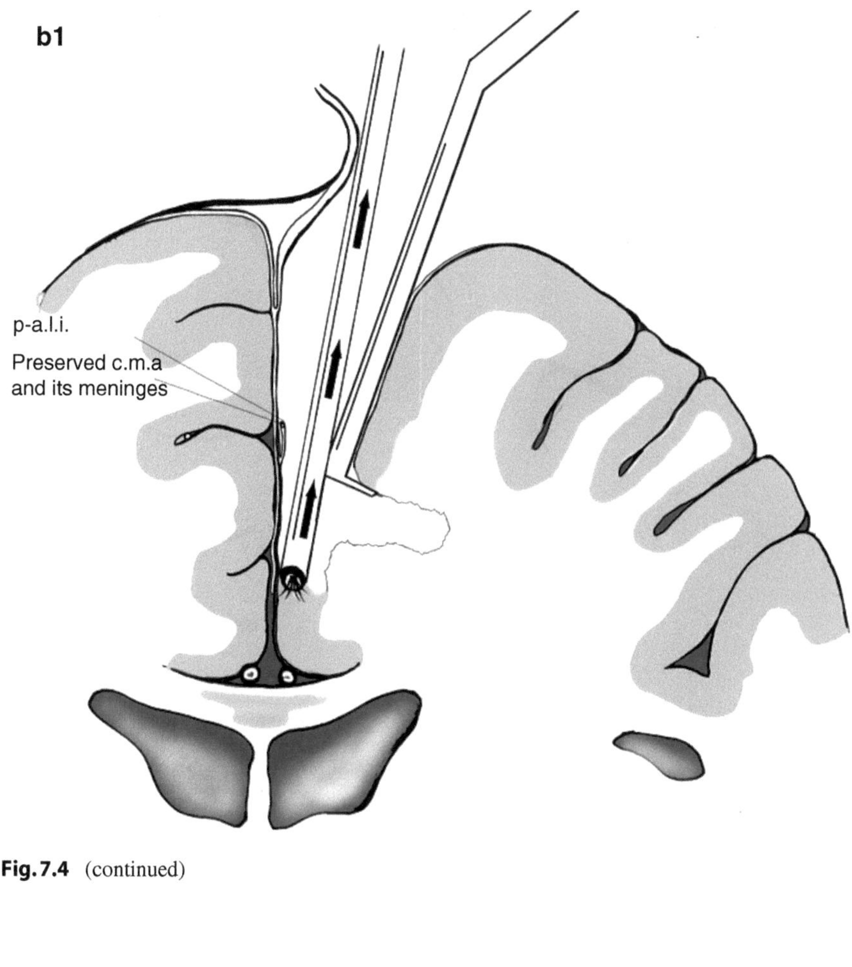

Fig. 7.4 (continued)

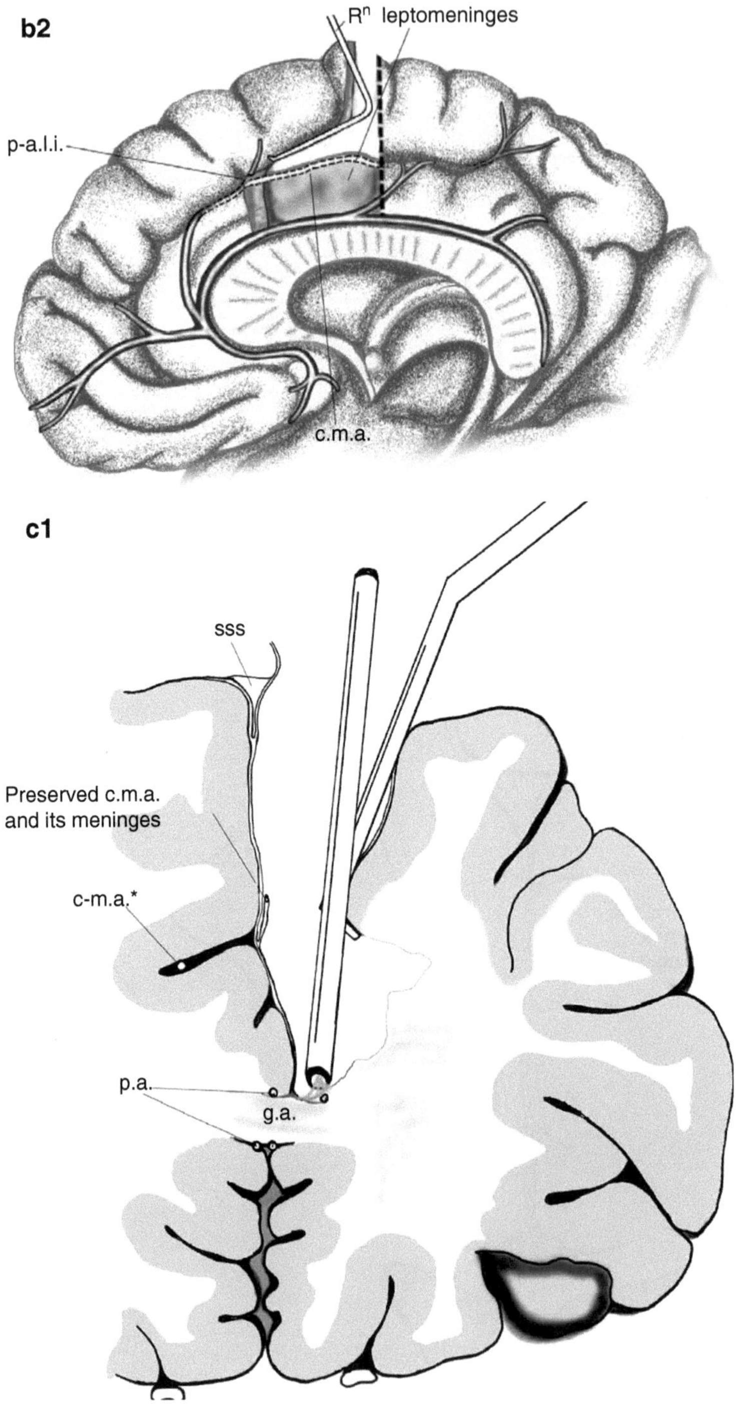

Fig. 7.4 (continued)

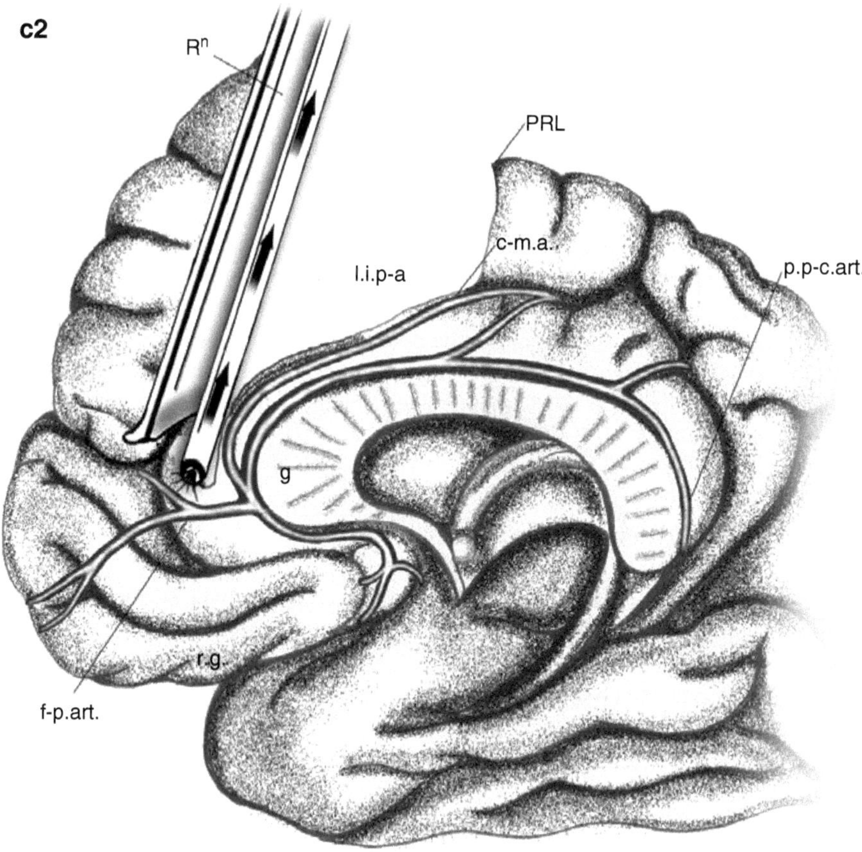

Fig. 7.4 (continued)

callosomarginal artery which was initially in the depth of the sulcus (Fig. 7.4a) has now been freed from any associated parenchyma as a result of subpial resection and, along with the leptomeninges overlying the sulcus and the pial meninges of the sulcus, which in fact remains covering it, is retracted medially (Fig. 7.4b1), and the ongoing subpial resection is carried inferiorly onto the cingulate gyrus. Figure 7.4b2 illustrates the advancement of the dissection/resection anteriorly through the initiation of a posteroanterior leptomeningeal incision ("p-a.l.i.") along the leptomeninges superior to the callosomarginal artery, i.e., by either separation by blunt dissection or piece meal subpial resection of the cortex down to the corpus callosum; at this juncture the ipsilateral pericallosal artery will be evident through the leptomeningeal barrier when the bottom of the cingulate gyrus is reached. Once the commitment to subpial resection has been made, the surgeon is not dependent upon identifying any further large arteries more inferiorly, in order to preserve them, as all these arteries will be preserved by virtue of their being outside the meninges, which are being used as a protective barrier in the subpial dissection. The subpial dissection will be completed inferiorly with the removal of gray matter down to and including that in the sulcus of the corpus callosum (Fig. 7.4c1). Figure 7.4b2, c2 also depicts the important aid of the superior fronto-lateral retraction of the freed portion of the corticectomy.

The subpial dissection/resection will be continued anteriorly until the proposed anterior margin of the corticectomy is reached. If the anterior margin is posterior to the genu of the corpus callosum, then, the same strategies shown in the subfigures of Fig. 7.4, can be used for conducting the anterior boundary (resection line). If the margin is anterior to the emergence of the callosomarginal artery from the pericallosal artery, then the leptomeningeal incision having followed just superior and parallel to the callosomarginal to the point will now similarly follow the pericallosal artery. In the case when this is the beginning of the isolation of the medial frontal cortex in a radical aFLY, then the remainder of the resection anteriorly is covered in Sect. 7.4.

7.2.6 Orbitofrontal Corticectomy

Orbitofrontal resections, i.e., corticectomies, may occasionally be performed for the removal of tumors. While they may also infrequently be a lone corticectomy in treating an epilepsy focus, yet, they most commonly accompany aTLYs in the management of intractable epilepsy. In these patients there is usually a structural lesion and usually the important part of the resection is the posterior cortex, i.e., the allocortex, which is so closely allied both morphologically and physiologically to the cortex of the anteroinferomesial temporal lobe. If there is to be an associated aTLY, then the latter should be carried out initially, as the orbitofrontal corticectomy is significantly more easily conducted after an aTLY, by virtue of the removal of the requirement for any mobilization of the anterior Sylvian fissure and/or retraction of the anterior temporal lobe. If the corticectomy is being carried out for the removal of a tumor, then its magnitude will be less than the usual corticectomy for the treatment of an intractable epilepsy focus, which usually involves the removal of the whole of the orbital cortical surface. The latter is what will be described in the following.

Figure 7.5 illustrates a coronal section through the posterior aspect of the orbitofrontal cortex, illustrating the much greater ease of performing an orbitofrontal corticectomy with the anterior temporal lobe having been removed (Fig. 7.5b), in contrast to that when the anterior temporal lobe is intact (Fig. 7.5a). The surgery is conducted through the anterior part of the Sylvian fissure and over the sphenoid wing of the temporal bone, which is the posterior floor of the anterior cranial fossa. If the anterior temporal lobe is intact, then retraction is required in order to achieve the easiest visualization of the posterior orbital cortex.

The easiest way of initiating the resection is to begin with the lateral incision in the leptomeningeal covering of the inferior frontal gyrus (IFG) over the area of the sphenoid wing and then extending this anteriorly and posteriorly as required. This lateral resection line is shown in Fig. 7.6a1 by the bold broken line. If the

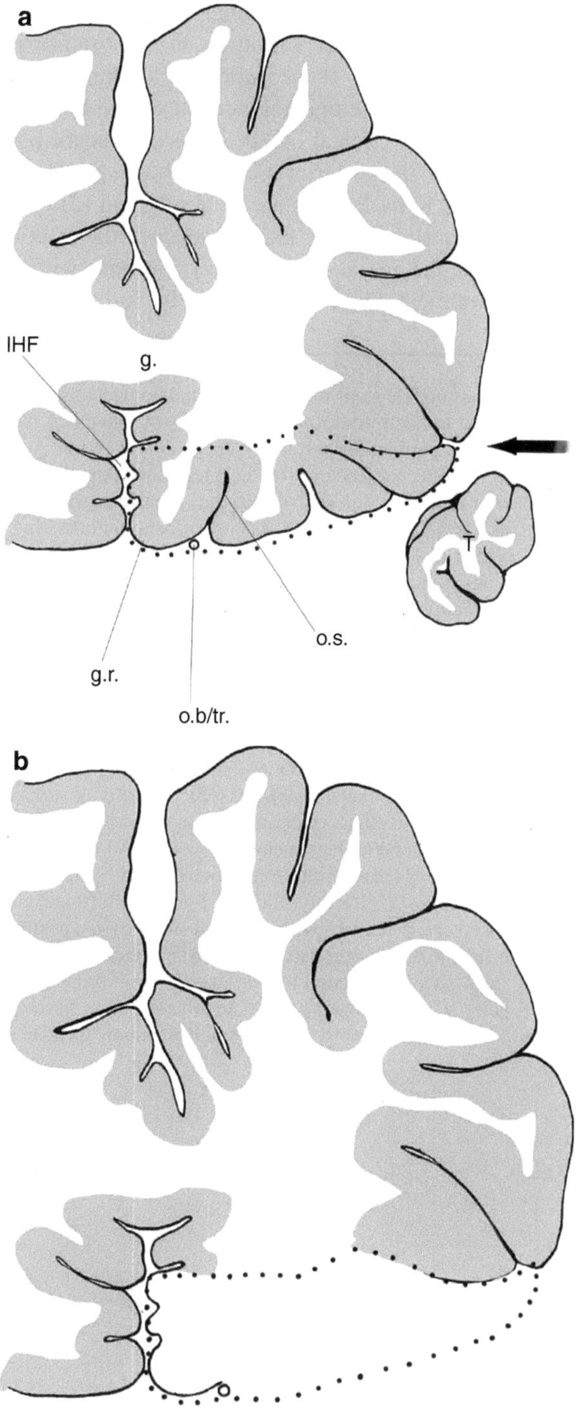

Fig. 7.5 Cross section of the posterior orbitofrontal cortex. A cross section of the posterior orbitofrontal cortex at a coronal level of the anterior temporal lobe: (**a**) intact orbitofrontal cortex and (**b**) a *dotted line* illustrating the removed orbitofrontal corticectomy. The *bold arrow* represents the location at which the surgery is initiated. *g.* genu of the corpus callosum, *g.r.* gyrus rectus, *IHF* interhemispheric fissure, *o.b/tr.* olfactory bulb and tract, *o.s.* olfactory sulcus, *T* anterior pole of the temporal lobe

corticectomy is to include the anterior frontal operculum in the dominant hemisphere, then there will be variations in its posterior incision depending upon the anesthetic being used. If the patient is awake, then Broca's area will have been localized and the posterolateral incision will be located in the most reasonable location to avoid any clinical compromise of speech. If the patient is under general anesthesia, then the posterior incisions should be (1) at least a gyrus anterior to what is determined to be Broca's area laterally and (2) one sulcus medial to the lateral surface inferiorly, e.g., the lateral aspect of the inferior surface. Figure 7.6b1 is a depiction of the initial lateroinferior incision, with the separation of the lateral periphery of the corticectomy (labeled by "orb-fr.c").

Fig. 7.6 The surgical steps in an orbitofrontal corticectomy. An illustration of some of the surgical steps used in a left orbitofrontal corticectomy. Note that the temporal lobe pole has been cut away, which is outlined by the finely *dotted line* (······) in A. (**a**) The proposed resection (*bold broken*) *lines* of the corticectomy on the lateral surface (**a1**) of the inferior frontal gyrus (*IFG*) and the posterior part of the inferior surface (**a2**) in the posterior orbital cortex. (**b**) The completion of the lateral resection line (**b1**); (**b2**) a coronal section, illustrating the medially directed subcortical resection line; (**b3**) the identification of the olfactory tract and the redirecting of the proposed leptomeningeal incision perpendicular to the PRL, just lateral and parallel to the olfactory tract (*bold dotted line*), thus establishing the medial boundary of the leptomeningeal resection. The two *fine arrows* at the anterior of the proposed medial resection line depict the two options of extending the membrane incision anteriorly to meet the anterior extent of the curvilinear lateral resection line (see text). (**c**) The completion of the leptomeningeal incisions and removal of the corticectomy specimen; the views illustrating this—the remaining medial leptomeninges and olfactory apparatus are illustrated in **c1**. (lateral view, showing the medial leptomeninges and olfactory apparatus in the depth), (**c2**). (the coronal view, showing again the olfactory apparatus and its associated inferior and medial leptomeninges), and (**c3**). (the inferior surface, similarly illustrating the base of the corticectomy, the olfactory parenchyma and the leptomeninges). *g.r.* gyrus rectus, *med.l.men.* medial (interhemispheric) leptomeninges, *l.r.l.* lateral resection line, *m.br.* midbrain, *m.r.l.* medial resection line, *orb-f.l.men.* orbitofrontal leptomeninges, *o.c.* optic chiasma, *ol.b.* olfactory bulb, *ol. tr.* olfactory tract, *ol.s.* olfactory sulcus, *orb-fr.c.* orbitofrontal cortex of the lateral periphery of the corticectomy, *orb.g.* orbital gyri, pre.g. precentral gyrus, *post.g.* postcentral gyrus, *PRL* posterior resection line, *R.f.* Rolandic fissure, *sb.r.l.* subcortical resection line, sb.c.w.m. subcortical white matter, *sp.r.l.* subpial resection line, *u.* uncus, ---- proposed resection line. *B* Broca's area, *FP* frontal pole, *IFG* inf. frontal g., *IHF* interhemispheric fissure, *ITG* inf. temp. g., *MFG* middle frontal g., *MTG* middle temp. g., *PG* parahippocampal g., STG sup. temp. gyrus

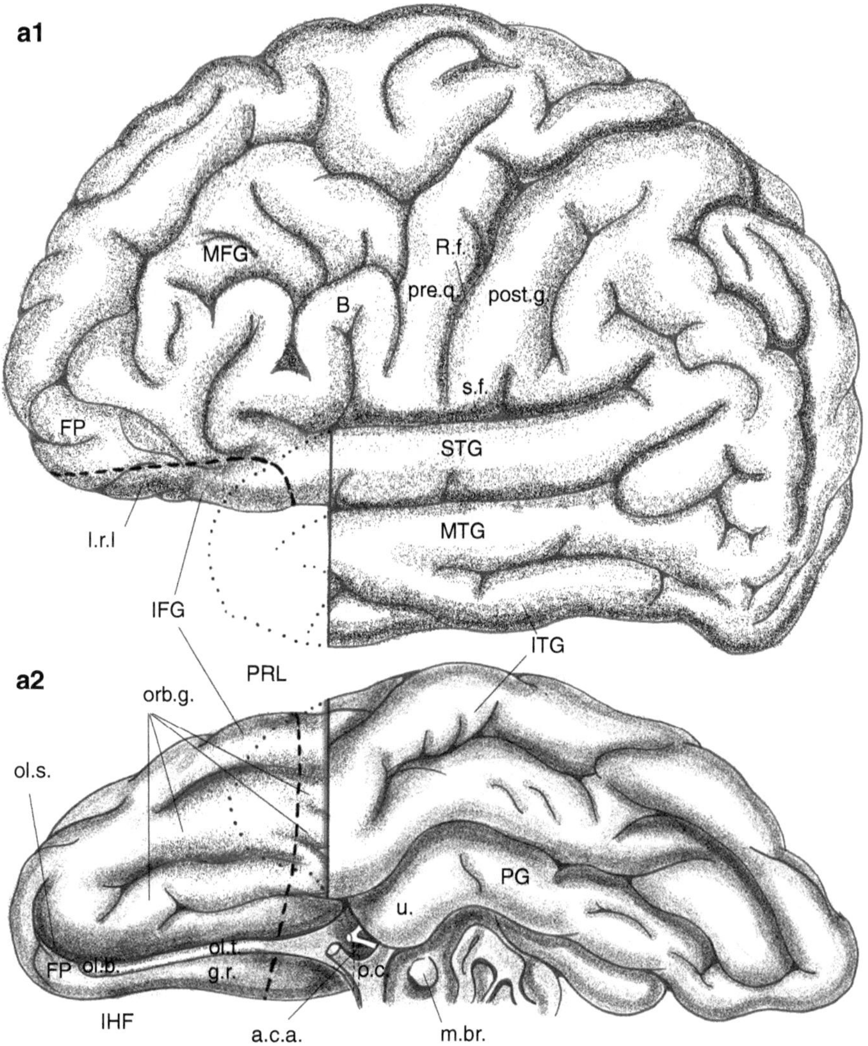
a1
MFG
R.f.
pre.g.
post.g.
B
s.f.
FP
STG
MTG
l.r.l
IFG
ITG
PRL
a2
orb.g.
ol.s.
PG
u.
ol.f.
FP
ol.b.
g.r.
p.c.
IHF
a.c.a.
m.br.

Fig. 7.6 (continued)

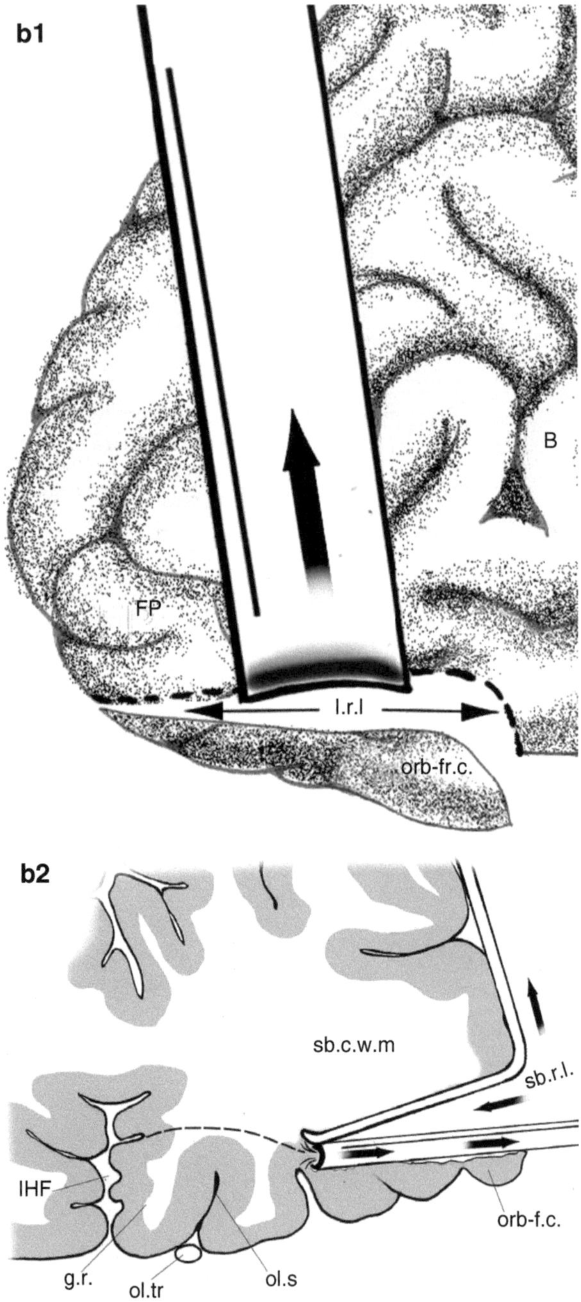

Fig. 7.6 (continued)

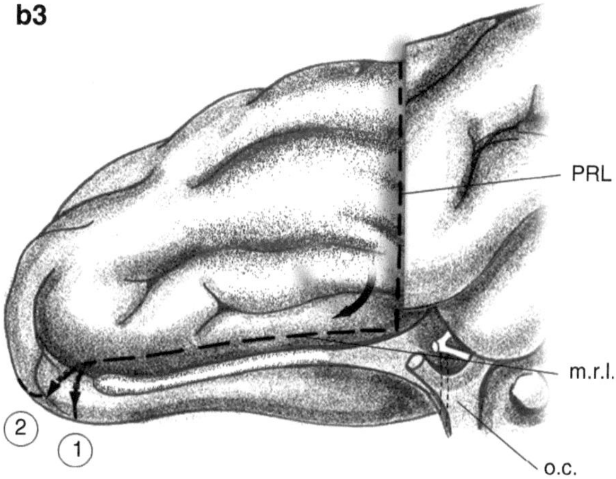

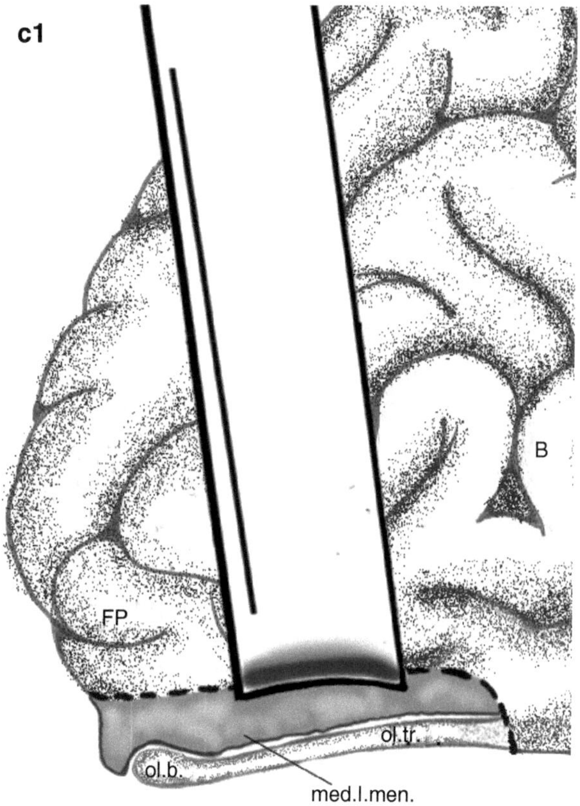

Fig. 7.6 (continued)

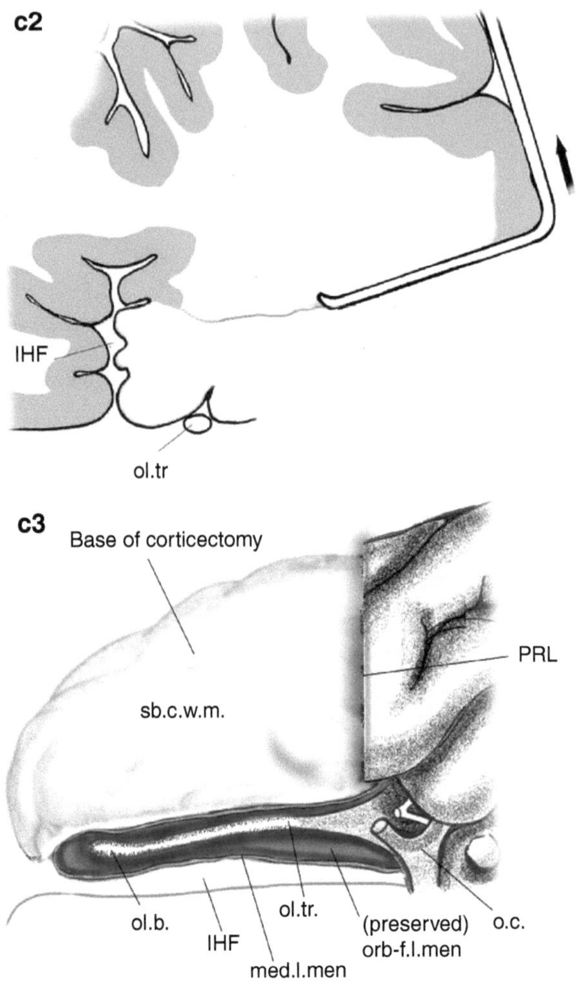

With the modifications noted in the foregoing, the corticectomy is carried out using the typical principles of subpial resection, leaving as healthy as possible the intact margins around the corticectomy. The initial lateral incision is best taken down on the inside of one of the horizontal sulci, when possible. The leptomeningeal margins are delineated, coagulated, and incised, as the resection is directed medially through the subcortical white matter, as superficially as possible, as described in Sect. 5.2. During the course of the medial dissection, there is an advantage in defining the posterior resection line (PRL), as it greatly facilitates visualization of the subcortical resection bed through retraction of the inferior frontal lobe. The retraction simply opens up the angle between the two subcortical surfaces, which result from the medially directed subcortical resection. The specimen becomes larger and "floppier" with each step of the ongoing resection. Thus, the more it is "freed" from its anterior and posterior limits, the greater is the visibility of the region of the surgery and the ease of separation of the two surfaces. These are freed, using typical leptomeningeal/parenchymal incisions when crossing gyri perpendicularly (see Sects. 5.5.2 and 7.2.5).

The subcortical medially directed dissection of the white matter is just deep to the gray matter in the depths of the orbital sulci and somewhat more superficially between the sulcal depths, e.g., deep to the body of the gyri, as illustrated previously in Figs. 5.2 and 5.3a. It is illustrated in Fig. 7.6b2. There are at least two sulci, usually shallow, between the lateral cortical incision and the medial extent of the corticectomy at the interhemispheric fissure.

One of the more important recognitions of the surgical anatomy for those unfamiliar with orbitofrontal corticectomies is that of the interhemispheric fissure (IHF). It is important to make this distinction so as not to enter the parenchyma of the contralateral hemisphere. There are three potential aids to making this recognition. First, just prior to reaching the fissure, the olfactory bulb and tract come into view, either directly or indirectly as seen through the leptomeningeal barrier. These are anatomically under, and usually attached to, the area of the olfactory sulcus. In other words, if they are visualized as a result of the subpial resection of orbit-frontal cortex over them, the olfactory sulcus has been passed and the next medial "sulcus" will not be a sulcus, but rather the IHF. This recognition may occur directly as a result of the repetitive lifting of the leptomeninges as a part of the methodology in the stepwise latero-medial PRL incision, which is the posterior boundary of the corticectomy. The bulb or tract is seen as a white cylindrical parenchymal ribbon of fibers, 2–3 mm in diameter, directly underlying and partially attached to the undersurface of the leptomeninges in the immediate vicinity of the olfactory sulcus. The next encountered sulcus medial to the olfactory bulb and tract is *always* the IHF.

The second potential help in recognizing the IHF is that it is not a pial covering but rather a leptomeningeal covering, and thereby it can be appreciated as being a much more resilient barrier than the thin, fragile pial covering of the sulci that have been passed on arriving at the IHF. The third and most clearly confident recognition is the absence of finding a typical sulcal depth. The resection to this point, as noted above, is kept as superficial as possible after reaching the depth of each sulcus. Thus, the depth of each sulcus, once identified as the resection proceeds medially, is reached by progressively resecting the gray matter more deeply, with its depth being recognized when there is no longer gray matter, e.g., it "disappears" as recognizable gray (matter) parenchyma (see Fig. 7.6b2). When the IHF is encountered, even if it is considered at that juncture to be a sulcus, it will be confidently recognized as the IHF by virtue of the fact that there is no such "disappearance" of gray matter as the surgeon is now progressing more superiorly with the subpial dissection, e.g., the end of the cortical gray matter, at about the level of the depth reached in the other sulci just exposed, does not occur. Therefore, this is highly likely *not* a sulcus, but rather the IHF. At this juncture the resection of the gray matter and its subcortical white matter should be resected sufficiently superior to satisfactorily reach certainty that it is the medial leptomeninges. Figure 7.6c illustrates the location of the olfactory bulb and tract in its usual position in close proximity to the olfactory sulcus on the underside of the medial aspect of the inferior orbital surface and only a very few millimeters lateral to the IHF.

Once the olfactory tract and bulb are recognized, they should be saved—a matter of pride to the experienced neurosurgeon, a matter of training for the novitiate! This is accomplished, once they come into view, by redirecting the leptomeningeal incision of the PRL from the latero-medial course, which had been utilized up to this point, to a posteroanterior course, roughly parallel to and a millimeter or so lateral to the olfactory tract. This is illustrated by the intermittent bold line and bold arrow in Fig. 7.6b3. The remaining part of the medial resection will now consist of pure subpial dissection. (This is very similar to the strategy used in other examples such as: (1) preclusion of entering the contralateral frontal lobe, during the course of a medical corticectomy, in the presence of an area of bihemispheric leptomeningeal adherence (Sect. 7.2.3); (2) the preservation of the integrity of the callosomarginal and pericallosal arteries in a posteromedial frontal corticectomy (Sect. 7.2.5); and (3) a radical aFLY (Sect. 7.4).) The leptomeningeal incision on the lateral side of the olfactory tract can be carried around the anterior aspect of the bulb to the interhemispheric fissure or simply carried on to the frontal pole; this is illustrated by the arrows and the circled 1 and 2, respectively. If the former is chosen, then at the IHF the leptomeningeal incision may be carried anteriorly to the anterior extent of the resection. Eventually the anterior part of this incision will become contiguous with the anterior latero-medial incision that was initiated at the infero-lateral incision, which was the start of the corticectomy.

Figure 7.6c diagrams the lateral view (c1), the sagittal (medial) view (c2), and the inferior surface view (c3) at the end of the resection. Figure 7.6c1 illustrates a lateral view in the depth of which is the (preserved) medial leptomeninges. Figure 7.6c3 illustrates the retained portion of the inferior surface leptomeninges lying superior to the olfactory parenchyma.

If the investigation leading to the orbitofrontal corticectomy suggests that some of the inferior aspect of the medial cortex should be removed, then 1–2 cm can easily be removed after the inferior corticectomy specimen has been removed, by simply proceeding superiorly, subpially, on over the interior of the medial leptomeninges with the aid of a small amount of retraction of the resection bed with a retractor such as that seen in Fig. 7.6c2.

7.3 Frontopolar Lobectomy

The simplest frontal resection is that of removal of the anterior frontal pole and will be referred to as a frontopolar resection or frontopolar lobectomy. This consists of removal of only the anterior part of the so-called prefrontal portion of the frontal lobe. It will involve removal of parts of the anterior dorsolateral, medial, and orbitofrontal cortices, arbitrarily as far posteriorly as perhaps half way to the genu of the corpus callosum. Thus, it will not normally involve the corpus callosum, any "eloquent" frontal cortical areas, e.g., Broca's, Rolandic motor, SMA, or the anterior horn of the lateral ventricle.

The principles of corticectomy are followed, utilizing sulcal boundaries whenever possible and maintaining the integrity of the white matter immediately beneath the cortical incisions, particularly around the peripheral incisions. The easiest sequence of incisions is to initiate the resection along the proposed dorsolateral cortical posterior resection line (PRL). There may be some argument about taking veins, but in general, any veins in the same coronal plain as the lobectomy may be included within the resected tissue. The safety of this is derived from the traditional general neurosurgical view that the anterior third of the superior sagittal sinus (SSS) can be sacrificed without penalty to the patient. Most of the arterial vasculature encountered in the resection represents end arteries in that their territories of irrigation are within the confines of the resection. This included the largest of these vessels, the frontopolar artery. The only exception to this generalization is the potential early branching of the callosomarginal artery from the pericallosal artery such that it is significantly anterior to the genu of the corpus callosum on the medial surface. In this case the artery is preserved in exactly the same way as described in an earlier section (Sect. 7.2.5) and will also be described in the next section (Sect. 7.4).

In the more radical frontopolar lobectomies, the medial PRL may follow the course of the pericallosal artery between the junction of the anterior communicating artery and the genu of the corpus callosum, and the inferior PRL may or may not involve removal of portions of the posterior orbitofrontal cortex. It is worth noting the immediately preceding section (Sect. 7.2.6) of orbitofrontal corticectomy. However, unlike the latter, the subcortical incision line, or lines, simply follows the posterior resection lines through the white matter of all three surfaces and thus completes a deep cross-sectional (coronal) incision. Being in front of the genu of the corpus callosum, there is no concern about entering the ventricle. It must be remembered, however, that resections for primary parenchymal tumors may include the ventricular wall and even the head of the caudate nucleus.

7.4 Radical aFLY

The radical aFLY involves the removal of the entire frontal cortex, excepting the so-called "eloquent" cortex, i.e., the motor cortex and Broca's speech area. The PRLs over the dorsolateral and medial surfaces will be the precentral sulcus in the nondominant hemisphere and in the dominant hemisphere, in addition to the precentral sulcus, the sulcus anterior to Broca's area in the frontal operculum as well. This operation is carried out under local anesthesia and neuroleptanalgesia. The eloquent cortex is identified by cortical stimulation as outlined in Chap. 4. The operation involves PRLs over the dorsolateral, medial, and inferior surfaces of the lobe. The most satisfactory initiation of the resection is over the dorsolateral surface of the lobe. However, after the latter is completed and carried over onto the medial and inferior surfaces, the best strategy is a coordinated alternating interconnected continuum of the PRLs of all three surfaces, as this greatly facilitates the ongoing retraction, which is so necessary for this operation. As the operation proceeds there is a gradually increasing bulk of the resection specimen, which requires retraction.

The earlier the initiation of all three PRL incisions and the deeper the incisions are, the greater is the mobility of the lobe and the much greater is the ease of retraction.

In those parts of the aFLY behind the genu, and thus behind the anterior parts of the frontal horn of the lateral ventricle, the subcortical white matter incisions should be kept as superficial as convenient, in order to retain a mantle of white matter over the ventricular wall. If the anterior extent of the ventricle happens to be entered, then the entry should not be widened, but rather effort should be aimed at preserving the integrity of the ventricular wall to as great an extent as possible, as the absence of significant amounts of blood in the ventricle usually results in a smoother post-operative course. In order to accomplish this, a relatively superficial dissection through the subcortical white matter, much like the strategy used in the course of a corticectomy (see Sect. 5.3 and Fig. 5.2), is necessary. When dealing with the eloquent cortex, the importance of initiating this subcortical incision promptly, in the case of pial and leptomeningeal incisions juxtaposed to the eloquent cortex, has been noted previously (see Sects. 5.5.3 and 7.2.2) and will be again noted further on (see Sects. 8.4.1, 8.4.2, and 8.7). Contrary to what was noted in the foregoing, the retraction of this posterior part of the lobe that overlies the ventricle may become more difficult at this point, as the preservation of maximal amounts of subcortical white matter leaves a thinner, less bulky, and more "floppy" cortical specimen. Certainly assistants, who can handle retractors well, provide a distinct advantage at this aspect of the resection.

The principles underlying the resection of the orbital and dorsolateral surfaces are as outlined in the foregoing sections. The incision in the dorsolateral precentral sulcus was noted in Sects. 5.5.3, 7.2.2, and 7.2.5 and is described in detail in Chap. 8. Once the depth of the sulcus is reached, the incision should not be deepened and particularly it should not be carried posteriorly. Either of these two practices, particularly the latter, can damage some of the efferent outflow of the precentral cortex and result in postoperative weakness. The same obtains in the case of Broca's area. Therefore, the resection of whatever gray matter is to be removed in the immediate vicinity of the precentral gyral parenchyma should be promptly followed by a shallow subcortical incision, taken anteriorly, for a centimeter or so (see Sects. 5.5.3, 8.1.2, and 8.4). That is to say, the step simply consists of carrying the incision over the initial centimeter away from the juxtaposed eloquently defined cortex as superficially as possible within the subcortical white matter (see particularly Sect. 5.3). The continuation of this strategy will also preclude the entry of the ventricle, which is helpful in the postoperative course.

The incision in the precentral sulcus on the medial surface is more complex than that on the dorsolateral surface because of the necessity of preserving the pericallosal and callosomarginal arteries, which irrigate the cortex behind the PRL. As outlined in the foregoing section (Sect. 7.2.5), the leptomeningeal incision is carried out from the dorsolateral PRL over onto the medial surface. As the medial PRL is extended inferiorly, it is of the utmost importance to recognize the presence of the callosomarginal artery, as it must be saved in order to preclude leg weakness as a postoperative neurological deficit. This artery is easily recognized if it is on the surface but more difficult if it is in a sulcus, which is often the case (see Fig. 7.4). Thus, the sulci encountered along the medial PRL, per se, should be exposed subpially in order to determine whether or not they contain arteries that should be preserved. If there is no such containment, then the sulcal pial investments can be coagulated and incised and subpial dissection continued inferiorly. A discussion regarding the surgical preservation of an artery that is identified at this point was discussed in Sect. 7.2.5 but will be mentioned again briefly here. The remaining part of the incision, once a "must-preserve" artery is found, down to the corpus callosum, must be conducted subpially; there is a transition in the surgery from a leptomeningeal/parenchymal to a subpial incision strategy. The safest and easiest way to achieve this is to initiate a posteroanterior leptomeningeal incision just superior (rostral) to the artery or to the sulcus in which the artery is found (see Fig. 7.4b, c) and parallel to it. From this point onward, the incision is conducted subpially with either piece meal or en bloc resection of the underlying cortex down to the corpus callosum, while at the same time gradually extending the leptomeningeal incision anteriorly. During this procedure the callosomarginal and finally the pericallosal arteries will be seen. By being subpial at this stage, the surgeon is not dependent upon identifying any larger arteries during the remainder of the incision, in order to preserve them, given that its overlying leptomeninges, which are now intact, will provide a protective barrier for them.

The foregoing example of transferring the surgical strategy from a leptomeningeal-parenchymal incision to a subpial resection was similar to the situations of dealing with the bihemispheric adherence of the leptomeninges on either side of the interhemispheric fissure (Sect. 7.2.3) and in preserving the olfactory apparatus in an orbitofrontal corticectomy (Sect. 7.2.6). It also enjoys some similarity to the procedure of "skeletonization" of *en passage* vessels in order to preserve their integrity during the course of a corticectomy (see Sect. 5.2).

Once the pericallosal artery and corpus callosum are identified, through the leptomeningeal barrier, the mesial cortex of the cingulate gyrus continues to be easily removed, down to and including the cortex in the corpus callosal sulcus, through gradually extending the leptomeningeal incision anteriorly. At the same time the subpial resection is continued anteriorly.

The leptomeningeal incision, paralleling the callosomarginal artery, will eventually reach the point where the latter branches off the parent pericallosal artery (see Figs. 7.4b, c). The incision line, which had followed the callosomarginal artery to this point, now follows the pericallosal artery in much the same way; this is clearly depicted in Fig. 7.7a. The subpial resection is continued until the genu of the corpus callosum is identified, which is most easily recognized by the gradual down turning of the pericallosal artery. Somewhere around this point, the frontopolar artery will become obvious and can be cauterized and incised (see Fig. 7.7b). It is *always* wise to follow this artery through subpial resection until it is certain that it is coursing anteriorly and is not a callosomarginal artery, which has an unusually anterior takeoff from the pericallosal artery. In the absence of bihemispheric leptomeningeal

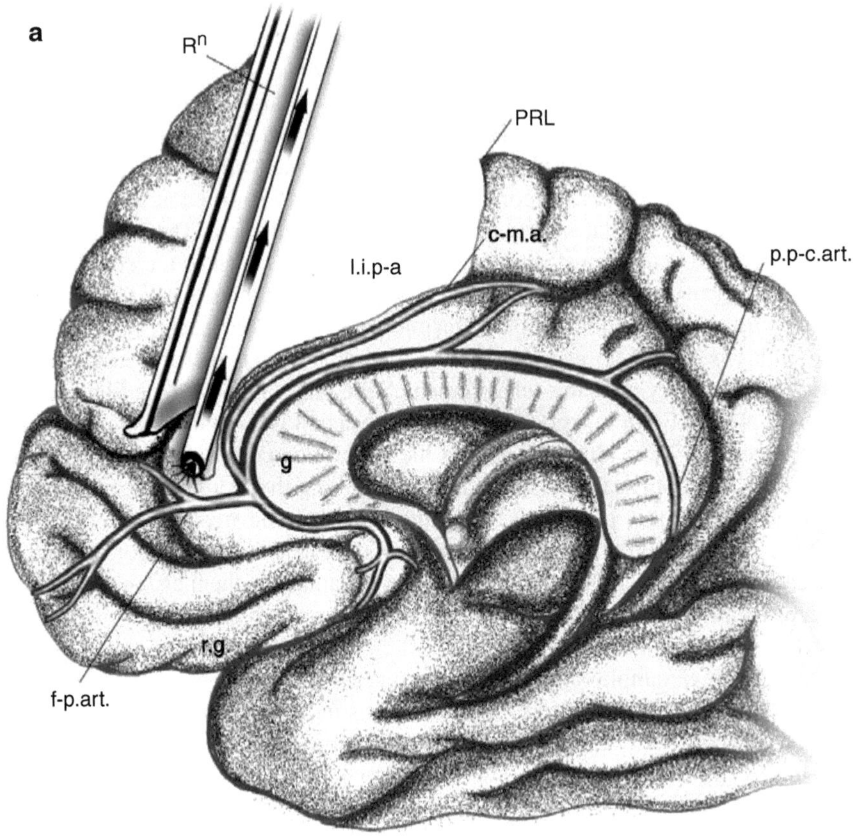

Fig. 7.7 Further steps in preserving the callosomarginal and pericallosal arteries. An illustration of the continuation of Fig. 7.4, which illustrated the preservation of the callosomarginal and pericallosal arteries in a right frontal posteromedial corticectomy. (**a**) Is the same as Fig. 7.4c2 in which subpial dissection/resection was employed to preserve the callosomarginal and pericallosal arteries, in the anterior medial frontal lobe. (**b**) Illustrates the remainder of the medial posterior leptomeningeal resection line which is simply anterior and parallel to the curvilinear course of the pericallosal artery between the genu of the corpus callosum and the region of the anterior communicating artery complex, eventually becoming continuous with the medial aspect of the PRL of the orbitofrontal cortical removal. *a.c.art.c.* anterior communicating artery complex, *c-m.a.* callosomarginal artery, *CC* corpus callosum, *f.p-art.* frontopolar artery (coagulated and incised), *g.* genu of the CC, *l.i.p-a* the longitudinal, posteroanterior leptomeningeal incision, parallel to and just superior to the callosomarginal artery, *o-t.g.* occipitotemporal (fusiform) gyrus, *p.a.* pericallosal artery, *p.p-c.art.* posterior pericallosal artery, *ph.g.* parahippocampal gyrus, *r.g.* rectus gyrus, R^n superior-lateral retraction of the partially separated frontal cortex, *PRL* posterior resection line, *u* uncus, *l* the area of the juncture of the medial incision and orbitofrontal PRL

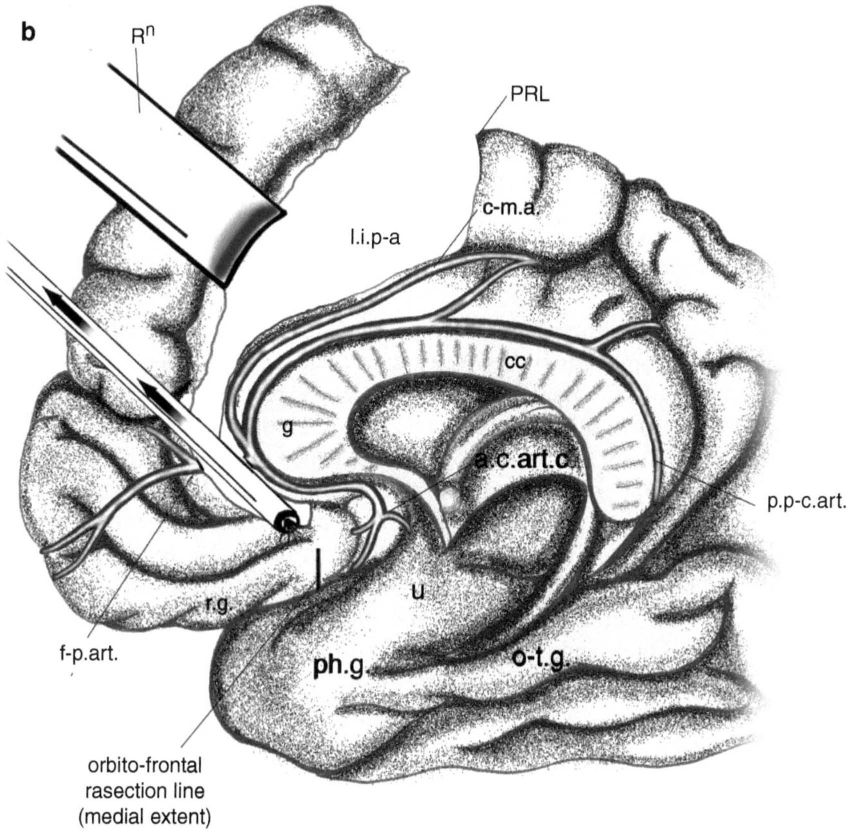

Fig. 7.7 (continued)

adherence (Sect. 7.2.3), the resection from this point onwards will return to a leptomeningeal-parenchymal incision and will follow a course parallel to and anterior to the pericallosal artery down to the region of the anterior communicating artery complex. In this area it forms a continuum with the medial end of the PRL of the orbitofrontal cortical resection (see Figs. 7.6a and 7.7b).

When the dorsolateral PRL is taken inferiorly (more laterally) and deepened, it will cross the frontal operculum superficially and then the anterior pole of the insula more deeply. The latter will involve the identification, coagulation, and incision of some very large arteries, which belong to the anterior trunk of the MCA and which branch out to irrigate the lateral basal and inferior dorsolateral cortices. This group of vessels is described by some as a "candelabra" arrangement of vessels (see, e.g., Nieuwenhuys et al. 1988). As the opercular area is further deepened, the lateral aspect of the inferior surface of the orbital cortex will be entered. At this point an orbitofrontal corticectomy is conducted, similar to that outlined in the foregoing section (Sect. 7.2.6). The dorsolateral and medial incisions in the subcortical white matter are angled anteriorly. They need only to be taken as far anteriorly as the genu of the corpus callosum in order to be anterior to the tip of the frontal horn of the lateral ventricle.

As noted in the orbitofrontal corticectomy, the inferior centimeter or two of the medial cortex can be easily removed as part of this corticectomy (Sect. 7.2.6). Greater amounts of the infero-medial cortex can be removed in the case of the radical aFLY in that the full thickness of the subcortical white matter will be gradually incised along the orbital cortex PRL, which provides further access to the medial cortex. The greater the infero-medial cortical resection can be achieved from beneath the lobe, the greater is the ease of conducting the resection of the remaining medial cortex from above, which often has to be undertaken piece meal between bridging veins to the superior sagittal sinus (SSS). Along with the progression of the surgical resection, not only does the disconnected cortex become larger in bulk and the retraction associated with it more difficult, but usually at some point the bridging veins to the SSS become a hindrance to the provision of satisfactory vision of the medical cortical resection bed and retard progress in establishing the inferior part of the medial incision. While occasionally the veins provide no impediment whatsoever, nevertheless this is the exception. When numerous and troublesome, these can be sequentially coagulated and incised, but only *after* as much of the arterial irrigation of the resected cortex as possible has been removed. The medial incision can usually be made to a reasonable extent by working between the bridging veins. This is less laborious if a significant amount of the resection has been achieved during the course of removal of the orbitofrontal cortex. There is nothing necessarily catastrophic about sacrificing the veins early, but the inability to abolish a significant arterial supply to the part of the lobe to be removed prior to the sacrifice of the venous drainage *will*, without doubt, become quickly associated with varying degrees of congestion, swelling, and not uncommonly even some venous bleeding, which can be very irritatingly troublesome! Thus, if the medial incision can be carried down to join the medial boundary of the orbital surface incision, before sacrificing the major venous drainage, then the venous oozing will be kept to a minimum. The removal of the veins aids greatly in the retraction required for finishing the resection, which usually involves the resection lines close to the medial and inferior surfaces at the pole.

The final resection bed should consist of the thick mantle of subcortical white matter surrounding the frontal ventricular horn and the peripheral olfactory apparatus, covered with a layer of leptomeninges.

7.5 Safe Limits of Resection

It is worth again outlining the means of measuring various areas of functional localization within the frontal lobe, using the small flexible rubber catheter, and making enough, usually 2–3, measurements to be certain of the reliability (repeatability) of the given measurement in cases when the patient is under local anesthesia. This is illustrated in Fig. 7.8. The dashed line is the distance between the frontal pole and the precentral sulcus. Both the bold and interrupted lines are simply illustrated examples of some interesting distances.

Some of the determinations are provided in Table 7.1 (also see Tables 6.1 and 6.2 in Sect. 6.6). While these do provide some rules of thumb when occasions might

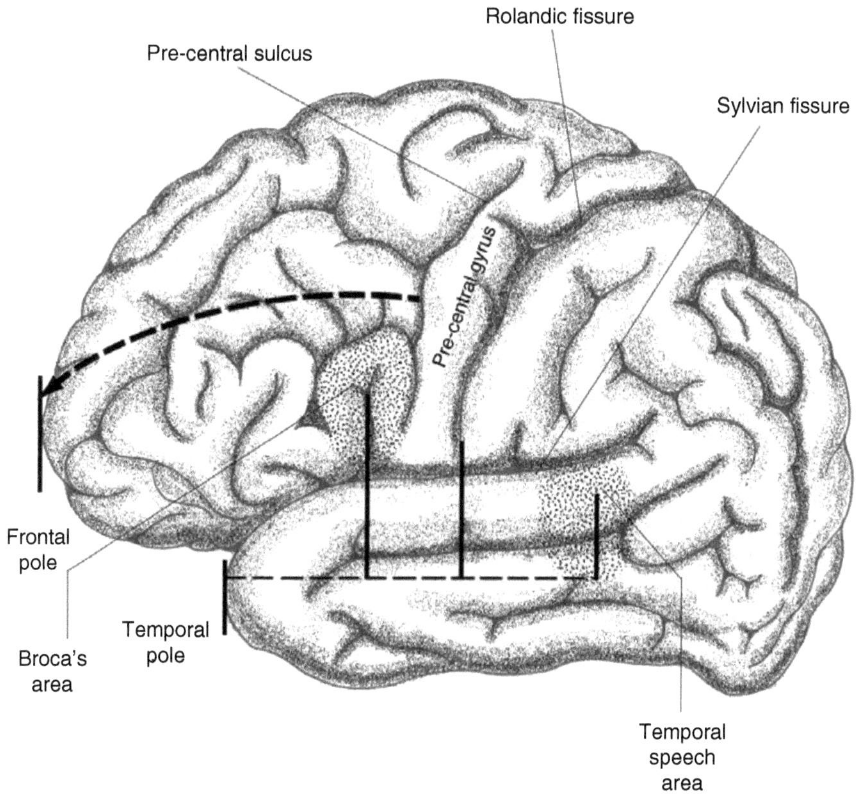

Fig. 7.8 Measuring, for cortical functional localization, over the dorsolateral surface of the hemisphere. Left (dorsolateral) hemispheric surface, exhibiting rough rules-of-thumb measurements, carried out by the use of a # 8 red rubber (pediatric, urinary) catheter. The latter is simply placed along the middle of the lateral surface and its tip is gently extended anteriorly until it reaches the point where it can no longer be extended. Each of these measurements was always the result of taking enough individual measurements, usually 2–3, to make certain of satisfactory (repeatability) reliability of the measurement (see text)

Table 7.1 Intraoperative measurements of various "eloquent" cortices from the poles of the temporal and frontal lobes

	Intraoperative measurements (cm)			
Anatomical designation	Distance behind temporal pole	Distance behind frontal pole	*n*	Range
Rolandic fissure	6.1	–	86	4.5–6.7
Temporal speech area	7.4	–	61	5.7–8.9
Broca's area	4.0	–	47	1.8–4.7
Precentral sulcus	–	11	20	8.8–13.6

arise unexpectedly under general anesthesia, I would still strongly adhere to the opinion that when such determinations might possibly be of importance in a surgical procedure, then it should be conducted under local anesthesia and determined by electrocortical stimulation, which is the gold standard for patient safety. Having said this, I am well aware of the tremendously important advances and contributions of functional magnetic resonance imaging (fMRI) over the last two decades, and hopefully in the future this will replace some of the necessity of using local anesthesia and neuroleptanalgesia!

As recorded in Table 7.1, the precentral sulcus is ~11 cm behind the frontal pole. The range of this measurement was 8.8–13.6 cm from the total of 20 such estimations. The distance to the Rolandic fissure will, of course, be simply the sum of that to the precentral sulcus (11 cm) plus the width of a typical gyrus (~1 cm), or therefore ~12 cm.

The temporal measurements are provided here with the frontal measurements, as not infrequently enough of the temporal lobe is exposed in frontal craniotomies, such that frontal measurements related to the temporal pole can also be determined. The junction of Rolandic and Sylvian fissures averages 6.1 cm behind the tip of the temporal pole, with a range of 4.5–7.3 from 86 measurements. Using the same approximate 1 cm width of a gyrus, the precentral sulcus will be on average ~1 cm less from the temporal pole than the Rolandic fissure and thus is ~5 cm behind the pole at the Sylvian fissure, and, reducing the value of another centimeter, Broca's area will be ~4 cm behind the temporal pole.

In this author's initial experience in the field of cerebral resections, the dictum was that any part of the telencephalon, with the exception of the so-called "eloquent" cortex, could be removed unilaterally with impunity. However, there are some practices that at least suggest that this is not quite so absolute. For example, the area just anterior to the motor leg area in the medial cortex that was initially shown to exhibit rather widespread movements, often bilateral, in mammalians (Munk 1881; Horsley and Schäfer 1888; Leyton Sherrington 1917; Vogt and Vogt 1919; Foerster and Penfield 1930; Foerster 1936) was, through the use of electrocortical stimulation, systematically investigated by Penfield who gave the name of the area "supplementary motor area" (Penfield 1950; Penfield and Welch 1951). He also disclosed that the movements made by its stimulation were not dependent upon the integrity of the Rolandic cortex and that it could be removed without deficit.

Further, it would now perhaps not be strictly applied to the basal ganglia, given that in the current twenty-first-century practice, apparently the frequency of bilateral stereotactic lesions being placed in forebrain deep gray matter in cases of movement disorders can be undertaken without unexpected postoperative neurological deficits.

Also, with respect to the foregoing, I cannot fail to note for the reader the outcomes of some cases of radical nondominant frontal lobectomies (usually for neoplasms) that I have conducted. For many years I, independently, was of the opinion that these could be carried out with complete impunity, with respect to postoperative deficits. The reason for this was what appeared to be perfectly neurologically intact postoperative patients. This was also reflected in the statement of Penfield and Rasmussen (1968, p. 192) who noted "Removal of very large areas, indeed of practically the whole frontal lobe on one side anterior to the precentral gyrus, results in an amazing lack of obvious defect. The patient walks, talks, and remembers. His disposition is little altered. There are no specialized functional zones here, the absences of which are easily recognized." However, over the ensuing postoperative courses of months and years, I feel certain that this notion cannot be applied to all such patients. The increasingly critical clinical follow-ups and neuropsychological assessments of these patients led me to the conclusion that at least some experience subtle and sometime significant deficits. This first became apparent to me personally when a young man, upon whom I carried out a radical nondominant aFLY for a middle grade glioma, was perfectly "normal" postoperatively from the view of his parents, his spouse, and a number of family members who actually worked in the health care service; I agreed fully with them. In spite of this, the surprise to all of us was that while he returned initially to his preoperative employment, he never achieved his preoperative quality in the workforce. Upon review many years postoperatively there is no doubt that one could detect subtle mental slowness, slowness that in retrospect we considered was probably present when he recovered from the operation but simply was not appreciated. Penfield and Rasmussen (1968, p. 193) went on to record in a patient who had a radical right aFLY for a glioma that she "demonstrated no alteration in behavior, except an 'impairment of those mental processes which are prerequisite to planned initiative.'" (The patient was actually Dr. Penfield's sister!)

In retrospect, it probably is fact that many such patients have in fact exhibited some slowness in mental responses in their early postoperative states. The reason for mentioning this here is not to suggest that such operative resections should not be done, if thought to be necessary, but rather to simply indicate that it is worth mentioning this potential postoperative state to the patient if understood and to the patients' family and caregivers. The obviousness of this is again not associated with clear-cut cognitive losses, but rather in subtle ways by the appreciation of small behavioral alterations, e.g., less alertness, less energetic deportment, less self-motivation, or some subtle incomprehensible feature that is "different" from their preoperative states. This has not been scientifically studied to my knowledge, and there have been insufficient critical numbers of neuropsychological assessments of these types of resections to provide certain satisfactory conclusions of whether the notion of such postoperative states is in fact understood. Once again, I remind the reader that the complications of epilepsy surgery have been very well covered by Pilcher and Rusyniak (1993).

In keeping with the foregoing consideration of "safe" limits of resection in the frontal lobe, it is perhaps important for the reader to be familiar with the article by the Montreal school relating to bilateral frontal corticectomies (Penfield 1947; Penfield and Steelman 1947; Penfield and Rasmussen 1968). In the early part of the twentieth century, Penfield conducted bilateral frontal corticectomies for psychoses and neuroses. A consideration of bilateral frontal corticectomies would unlikely occur again, but there could be the equivalent of such if a traumatic lesion occurred in one hemisphere and potential surgery, for whatever reason, was suggested for the other hemisphere. If one were confronted with such a circumstance, it would be of some importance to have been aware of the safety or lack of safety as available in these articles by Penfield and his colleagues. Penfield showed that bilateral corticectomies of the very anterior lateral frontal cortex or orbitofrontal cortex might be carried out harmlessly. This is illustrated by the broken line in Fig. 7.9. This was

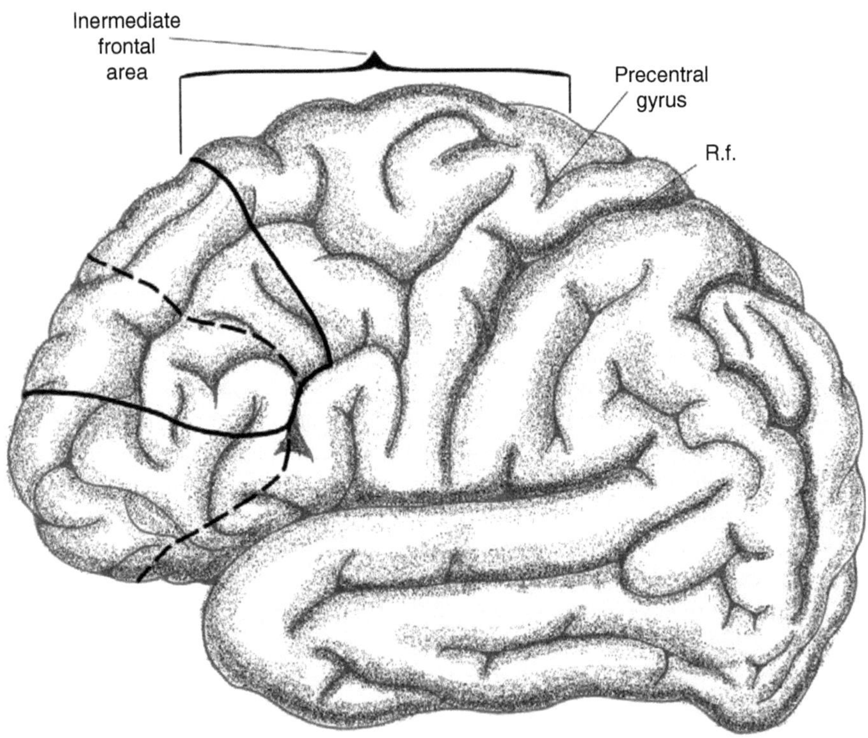

Fig. 7.9 Redrawn figures of Penfield's (1947) "bilateral frontal gyrectomy." This figure illustrates the experiences of Penfield, in an early era, when he conducted corticectomies in both frontal lobes. He observed that such "posterior superior" frontal cortical resections, if removed bilaterally, often resulted in prolonged postoperative mental confusion, incontinence, repetitive automatic movements, and apathy or stupor (see text). The *broken line* depicts the cortex that can be resected bilaterally without causing a postoperative deficit. The *solid line* of areas more posteriorly located, which removed bilaterally led to significant postoperative deficits (Redrawn, with permission, from Penfield (1947))

Table 7.2 Safety in resections of the frontal lobe

Area (frontal lobe)	Safety of resection			Postoperative course		
				Deficit		
	Safe	Unsafe	?	Transient	Permanent	Uneventful
Broca's area	–	√		–	Aphasia	–
Conservative aFLY (<8 cm)	√	–		–	–	√
Radical aFLY	–	–	√	? Transient weakness and/or aphasia	? Subtly impaired cognition especially planning	–
Bilateral orbital corticectomies	√	–		–	–	√
Bilateral polar corticectomies	√	–		–	–	√
Bilateral posterosuperior corticectomies	–	√		? √	Altered consciousness, impaired cognition, ? apathy	–

still evident 20 years later when Penfield and Rasmussen indicated that "One of the surprising results .... was the fact that bilateral ablation of these [orbitofrontal] surfaces had remarkably little effect ..." (1968). Penfield used a label of "intermediate frontal area," which involved a significant portion of the latter half of the frontal lobe; this area is outlined in Fig. 7.9 by a parenthetic symbol. Later he carried out bilateral frontal cortical resections (the bold lines in Fig. 7.9) that extended more posteriorly than those involving the frontal poles; they encroached on his "intermediate frontal area." These gave rise to increasing risks of significant postoperative cognitive impairments (Penfield 1947).

Table 7.2 provides a brief review of what can and what cannot be resected with safety in the frontal lobe.

References

Foerster O. The motor cortex in man in the light of Hughling Jackson's doctrines. Brain. 1936;59:135–59.

Foerster O, Penfield W. Der narbenzug am und im gehirn bei traumatischer epilepsie in seiner bedeutung für das zustandekommen der anfälle und für die therapeutische bekämpfung derselben. Z Neurol Psychiatry. 1930;125:475–572.

Horsley V, Schäfer EA. A record of experiments upon the functions of the cerebral cortex. Phil Trans. 1888;179:1–45.

Leyton ASF, Sherrington CS. Observations on the excitable cortex of the chimpanzee, orang-utan, and gorilla. Q J Exp Physiol. 1917;11:135–222.

Munk H. Über die Functionen der Grosshirnrinde. In: Hirschwald A, editor. Gesammelte Mittheilungen aus den Jahren, mit Einleitung und Ammerkungen, Berlin. 1881; 1877–80.

Nieuwenhuys R, Voogd J, van Huijzen C. The human central nervous system: a synopsis and atlas. 3rd ed. New York: Springer; 1988. p. 37.

Penfield W. The supplementary motor area in the cerebral cortex of man. Arch Psychiatry Zeit Neurol. 1950;185:670–4.

Penfield W. Bilateral frontal gyrectomy and postoperative intelligence. Chapter XXIII – Symposium on Gyrectomy, Part 1. Res Publ Ass Nerv Ment Dis. 1947;27:519–34.

Penfield W, Rasmussen T. The cerebral cortex of man: a clinical study of localization of function. New York: Hafner Publishing Company; 1968. 248 pp.

Penfield W, Steelman H. The treatment of focal epilepsy by cortical excision. Ann Surg. 1947;126:740–62.

Penfield W, Welch K. The supplementary motor area of the cerebral cortex: a clinical and experimental study. AMA Arch Neurol Psychiatry. 1951;66:289–317.

Pilcher WH, Rusyniak WG. Complications of epilepsy surgery. Neurosurg Clin N Am. 1993;4:311–25.

Rasmussen T. Characteristics of a pure culture of frontal lobe epilepsy. Epilepsia. 1983;24:482–93.

Vogt C, Vogt O. Allgemeinere Ergebnisse unserer Hirnforschung. J Psychol Neurol. 1919;25:273–462.

Wennberg R, Quesney F, Olivier A, Rasmussen T. Electrocorticography and outcome in frontal lobe epilepsy. Electroencephalogr Clin Neurophysiol. 1998;106:357–68.

Rolandic Surgery 8

8.1 Physiology and Surgical Anatomy of the Rolandic Cortex

8.1.1 Physiology

As noted in the previous chapter, in keeping with a tenet of Dr. Theodore Rasmussen (personal communication), the Rolandic cortex is being considered as an independent entity, because of its obvious physiological differences from the more anteriorly situated frontal cortex and its more posteriorly situated parietal cortex. I suppose it is reasonable to include the fact that (Brodmann 1903; Garey 1994) recognized sufficient differences in their morphological characteristics that he assigned different morphological numerical areas to the precentral cortex (Area 4) and the postcentral cortex (Areas 3, 2, and 1). A knowledge of the anatomy and the physiology of the Rolandic cortex aids in the understanding of a number of surgical decisions in dealing with seizure disorders pertaining to it or its immediately adjacent environs.

The physiological concept pertaining to the mammalian cerebral cortex is that of functional units, or columns, of cells arranged perpendicular to the surface of the cortex and probably being something of the order of 0.5–1 mm in diameter. These columns (functional units) are loosely connected to one another. The integration within a column is reflected in the subcortical output of that column. The immediately subcortical U-fibers and the intracortical nerve nets joining the columns to their neighbors provide an intracortical conduction system parallel to the surface of the gyrus. Thus, at least theoretically, a cortical incision, perpendicular to the surface of the cortex, would be less damaging to the physiological role of that cortex than one parallel to the surface (see Colonnier 1966).

J.P. Girvin, *Operative Techniques in Epilepsy*,
DOI 10.1007/978-3-319-10921-3_8

8.1.2 Anatomical Considerations

Anatomically the afferent and efferent fibers of the cortical columns join and leave, respectively, the precentral and postcentral gyral cortex and traverse the subcortical white matter, forming part of the corona radiata, to reach the genu and posterior limb of the internal capsule. When surgery involves subpial dissection/resection of the cortex adjacent to the pre- and postcentral cortices, then the course of the inflow and outflow of the immediate subcortical connectivity becomes an important surgical anatomical consideration. Figure 8.1 outlines two parasagittal (anteroposterior) sections through the Rolandic region, one just above the Sylvian fissure (Fig. 8.1a) and one just lateral to the interhemispheric fissure (Fig. 8.1b), in other words one in the inferior Rolandic region and one in the superior Rolandic region, respectively.

In the superior part of the Rolandic cortex, the relationship between its surface location and its connectivity is less striking and even somewhat reversed when compared to the inferior Rolandic cortex, as the Rolandic fissure and its associated cortices angle posteriorly in their courses from the inferior Sylvian fissure to the superior interhemispheric fissure. In a series of coronal sections, the difference between its junction with the Sylvian fissure and that of its junction with the interhemispheric fissure is as much as 3–4 cm in an anteroposterior direction. In other words the superior dorsolateral Rolandic cortex at the interhemispheric fissure (IHF) is ~4 cm posterior to the inferior Rolandic cortex at the Sylvian fissure. Given the foregoing and given that the main connectivity of the Rolandic cortex is to the posterior limb of the internal capsule, which is significantly posterior to the inferior Rolandic area, the fibers leaving the inferior Rolandic area must proceed significantly more posteriorly in order to reach the posterior internal capsule than the superior cortex. This is illustrated in Fig. 8.1a. From this figure it can be appreciated that an extension of a straight perpendicular incision inferiorly in the depth of the postcentral gyrus would significantly interfere with that connectivity and thereby with the maintenance of the clinical function represented in its fibers. Such would not be as significant were the incision made in the depth of the *pre*central sulcus. Similarly, in neither the precentral nor the postcentral sulci near the IHF would such an incision result in such interference in the Rolandic connectivity nor the resulting associated clinical impairments, as the fibers are not sweeping as significantly posteriorly in their subcortical courses. These differences are illustrated in the diagrams in Fig. 8.1a, b, which portray the direction of the course of the fibers of connectivity. This figure depicts similar important surgical anatomical features in subpial resection techniques in cortex adjacent to the so-called eloquent cortex, such as those demonstrated in Figs. 5.3 and 7.2 in Sects. 5.5.3 and 7.2.2, respectively. These latter figures point out the importance of going no deeper than the gray matter in the depths of sulci immediately adjacent to the eloquent cortex. In Fig. 8.1a, b the broad arrows at the bottoms of the pre- and postcentral sulci

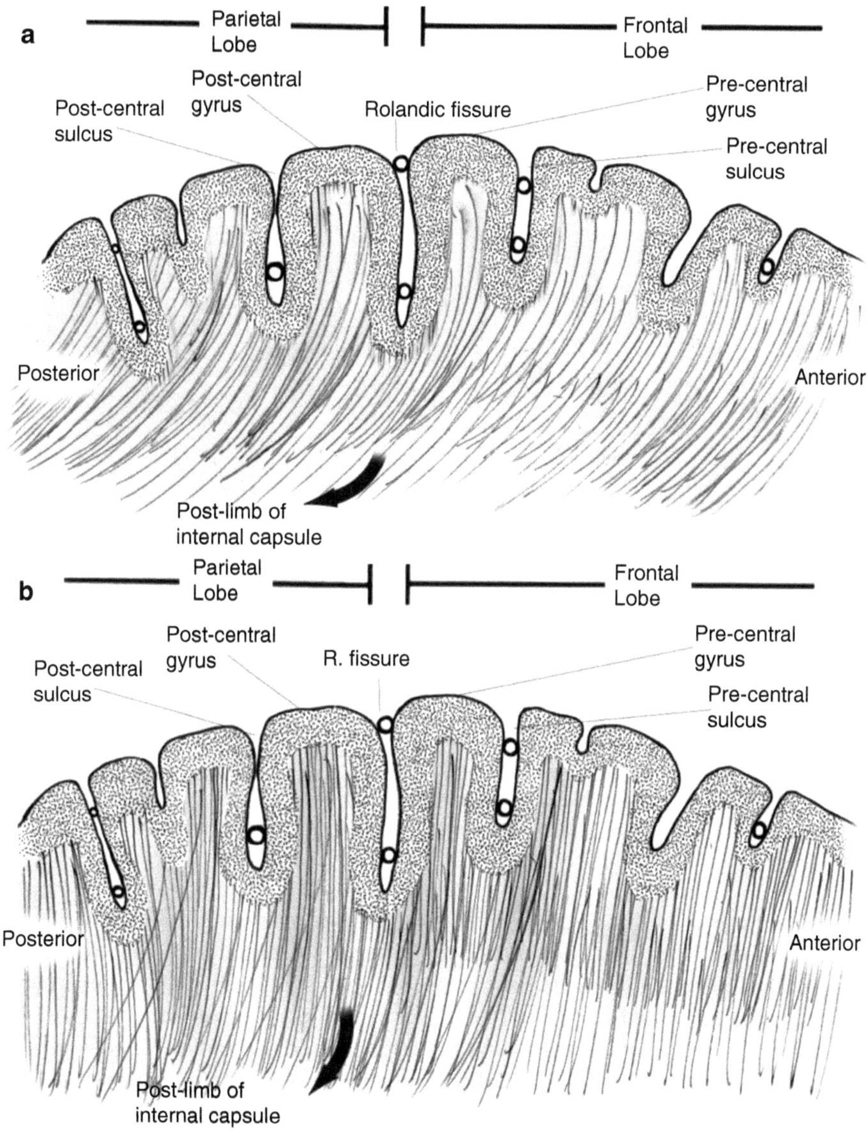

Fig. 8.1 Illustration of the neural connectivity of the Rolandic cortex. Anteroposterior (sagittal) sections through the Rolandic cortex, illustrating the course of the connectivity of both the precentral (motor) and postcentral (sensory) cortices in the immediate subcortical white matter. (**a**) The anteroposterior (parasagittal) section is through the Rolandic region just above the Sylvian fissure. (**b**) This anteroposterior section is just medial to the interhemispheric fissure. The *broad arrows* designate the sweeping path of the Rolandic fibers upon leaving the cortex (Redrawn, with permission, from Girvin (1991))

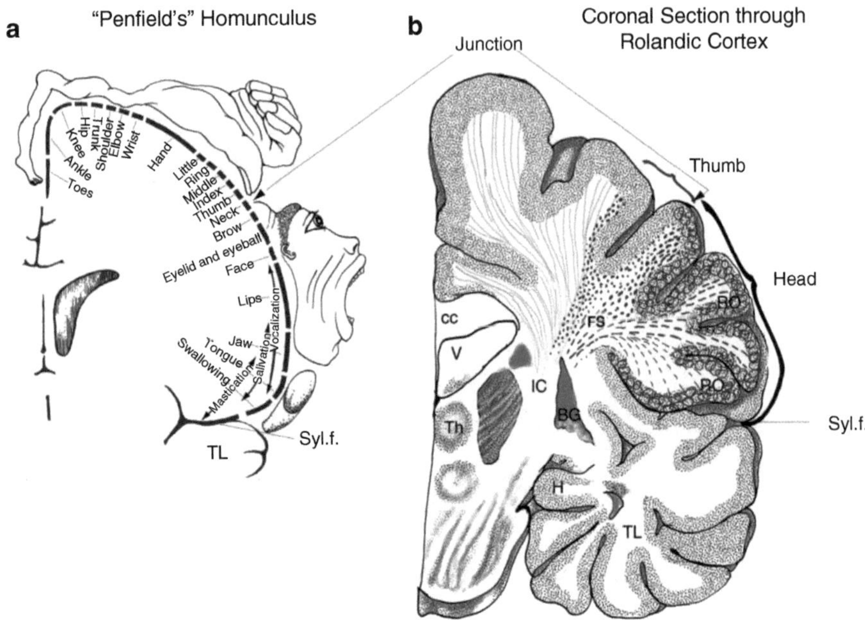

Fig. 8.2 Coronal section through the Rolandic cortex. Coronal section through the Rolandic cortex. (**a**) Illustration of the Penfield homunculus, depicting the relative proportions of the cortex representing the various motor and sensory functions of the body. (**b**) Illustration of the cortical efferent pathways of the inferior Rolandic cortex into the subcortical white matter and internal capsule. *BG* basal ganglia, *cc* corpus callosum, *FS* frontal stem, *H* hippocampus, *IC* internal capsule, *junction* junction of the thumb and head representation in Penfield's homunculus (**a**) and in human cortex from electrocortical stimulatory mapping (**b**); *Syl.f.* Sylvian fissure, *Th* thalamus, *TL* temporal lobe, *V* lateral ventricle

disclose the path of the fibers, either leaving or proceeding to the Rolandic cortex and going to or coming from the mid- to posterior internal capsule and the thalamus of the motor and sensory fibers, respectively. It is illustrative of the importance of not violating the subcortical white matter immediately below the bottom of the postcentral sulcus. Rather, any continued resection should be directly posterior, as noted in the foregoing, as superficially as possible and directed *away from* the eloquent cortex.

The foregoing is primarily of importance in the resection of the inferior Rolandic cortex (*vide infra*, Sect. 8.4), which is probably the commonest operation associated with the Rolandic cortex, as it is used in general neurosurgery probably to a greater extent than in specialized epilepsy surgery. Figure 8.2a represents a cartoon coronal section through the Rolandic cortex, outlining Penfield's homunculus. Figure 8.2b is an illustration of a coronal section through the same area. The primary reason for this illustration is to bring attention to what I call the "frontal stem," which is the frontal counterpart to the temporal stem, which is so important in the conduct of an aTLY. It can be appreciated that the frontal stem (FS) in Fig. 8.2b represents an orderly, and indeed intuitively predictable, layering of the fibers subserving the Rolandic opercular cortex (ROC) in which its most inferolateral component is that of the inferomedial ROC embedded in the Sylvian fissure at its junction with the insula (I). Proceeding more superomedially within the FS are the fibers subserving progressively more superior functional components of the ROC within the head, e.g., tongue → jaw → lips → face → eyes, etc. Continuing on in the FS, the components of the head are followed by those of the hand, beginning with the thumb, e.g., thumb → index finger → middle finger → ring and small fingers → hand, etc. It is this junction (see "junction" in Fig. 8.2a, b) between head and thumb within the inferior Rolandic cortex, as well as the subcortical junction of the neuronal efferent outflows between those fibers on either side of the cortical junction, which is of importance in the inferior Rolandic corticectomy (Sect. 8.4).

Another anatomical feature of the Rolandic cortex pertains to the variability of the positions of the homunculi that can occur. The surgeon should be aware of this variability, but given that these operations are, or should be, conducted under local anesthesia, they are rarely of significance other than this awareness. One variation is that which can exist between the representation of the motor and sensory homunculi across the Rolandic fissure. In the common neuroanatomical textbooks, there is usually no reference to potential asymmetry that may exist between the two homunculi, with respect to the pre- and postcentral gyri. That is to say, the reader of the text book usually comes away with the notion that the two homunculi are perfectly symmetrical in that the motor and sensory representations of each part of the body across the Rolandic fissure are juxtaposed in the precentral and postcentral gyri, as illustrated in Fig. 8.3a. In general, this is the case or very close to the case regarding symmetry, with any asymmetry amounting to simply a differential of a few millimeters. However, on occasion the asymmetry may amount to several millimeters, such as illustrated in Fig. 8.3b, and if the surgeon is not aware of this possibility, it may lead to a search for a presumed error of some kind, e.g., such as faulty stimulation, presumed errors in interpretation of responses, etc.

The only instance where this asymmetry could be of significance is in the resection of the inferior Rolandic cortex. The superior border of this resection is the junction between the inferiorly situated head area of the homunculus and the more superiorly situated thumb area. This junction is the most important border of the operative procedure of inferior Rolandic corticectomy. The junction of the sensory homunculus in the postcentral gyrus cannot be used as the superior border, based on the assumption that the motor homunculus is symmetrically located anteriorly across the Rolandic fissure. For example, if the asymmetry was such as outlined in Fig. 8.3b and the border of the corticectomy was at the junction identified in the postcentral gyrus, then the thumb area of the precentral gyrus would either be partially removed or completely removed with the clinical postoperative counterpart of a paresis or paralysis of the hand. This depicts the importance of utilizing the junction of the motor homunculus rather than that of the sensory homunculus for

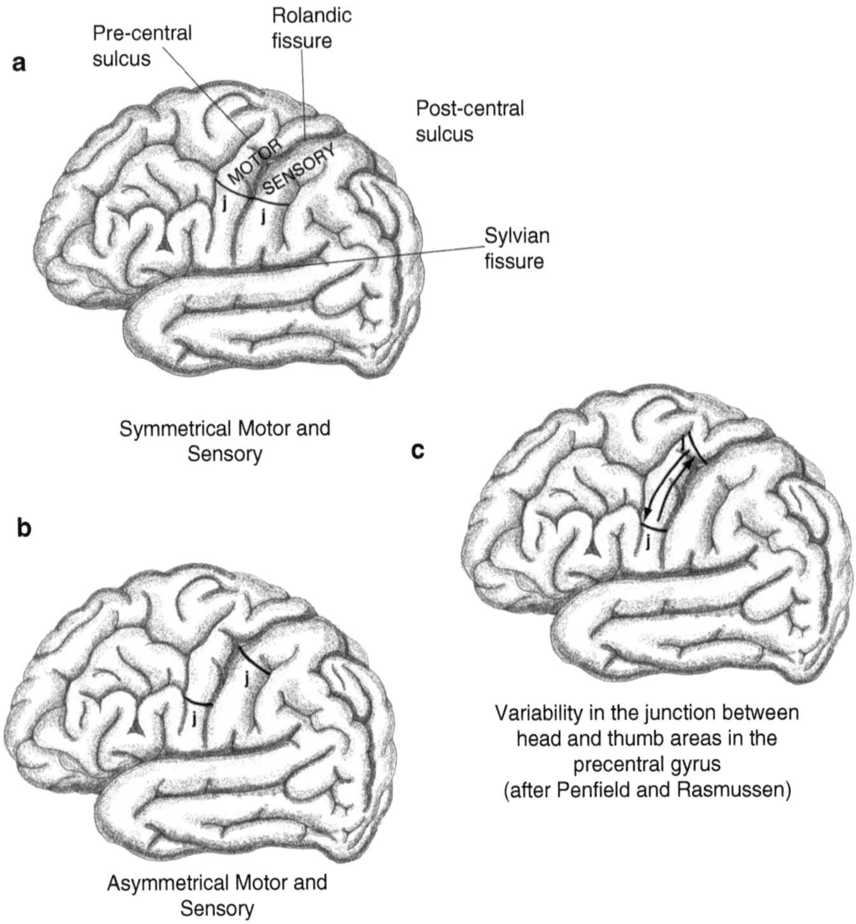

Fig. 8.3 Illustrations of the variation in the relationships of the sensory and motor homunculi. Left hemisphere, dorsolateral surface, illustration of the potential variability in relationships of the homunculi of the Rolandic region. Illustration of (**a**) symmetry and (**b**) asymmetry of the junctions between the head and thumb segments of the motor and sensory homunculi. (**c**) Illustration of the variability of the junction of the head and thumb segments of the homunculus along the precentral gyrus, e.g., between the Sylvian fissure inferiorly and the interhemispheric fissure superiorly (see text). *j* junction of the head and thumb segments of Penfield's homunculus; the *arrows* in (**c**) demonstrate the wide range over which the junction of the thumb and head and neck areas of the motor homunculus might be found

identifying the superior border of an "inferior Rolandic corticectomy." This circumstance would only be a potential problem if the motor thumb area could not be found, which, as noted earlier, is not necessarily rare. In the final analysis, any concern at all can, of course, be simply precluded by the operation being conducted under local anesthesia with continual clinical monitoring of thumb function.

Penfield and Rasmussen (1968, p. 47) noted that: "The relative size of the motor face, arm, and leg areas varies considerably. The face area may be large and extend to within 4 cm. of the midline, or it may be so small that thumb responses are elicited 2 cm. above the fissure of Sylvius. A similar variability exists for the leg area. It may be entirely located on the mesial surface of the hemisphere or it may extend well out onto the lateral surface for a distance of up to 3 cm." This exemplifies the extreme variability of the human motor cortical homunculus along the precentral gyrus, which Penfield and Rasmussen concluded was a representation in which "scientific accuracy is impossible" (p.56). This is illustrated in Fig. 8.3c. This variability is one that I have also observed (*vide infra*, Sect. 8.7).

Before leaving the physiology and anatomy of the Rolandic cortex, it should be noted that, unless fMRI eventually can clearly outline the Rolandic cortex, the surgeon must be aware that only through local anesthesia in the awake patient with electrocortical stimulation can the Rolandic fissure be *confidently* identified. I would agree with Penfield who stated "there is no way of determining the central fissure in a living patient except by stimulation because of the great variability in cortical pattern, especially in pathologic conditions." (1938, p. 242)

8.2 Surgical Strategies for Treating Rolandic Seizures

The strategies involved in the surgery of the Rolandic region depend to some degree upon whether the main objective is the removal of an epileptogenic focus, the removal of a lesion causing epileptic seizures, the removal of a lesion that may not be associated with epilepsy, or some combination of more than one of the preceding reasons. Every neurosurgeon is trained to accept the philosophy, when dealing with the eloquent cortex, e.g., speech, visual, and Rolandic cortex, that almost never will one sacrifice this cortex, if the function it serves is intact. For example, unless the patient has a hemiplegia or monoplegia, the precentral gyrus would never be removed. Thus, dealing with neurosurgical problems associated with this cortex, that philosophy would always be paramount in any considerations of the neurosurgical management of such problems.

Given the foregoing, the Montreal school, under the tutelage of Dr's Penfield and Rasmussen, in dealing with intractable seizures arising in the Rolandic cortical regions, would often choose to carry out what they referred to as "peri-Rolandic" corticectomies. In these cases the cortex immediately adjacent to the Rolandic cortex, e.g., in the posterior frontal cortex and/or the anterior parietal cortex, would primarily define the resections. Dr. Rasmussen felt that the peri-Rolandic corticectomy was a strategy that could reduce the "epileptic tendency" to the point of at least making the intractable seizure disorder more easily treated medically. Usually the precentral or postcentral sulcus will form one of the peripheral borders of these corticectomies, except where the speech areas were in the dominant hemisphere.

A second strategy of the Montreal school was the removal of the inferior Rolandic cortex, i.e., that below the thumb area in the homunculus of the precentral gyrus. In this case the head and neck motor representation would be removed. The removed cortex represents primarily axial motor innervation, which is known to be bilateral, and hence usually does not result in a significant permanent neurological deficit (Rasmussen 1987).

The third strategy is the use of multiple subpial transections (MSTs), an operation that was introduced more recently (Morrell 1973; Morrell et al. 1989). These will be discussed in more detail later (*vide infra*).

8.3 The Peri-Rolandic Resection

Early on in the history of epileptic surgery, Rolandic seizure disorders were considered to be inoperable because neurosurgeons were unwilling to accept permanent neurological deficits in patients, which were purely attributable to the surgery. As noted in the foregoing, the Montreal school developed more acceptable attempted strategies in dealing with cases of clear-cut intractable sensory or motor seizures arising in the Rolandic area in cortex pertaining to the extremities. The initial attempt dealt with the use of the so-called peri-Rolandic resection. The peri-Rolandic resection consists of removing non-eloquent, or as Penfield called it, "dispensable," cortex in the vicinity of the identified focus within or adjacent to the Rolandic cortex. The rationale for this type of resection had its origin in the empirical notion that a certain critical mass of neurons was responsible for chronic epilepsy and that the mass might be significantly larger than what was determined by the electroencephalography (EEG) or the intraoperative electrocorticography (ECoG) at the time. A further extension of this notion was that because of the small size of seemingly involved segments of the Rolandic cortex in contrast to the adjacent non-Rolandic cortex, a significant portion of this critical mass might be situated outside of the Rolandic region, per se, intuitively considered to be in the immediate vicinity of the segment of the Rolandic cortex that was demonstrated to be the focus. Further, it was well appreciated at the time that epileptic foci may be extra-Rolandic, but yet present clinically, through the spread of epileptic electrical activity, as Rolandic seizures.

The difficulty of surgically treating such seizures was all too well known at the time, and certainly the intractable sensorimotor seizures were the most resistant to satisfactory surgical management. While the strategy of the use of the peri-Rolandic corticectomy was not as effective as many other corticectomies or lobectomies, nevertheless it sometimes converted a sensorimotor intractable seizure disorder into a satisfactorily medically managed seizure disorder. However, it must be noted that in many cases it simply added to the failures and woes of dealing with intractable central seizures. For those who toiled with these patients, the introduction of the operation of MSTs was enthusiastically received and endorsed.

The peri-Rolandic surgical strategy consists of the removal of the cortex immediately adjacent to the pre- and/or postcentral gyri, i.e., the posterior frontal and/or the anterior parietal cortex, respectively. Thus, they really consist of simple frontal and/or parietal corticectomies—simple other than for the requirement of very careful removal of the non-Rolandic cortex bordering on the Rolandic cortex without injuring the latter, the principles of which are outlined in Sects. 2.2.6, 5.2, 5.3, 5.4, and 8.1.2. Since the operations necessitate the accurate identification of the pre- and postcentral gyri and sulci, they are conducted under local anesthesia, with ECoG facilitated identification of the location of any epileptogenic activity. While the characteristics of the semiology of the seizures may often give the surgeon some indication as to where any extra-Rolandic epileptogenicity might be centered, nevertheless the gold standard for this determination, under these circumstances, was the ECoG.

In the case of the frontal corticectomy, the cortex involved is the posterior part of the so-called premotor area, which includes the supplementary motor area (SMA), which is that cortex immediately in front of the precentral sulcus, primarily on the cortex of the medial surface. The resections are carried out using all the principles of subpial dissection, as applied to corticectomy (*vide supra*, Chap. 5 and Sect. 2.2). In the case of removals of the SMA, attention must be directed to the preservation of the callosomarginal artery, as outlined in Chap. 7 (Sects. 7.2.5 and 7.6), dealing with the removal of the mesial cortex in the posteromedial frontal corticectomy and radical aFLY, respectively.

In the case of the extra-Rolandic parietal corticectomy, the resection is conducted as noted in the foregoing in accordance with the principles laid out in Chap. 5 and Sect. 2.2 and with reference to the resection of the parietal cortex, as outlined in Chap. 9. As noted earlier (*vide supra*, Sect. 8.1.2), any deepening of the subpial incision at the bottom of the postcentral sulcus should be carried out very cautiously and with ongoing clinical examination of the sensory function represented in the immediate vicinity of the surgery in order to preclude the risk of compromise from impingement upon the postcentral gyrus at the point of surgery.

8.4 Inferior Rolandic Corticectomy

8.4.1 Vicissitudes of the Inferior Rolandic Corticectomy

Gradually increasing experience, particularly in the hands of Dr.'s Penfield and Rasmussen of the Montreal school, with Rolandic epilepsy led to the evolution of the awareness that the inferior Rolandic cortex usually could be sacrificed without the production of an unwanted neurological deficit. The evolution resulted in the now accepted fact that the entire Rolandic cortex in the suprasylvian region, below the thumb area, can be removed without deficit. This has been intuitively attributed to the fact that much of the head musculature, e.g., face, pharynx, larynx, and neck, has bilateral cortical innervation whereby the loss of one of the two innervations usually can be tolerated without the production of a permanent deficit (Penfield and Rasmussen 1950, 1968; Penfield and Jasper 1954; Penfield and Roberts 1959; Rasmussen 1975a, b; Lehman et al. 1994). This perhaps might have been predicted from the knowledge that in the majority of strokes from occlusion of the middle cerebral artery, the monoplegic upper limb is not accompanied by a permanent significant deficit in the head and neck. When minimal dysarthria or facial paresis occurs, they often disappear within a few days. This is not dissimilar to uncommon such deficits following the inferior Rolandic corticectomy.

Once again this resection must be conducted under local anesthesia and with intraoperative electrocortical stimulatory mapping of the Rolandic area. The latter must delineate the point of transition, within the homunculus, between the head and neck representation and the representation of the thumb. The homunculus is shown in Fig. 8.2a and depicted in the coronal illustration of Fig. 8.2b. Electrocortical stimulation is used with the objectives of defining the Rolandic cortex and the determination (localization) of the junction between the head and thumb segments of the pre- and postcentral gyri. The more important of these two junctions is that over the precentral gyrus, as noted earlier. It is not uncommon to *not* find a clearly defined thumb area. In these cases the area is assumed to be somewhere in the depths of the Rolandic fissure. It is in these cases when ongoing, very careful clinical monitoring of thumb function during the conduct of the corticectomy is most important in order to thwart a surprise postoperative deficit.

When operating on, or in the immediate vicinity of, the eloquent cortex, even with gentle manipulation, low-current bipolar coagulation, and restrained retraction, a *transient* clinical compromise of the function of that cortex often occurs. It may begin to occur as early as 15–20 min after the resection. This timing is very similar to that seen from simply retracting the eloquent cortex. For example, in the retraction of the parasagittal cortex for the removal of a falx meningioma—an observation that will be appreciated by those surgeons who operate under local anesthesia in circumstances where retraction of the eloquent cortex is required—the greater the force of the retraction, the earlier will a clinical deficit show itself and the greater will be the deficit. With moderate retraction there may be the onset of associated alteration in the function of the retracted cortex within 15–20 min. With removal of the retraction, the function usually returns within 20–30 min. Thus, if achieving the incision takes longer than this period of time, there is a possibility that the function of the thumb and hand may be lost before the incision is completed. Under these circumstances the surgeon has lost all of the advantage that led to the operation being done under local anesthesia, e.g., the ability to conduct the resection using the clinical monitoring of the function of the extremity *during* the surgery. If the function is lost, then the completion of this strategically important part of the operation would have to be carried out without any clinical monitoring and thus without knowledge of whether a potential deficit was being added to or completed as a result of the further surgery. Take-home message? Conduct this part of the operation without haste! Once this has been completed in the absence of a deficit, then any deficit that subsequently develops will *always*—well *nearly* always—be self-limited, i.e., will be transient, not permanent.

Another critical factor in the inferior Rolandic corticectomy consists of the preservation of the arterial vessels of passage whose final cortical irrigations are those of more superiorly situated Rolandic cortex, e.g., the upper extremity representation. Most of these *en passage* vessels can be seen superficially, emerging out of the Sylvian fissure and coursing over the inferior Rolandic cortex to reach more superior irrigation fields above the superior extent of the corticectomy. However, occasionally vessels of passage will enter beneath the surface of the gyri, coursing over the insula, reaching vertical sulci or the Rolandic fissure in the Sylvian fissure in which they may travel for varying distances before emerging onto the surface of the Rolandic cortex. These, therefore, will not be so apparent. The preservation of these *en passage* vessels, which of course travel in the subarachnoid space and hence are outside the pia, is achieved either by simple subpial dissection and/or through the process of "skeletonization" (as outlined in Sect. 5.2). The latter is sometime necessary when the vessel courses over the middle of a gyrus, but in general most of the isolation can be achieved by simple subpial resection. This often also requires that the resected cortex be taken out piece meal.

The final point to reemphasize is that if there is a marked difference between the pre- and postcentral gyral junctions of the head/neck and thumb the superior incision line is that over the precentral gyrus.

Figure 8.4 illustrates the dorsolateral surface of a left temporal lobe after the completion of an inferior Rolandic corticectomy and the preservation of the three *en passage* arteries whose courses were across it. The three arteries are included to simply exhibit the various ways in which the arteries achieve and cross the proposed

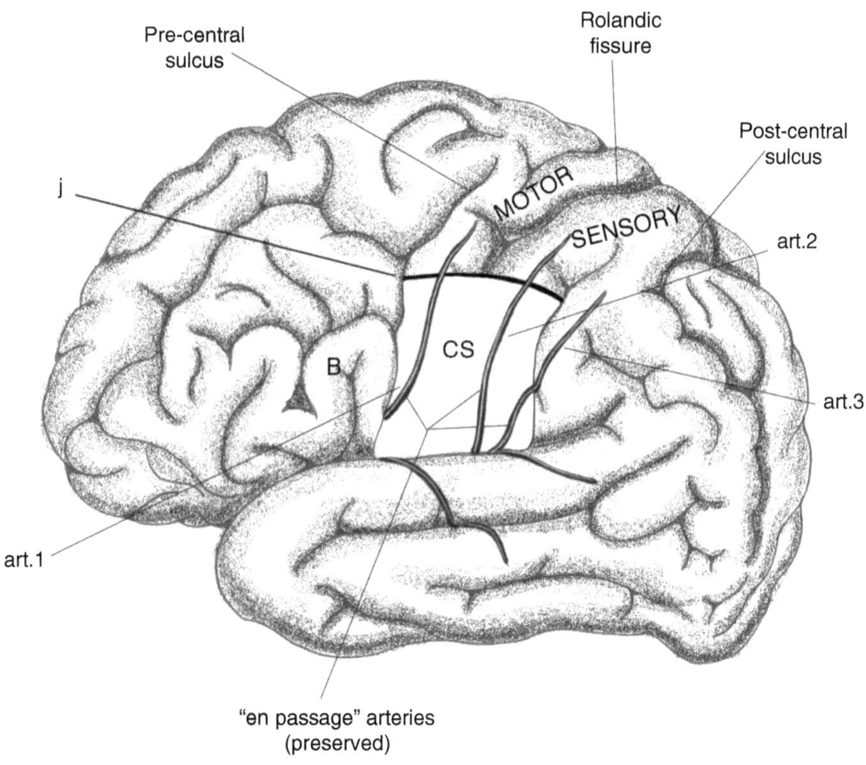

Fig. 8.4 Dorsolateral surface illustrating *en passage* arteries after completion of an inferior Rolandic corticectomy. The dorsolateral surface of the left hemisphere illustrating the completion of the inferior Rolandic corticectomy (CS) and the preservation of three en passage arteries. Each of the en passage arteries (*art.1–3*) has some differences from one another (see text). *art.1–3* en passage arteries, with respect to the corticectomy, arteries, *CS* inferior Rolandic corticectomy (completed), *j.* junction between the head/neck and thumb areas of the homunculus (see text)

corticectomy. The furthest left artery (art.1) emerges from the inferior precentral sulcus, crosses the CS, and irrigates the superior Rolandic cortex. The middle of the *en passage* arteries (art.2) follows the more typical course of the *en passage* arteries that require preservation in the conduct of an inferior Rolandic corticectomy. It emerges from the Sylvian fissure and then courses superiorly over the full caudal-rostral extent of the corticectomy area to irrigate the Rolandic cortex superior to the superior boundary of the corticectomy. The third artery (art.3) emerges from the Sylvian fissure and crosses the inferior part of the corticectomy to supply the parietal lobe cortex. In this particular case the likelihood is that arteries 1 and 3 would probably need little or no skeletonization.

8.4.2 The Corticectomy

Preparatory to the initiation of the surgery of the corticectomy, per se, will have been the identification of the homuncular junction of the head/neck and thumb by electrocortical stimulation, the skeletonization of any obvious *en passage* arteries over the proposed area of the corticectomy, and an able team member to begin the clinical monitoring of the patient's hand function, particularly when the incision at the homuncular junction is conducted.

The initiation of the corticectomy can be made anywhere. However, there is some advantage in initiating it just above the Sylvian fissure as some of the vessels irrigating only the corticectomy cortex may be sacrificed early on and will thereby decrease the vascularity of the remaining corticectomy incisions. Figure 8.5 outlines the coronal anatomy of the Rolandic cortical cross section and the various strategies of the corticectomy. Starting at the Sylvian fissure engenders the same philosophy as discussed in the initiation of the aTLY in the STG and sacrificing the vessels emerging from the Sylvian fissure feeding the anterior temporal lobe early (Sect. 8.6.2.4). With the confident awareness of the vessels that clearly will be sacrificed as part of the inferior Rolandic corticectomy, then the leptomeninges are coagulated ~2–3 mm above the Sylvian fissure (see incision line, – – – A, in Fig. 8.5b), incised in between any arteries to be sacrificed, some parenchyma removed from around the arteries, which are then picked up, coagulated, and incised. This is exactly the procedure followed in the initiation of the aTLY (in the STG). Any *en passage* vessels that require skeletonization should be skeletonized at this point. [The reason for making certain that the skeletonization is done now is that it reduces the likelihood of possibly prolonging any later surgery during or *after* the initiation of the incision of the superior margin (i.e., junction) of the corticectomy and *before* the surgery has been completed in that area; the concern of this eventuality has been outlined in the foregoing Sect. 8.4.1].

Figure 8.5a illustrates the junction of the head/neck and the thumb area in the inferior Rolandic cortex and the courses of the axons leaving the segments of those areal representations of the homunculus into the frontal stem. Once the suprasylvian incision is completed, the subpial resection is initiated along the inferior limb of the Rolandic operculum to the insula (see ↑↑↑→ directional designation in Fig. 8.5b),

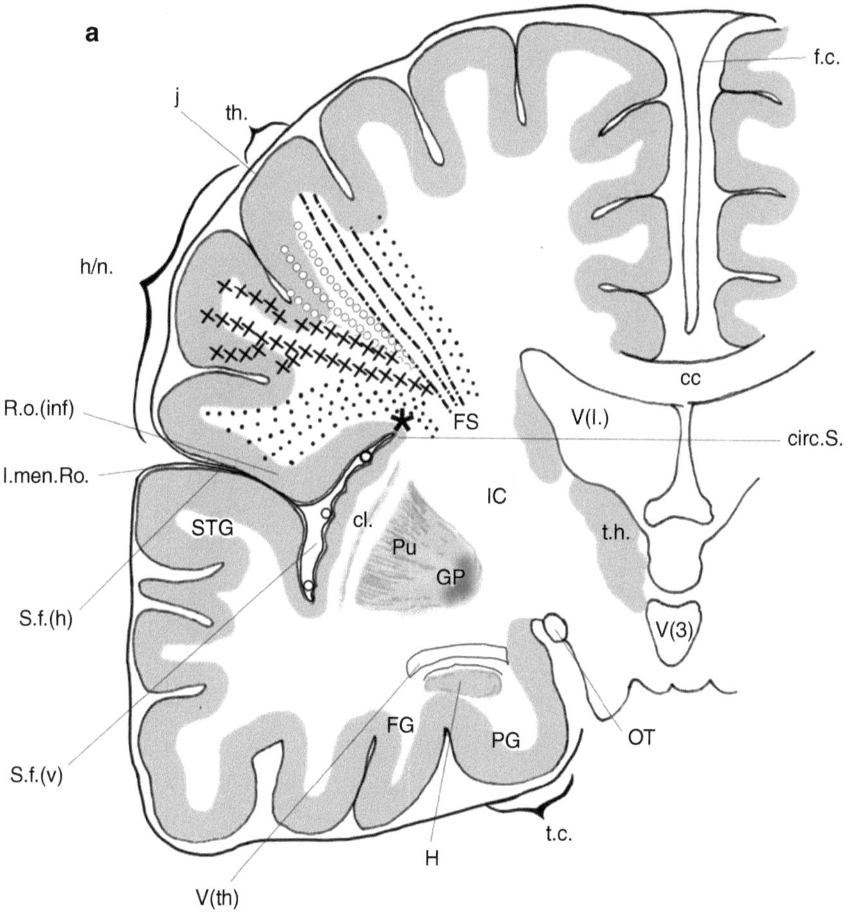

Fig. 8.5 The corticectomy of the inferior Rolandic cortex. Illustrations of the Rolandic cortex involved in an inferior Rolandic corticectomy. (**a**) The coronal section (similar illustration to Fig. 8.2b); note particularly the frontal stem and the layering of the connectivity of the various segments of the homunculus through the subcortical white matter and frontal stem; (**b**) the same figure as (**a**), primarily indicating the arrows outlining the incisional lines of the corticectomy; (**c**) the same coronal diagram after the removal of the corticectomy. *circ.S.* superior aspect of the circular sulcus of the insula, *cc* corpus callosum, *cl.* claustrum, *CS* corticectomy area, *f.c.* falx cerebri, *FL* frontal lobe, *FG* fusiform gyrus, *FS* frontal stem, *GP* globus pallidus, *h/n* head/neck area of the homunculus, *H* hippocampus, *IC* internal capsule, *j.* junction of the homuncular head/neck and thumb areas, *l.men.Ro.* leptomeningeal investment of the inferior surface of the Rolandic operculum, *OT* optic tract, *PG* parahippocampal gyrus, *Pu* putamen, *R.o.(inf.)* inferior surface of the frontal operculum (superior surface of the horizontal limb of the Sylvian fissure), *STG* superior temporal gyrus, *S.f.(h)* Sylvian fissure (horizontal limb), *S.f.(v)* Sylvian fissure (vertical limb), *t.c.* tentorium cerebelli, *t.h.* thalamus, *th.* thumb area of the homunculus, *V(3)* third ventricle, *V(l.)* lateral ventricle, *V(th)* temporal horn of the lateral ventricle, – – – ∪ the incision line ~ 2–3 mm above the Sylvian fissure, ↑↑↑→ the direction of the initial subpial resection in the Rolandic operculum, ●●●● the superior incision line, in the subcortical white matter, of the corticectomy, * the medial juncture of the inferior frontal opercular cortex and the insula

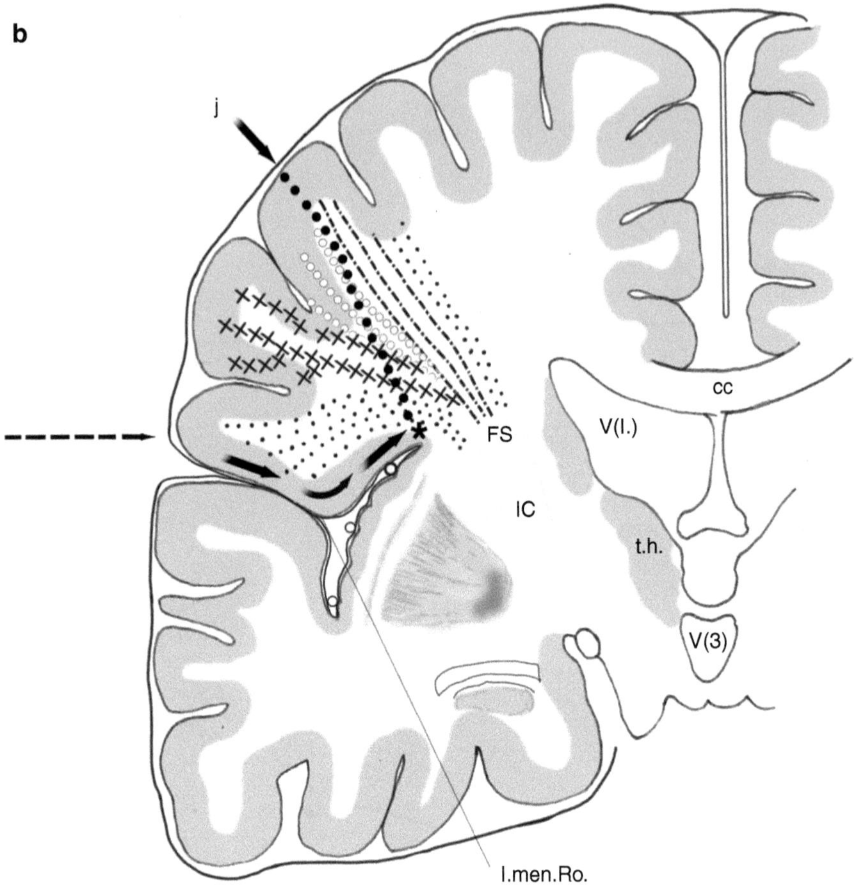

Fig. 8.5 (continued)

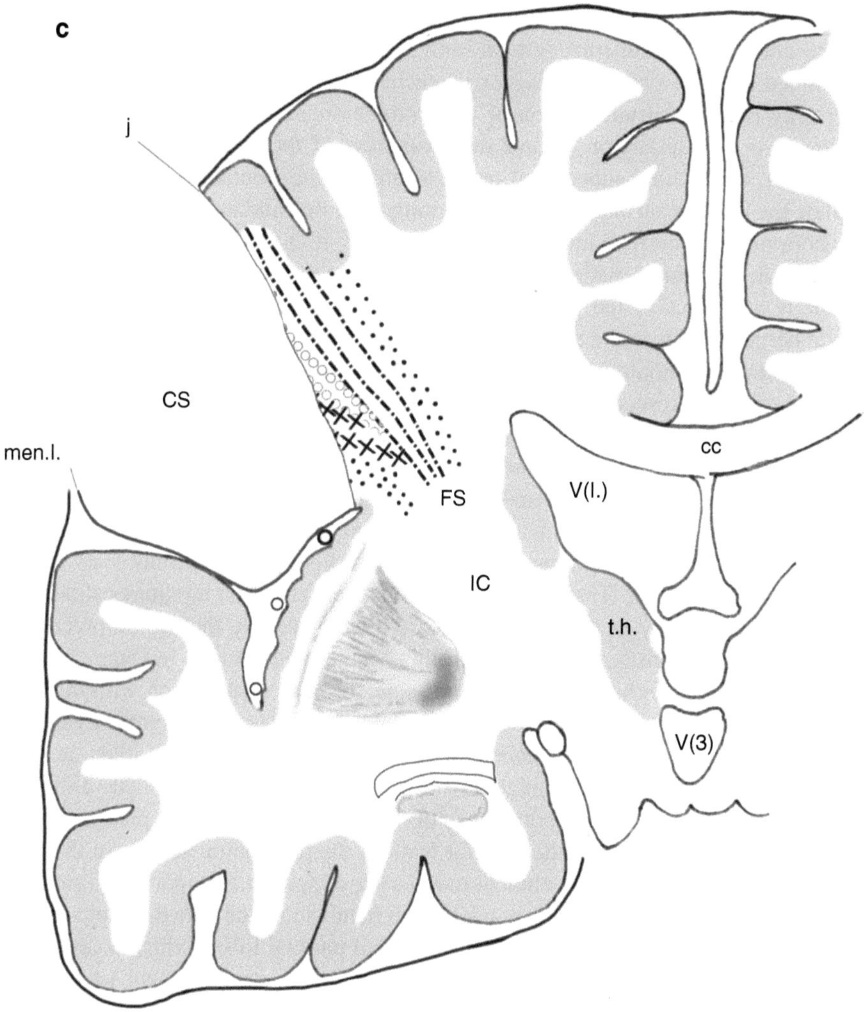

Fig. 8.5 (continued)

i.e., the superior cortex of the horizontal limb of the Sylvian fissure and then into the lateral cortex of the superior vertical limb of the Sylvian fissure. This resection is continued until the end of that cortex is reached, recognized by the end of any further gray matter, the termination of the leptomeningeal investment that has been followed in the dissection, and/or the awareness of the insula (*). This point is important, as the final subcortical incision through the frontal stem, which in fact will be the inferior surface of the corticectomy, will be conducted to that point from the bottom of the cortical incision at the head/neck-thumb junction.

Now the incision is made in the junction between the head/neck and thumb areas of the homunculus of the precentral gyrus; as shown in Fig. 8.5b the incision is made perpendicular to the surface, and at the bottom of the gray matter of the cortex, it is then immediately angled in a line to the point where the end of the Rolandic cortical opercular resection ended at the insula (*). This line is illustrated in Fig. 8.5b (see ●●●● line). Also, during this part of the surgery, there must be continual ongoing clinical monitoring of the patient's hand function, particularly the thumb. Therefore, as outlined in this and previous chapters, the incision is carried both superficially and "away" from what is the eloquent cortex. In this case the "eloquent cortex" is actually the superomedial frontal stem fibers of the connectivity of the hand, which are at risk. This resection and whatever retraction it requires should be conducted as quickly as it can be done carefully, especially that in the precentral gyrus, for the reasons outlined earlier in this chapter and detailed in Chap. 5 (Sect. 5.5.3). Figure 8.5c exhibits primarily the same coronal cross section with the now absence of the parenchyma of the corticectomy; only the leptomeningeal investment of the inferior surface of the Rolandic operculum remains. Figure 8.4 illustrates the removal as seen from the dorsolateral surface of a left hemisphere. The corticectomy, of course, will include both banks of the Rolandic fissure, the posterior bank of the precentral sulcus and the anterior bank of the postcentral sulcus. In the case of the dominant hemisphere, clinical monitoring of speech is important during the resection of the latter two. In the nondominant hemisphere the peri-Rolandic cortex, juxtaposed to the corticectomy in the frontal and parietal lobes, which is identified as being epileptogenic by ECoG, is often resected as an additional part of the surgery.

In the case where a confident junction between head/neck and thumb cannot be determined because of the lack of thumb responses, it is reasonable to initiate the incision in roughly the same area or just below it, coincident with very good clinical monitoring in the awake patient. It is this eventuality where the latter is most important. If the incision can be achieved without a suspicion of altered weakness of the thumb, the remainder, still carefully clinically monitored, can nearly always be carried out uneventfully.

In order to provide the verification of the foregoing few pages, regarding the inferior Rolandic corticectomy, I will note a paragraph in one of the letters that I received from Dr. Rasmussen: "The cortex of the sensory and motor face area in the dominant hemisphere can be removed completely without producing a lasting dysphasia. It is essential, of course, that the excision be carried out with great care to avoid touching the adjacent banks of the anterior and posterior speech convolutions and to avoid any interference with their blood supply, and also to avoid jiggling the underlying white matter which might interfere with projection fibers from the two speech areas. I have been particularly interested in this group of patients because it shows quite clearly in my opinion that the integration between the functions of the anterior and posterior speech centers is carried out by means of some sub-cortical region rather than via cortical connections on the surface."

8.5 Superior Rolandic Corticectomy

The realization of the ability to remove the inferior Rolandic cortex with impunity has really led to the distinction between this part of the Rolandic cortex and the more superiorly located cortex, which subserves appendicular function (arm and leg), which cannot be removed without producing a permanent deficit. The realization of this distinction really gives rise to two Rolandic cortices from the point of view of surgical license, an inferior and a superior.

As already noted, the superior Rolandic cortex, historically, has shared in common with the language cortex and the primary visual cortex the group of areas that are inviolate to the surgeon's scalpel and hence have not been amenable to surgical intervention, with a single exception. The exception consists of those instances in which structural lesions have significantly compromised the function of the (eloquent) cortical area, the seizures are significantly intractable, and the patient and her/his caregivers clearly accept that the potential benefit of the surgery is much greater than the risk of its conduct. Thus, if the function is such as to render the arm or leg severely impaired and considered to be permanent and that the added impairment from removal of the cortex is judged to be relatively insignificant, compared to the relief of seizures, then resection of this otherwise "eloquent" cortex is perfectly reasonable, when full understanding of the patient is part of the preoperative discussion.

Much of the foregoing discussion has changed and is only acknowledged historically, as a result of the introduction of the operation of multiple subpial transections (MSTs) by Morrell in 1973.

8.6 Multiple Subpial Transections

8.6.1 Cortical Microanatomy: The Rational for MSTs

Although the technique of MSTs was noted by Morrell in 1973, it gained recognition through further articles by the Chicago group some years later (Morrell et al. 1989; Whisler 1995). It consists of a number ("multiple") of intracortical incisions beneath the pial ("subpial") membrane, resulting in "transections" of the subpial parenchyma, which extend across a cortical gyrus (or gyri). They suggested that the transections, perpendicular to the cortical surface, should be something of the order of 5 mm apart, to a depth that includes the full thickness of the cortex. While these suggestions were based on some experimental data, nevertheless there was a reasonable amount of arbitrariness to their suggested parameters of the operation. The rationale of the transections is that they interrupt the *intra*cortical connectivity, or the immediately situated subcortical U-fibers that traverse the area in which the incisions are made, and thereby impede, or abolish, the *intra*cortical spread of epileptic activity that is parallel to the cortical surface. The cellular anatomy of the cortex is such that the functional units are primarily vertically oriented (Colonnier 1966).

For an understanding of the rationale for the use of the treatment of multiple subpial transections, the reader must have some knowledge of the intracortical anatomy and physiology of the cerebral cortex. It was upon these bases, derived from observations on experimental animals, that Morrell and colleagues recommended the operative rationale for the operation. The cortical anatomy underlying the rationale for the operation was briefly covered earlier in this chapter (Sect. 8.1.1). These will be briefly enumerated. They include the following: (1) the functional units of the neocortex are columns of cells, perpendicular to the cortical surface; (2) the simultaneous discharge of a critical mass of neurons is required for the genesis of epileptic discharge; (3) horizontal propagation, i.e., parallel to the surface, occurs in the cortex and is a significant part of the spread of epileptogenicity; (4) "Cortical islands greater than 5 mm in width, or horizontal connections of greater than 5 mm, can support paroxysmal discharge" (Morrell et al. 1989); (5) pure vertical incisions in the cortex interfere minimally with cortical function, ostensibly because of the columnar arrangement of functional units; (6) subpial transection in isolated slabs of the cortex interfere minimally with normal electrocortical activity; and (7) transections of the cortex can be carried out with minimal cortical vascular injury, in that the vasculature consists of vessels coursing into the cortex from the pia and perpendicular to it.

8.6.2 The Technique

The initial instrumentation, now used for MSTs, had been used for many years in experimental animals, for creating what are called "isolated slabs" of the cortex in order to study the characteristics of pure cortical properties (Burns 1949, 1950, 1951). The isolated slabs, under these circumstances, typically have a rectilinear dimension, roughly 10×15 mm and a depth just greater than the cortical mantle. Classically the instrumentation for the production of the slab consisted of a length of platinum (Pt) wire, which was modified for the experimentation, one end of which is heated until a small ball is formed at the end of the wire. Figure 8.6a demonstrates the straight piece of Pt wire with the expanded, "balled" end. It is then bent (Fig. 8.6b) at a 90° angle, a distance from the tip that is just slightly greater than the depth of the cortex to be transected, i.e., ~3–5 mm. This first segment is that which actually transects the cortical layer. A second bend is then made a further distance from the first bend (Fig. 8.6c), thus creating a second segment. The bend is made in the same parallel, with respect to the wire, as the initial bend at 90°. The result is that the remaining wire is parallel to the initial segment. The length of the second segment will represent the length of the proposed incision. In the experimental

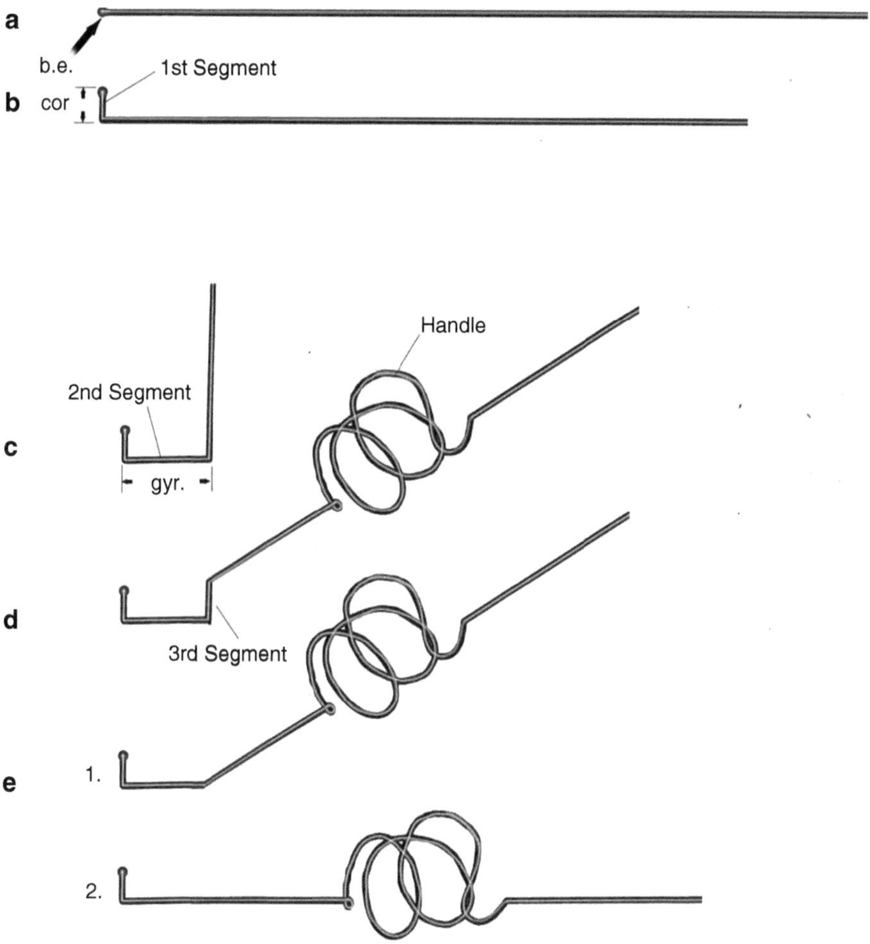

Fig. 8.6 Instrumentation for the conduct of MSTs. Illustration of the type of instrumentation used for the production of MSTs. (**a**) The initial length of wire with a "balled," or polished, end; (**b**) the first bend, which is made at an angle of 90°, such that the resulting initial segment represents the ~ depth of the (cortical) incisions of the MSTs; (**c**) a second bend is made at 90° in the same parallel as the initial, but in the opposite direction; this gives rise to a second segment between these two bends, the length of which is approximately the length of the proposed incision, e.g., about the same dimension as the width of a gyrus, i.e., ~10–12 mm; (**d**) a final bend is made in the same parallel at ~45° such that the third segment is the same length as the first segment; a few centimeters further along the length of the remaining wire (e.g., 5–15 cm) an alteration in the wire, usually a group of bends are made over the course of a few centimeters in order to fashion a type of "handle which is mandatory in the ability to use the instrument (see text)"; (**e**) a miscellany of MST transectors (see text). *b.e.* "balled" end of wire (see text), *cor.* the first bend is made such that the first segment is just slightly greater than the thickness of the cortex, *gyr.* the second segment is roughly the length of the width of a gyrus, e.g., 10–12 mm

animal (cat) in which the technique was devised, its length was the length of a side of the rectangle of the "isolated slab" of the cortex. In the human cortex its length is roughly the width of the gyrus, i.e., ~1 cm. A further bend is made (Fig. 8.6d), creating a third segment, which is the same length of the first segment, e.g., roughly the thickness of the cortex being transected. This bend is at something of the order of 45°. Finally, 5–15 cm further along the wire, some type of "handle" is created, which is mandatory for the control of the instrument when making the subpial transections. It is also shown in Fig. 8.6d. Without such a handle the wire tends to rotate in the fingers of the surgeon with the manipulation required for the transection. Thus, this handle is often best fashioned with bends that are even perpendicular to one another.

The technique involves a punctate penetration of the leptomeningeal cortex at a point where the transecting incision is to be initiated; the point is placed at the junction of the sulcal and exposed surfaces. This can usually be easily achieved with the use of a small (? # 25) hypodermic needle (Fig. 8.7A.a, b). The balled end of the wire is then gently introduced through the puncture site in the direction of the incision, keeping the ball applied to the underside of the leptomeninges, i.e., subpial (see Fig. 8.7b). The wire is then rotated such that the "heel" of the first bend is depressed into the cortex through the punctate hole, while maintaining the balled end juxtaposed to the underside of the leptomeninges (Fig. 8.7c). This ball can be visualized through the leptomeninges, as during this maneuver it will move somewhat in the direction of the proposed MST. This maneuver will also allow the heel of the transector, as it is depressed, to put an incision into the cortex beneath the stab incision. By continuing to gently push this segment in the appropriate direction, the transection through the depth of the cortical mantle (the length of the segment) will be made (see Fig. 8.7d). The depth, of course, can be continually monitored by visually keeping the balled end of the instrument juxtaposed to the undersurface of the leptomeningeal investment of the summit of the gyrus during its travel. (In experimental animals the rectilinear "isolated slab of the cortex" requires two punctures, in opposite angles of the rectangle, from each of which two sides of the rectangle are created. Although not pertinent to the MSTs under consideration here, nevertheless the final isolation of the experimental slab of the cortex in an animal requires the instrument to be placed in one of the transecting positions and then rotating it in the same position, parallel to the surface, thus undercutting the rectangle and creating the isolation of the cortical slab. In the operation of MSTs in human epileptogenic cortex, only the transections are made.)

Fig. 8.7 Demonstrations in the steps of surgical MSTs. Demonstrates the steps in conducting a subpial transection. (**A.a**) The surface of a gyrus in which punctate stab incisions are made with a #25 hypodermic needle in one edge of the gyrus, e.g., at the juncture of the summit of the gyrus at the sulcus; (**A.b**) a coronal section showing the stab incision through both membranes of the leptomeninges; (**b**) a coronal section in to which the transector has been introduced through the stab incision, maintaining the ball (o polished) end of the wire up against the undersurface to the leptomeninges; (**c**) the instrument is then depressed and slowly pushed across the gyrus, with the polished end juxtaposed to the underside of the pial membrane of the gyrus; (**d**) eventually the whole of the third segment of the transector will reach the punctate incision and will drop in through it (see text)

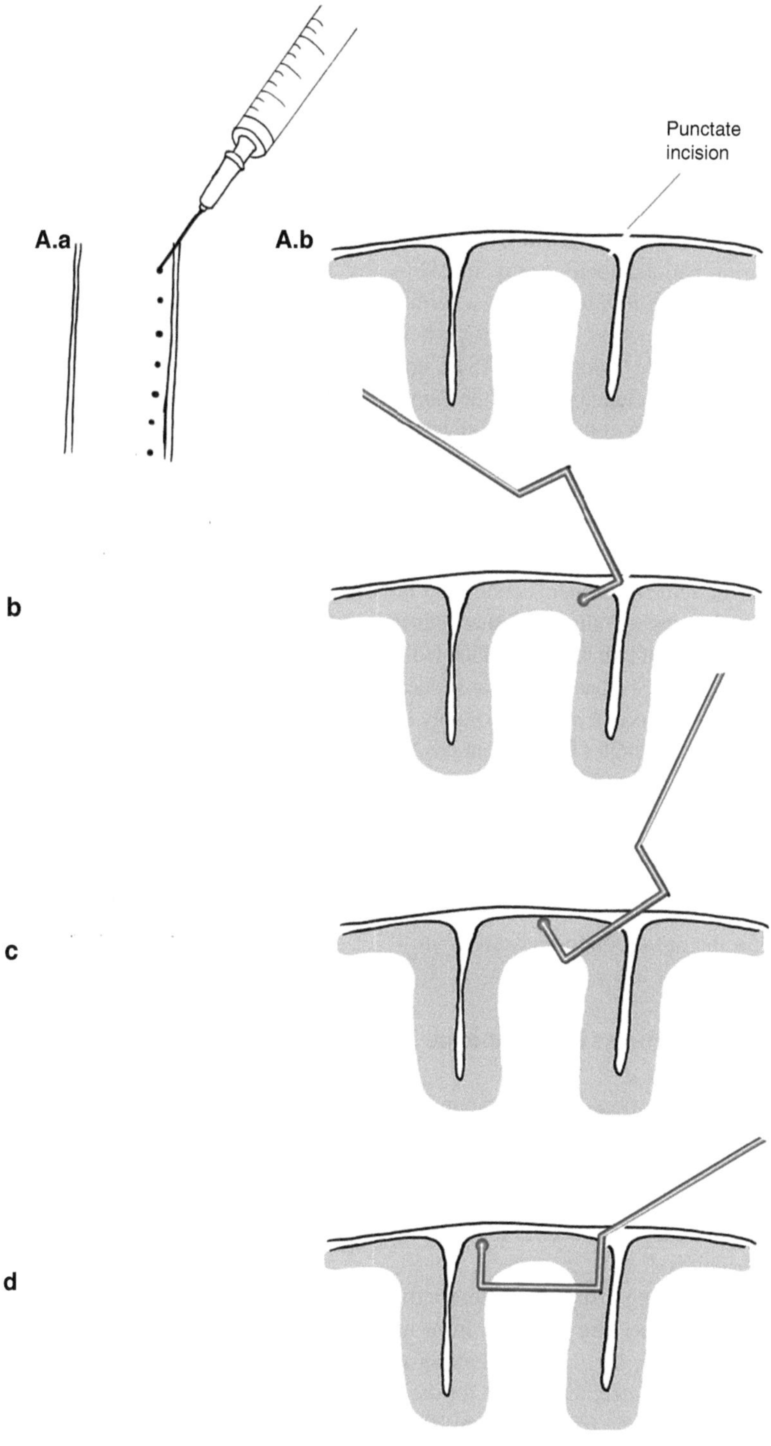
A.a
A.b
Punctate
incision
b
c
d

The transections are simply unidirectional subpial incisions perpendicular to the gyrus and its associated sulci. In Fig. 8.7A.a a number of dots, approximately 5 mm apart, are illustrated along the summit of the gyrus at the junction with the sulcus. These are simply those that have been judged to be the epileptogenic cortex that is to be transected and thus in each the steps in the foregoing test are simply repeated in each of them. The rather remarkable minimalist effect of these incisions is worth briefly reviewing here with a clinical case. I had as a patient a young teenage girl with intractable left parietocentral seizures, from a low-grade glioma, upon whom I had performed a superior parietal lobulectomy in 1986. Her postoperative seizure-free period of 3 years then ceased, and in 1990 a further parietal cortical resection was undertaken with much less success and in 1992, when her seizure frequency rose to 5–15 per day, she underwent the operation of MSTs, under local anesthesia. Eleven MSTs were carried out, which included seven in the thumb to toe area of the postcentral gyrus and four in the forearm area of the precentral gyrus. Rather to my surprise she had no difficulty in walking and using her hand well the following day! Her postoperative course speaks to the fact that the operation can be rather innocuous. She has had a normal neurological examination since that time. It is now 22 years since the MST operation, during which time her first anti-epileptic drug (AED) was removed and then during the beginning of the removal of her second (and last) AED in 1997 she had three small ~ one minute episodes of "slight lightheadedness" and "things looked far away from her" over the course of two months, which led to her being returned to the dosage of 200 mg of Tegretol t.i.d. She had a peculiar sudden onset of numbness in her left hand in 2009, 12 years later, thought to have possibly been an ischemic event, but the investigation was perfectly normal. (This patient has had a remarkable, nearly 22-year seizure-free course. It should not be construed as indicating that this has been the typical result of MST surgery, for such is not the case; however, it does indicate how effective the use of MST surgery can be and how much the human Rolandic cortex can be transgressed without a resulting impairment. I have wondered whether the MSTs having been conducted down the sulcal surfaces as well as the gyral surfaces could have been responsible for the post-operative seizure control!).

8.6.3 Variations in Technique

The ideal MST operation would consist of the maximum number of MSTs that can be performed, within the epileptogenic cortex, without the production of an unwanted neurological deficit. In other words, the optimal operation will consist of the interruption of as many intracortical connections as possible, short of creating a neurological deficit. There is really no truly scientific evidence as to how this ideal is best achieved.

The transecting instrumentation for the conduct of the MSTs is not terribly sophisticated and in fact can be made from many of the wire materials that exist in any operating theater, e.g., coarse stainless steel sutures, hypodermic/spinal tap needles, stylets from long needles, stylets for the probing of wounds, etc. Ideally the "transectors" could be made from platinum (Pt) with the end of the wire being heated to the point of melting and thereby producing a small ball at its end, as outlined above (Fig. 8.6) in the case of producing the isolated cortical slabs in experimental animals.

However, the balled end of the Pt wire can be substituted by simply using a fine metal file to remove the sharpness of the ends of the array of hospital metals noted in the foregoing. With good attention paid to the filing of the end can be made just as smooth as the ideal Pt balled end, especially with it being polished with very fine sandpaper. The initial segment is made about 3–5 mm in length (Fig. 8.6b), to correspond to the depth of the cortex that is to be transected. The second segment (Fig. 8.6c) is then fashioned to cover the length of the transection. In the case of gyri, this will be something of the order of the width of the gyrus, i.e., ~10±2–3 mm. It will be longer in length in some instances, such as including the sulcal cortex in the transections. When using such wire the "handle" can be made out of a number of overlapping bends in the wire at the appropriate area along the course of the wire (see Fig. 8.6d). This will be determined by the amount of length of the wire from the second bend that provides a comfortable manipulation as determined by the surgeon.

Taking the lead of Morrell and his colleagues, most surgeons who use the operation develop their own method. I was biased by Burns introduction of the isolated slab in cats, as I earned my graduate degree under him while he was at McGill University. However, as I have indicated many times, we choose methods through our many channels extending from residency to staff consultants. For example, with respect to MSTs Wyler and his colleagues use their MST instrumentation a reverse of 180° from what was Morrell's use, which I have described in the foregoing; instead of moving the point along the underside of the pial membrane, they use the point end downward, as they believe that this is safer (Wyler et al. 1995; Wyler 2001). Thus, there is also potential variation with respect to the parameters of the technique including: (1) the depth of the incisions below the surface, (2) the distance between the transections, (3) the number of transections, (4) the involvement of the sulcal cortex in the transections, and (5) the interruption of the subcortical U-fibers, especially those at the bottom of sulci. Again, it must be reiterated and emphasized that so far as I know there has been no significant systematic scientific investigative study that answers these queries with absolute certainty.

I will outline briefly my own practice—again, not arrived at scientifically, but rather simply by continuing to be more radical, through increasing experience with the operation. I cannot say that mine is any better than others and in fact I cannot say confidently that the more radical recent MSTs have achieved better outcomes! Since, I have always operated under local anesthesia, I have had the advantage of continual clinical monitoring during the procedures involving MSTs. Under these circumstances the limit of the radicalism of the parameters of the MSTs, in any given operation, has been heavily dependent upon the ongoing clinical neurological monitoring following each transection. Hence, in the absence of a significantly developing neurological deficit, the procedure is continued, the endpoints being the apparent development of a possible deficit, or the achievement of the premeditated planned cortical coverage of MSTs. Given the foregoing noted potential limits of the procedure, my own practice is to carry out the usual transections, approximately 5 mm apart over the surface cortex identified as being part of the epileptogenic focus.

In addition to the foregoing surface transections, I have chosen to also include the sulcal cortex. This requires an extra stab incision, so that each of the sulci, at either side of the gyrus, can be approached. The latter is far less straightforward than the surface cortex, primarily because of the lack of the visually monitored and guided transection, which is available in the case of the surface of a gyrus. However, in addition to this loss of visual observation, the sulcal transection of the subpial cortex is blind to the surgeon. Further, the only membrane of use in the sulcal cortical transection is the pial membrane, a considerably finer membrane than the leptomeningeal membrane over the summit of the gyri. Thus, in the sulcal transections the surgeon is entirely dependent upon the mechanical "feel" of the transector against the pial membrane, without any certain knowledge of the depth of the sulcus! When the sensitivity becomes vague or truly difficult to appreciate, then my practice has been to stop at that point. When the transector is being withdrawn, it must be done so in a very, very slow gentle manner, as it can get caught on the pial meningeal investment at the depth of the sulcus. However, if one chooses to include the sulcal cortex, then the transector may be altered physically; there are some suggestions of alterations noted in Fig. 8.6e. For example, that in Fig. 8.6e2 exhibits a transector with one bend in it. This can be used either way around in the sulcus. If there is concern about getting the balled end caught in the depth of the pial membrane, then it can be turned around and thus the balled end will then be at the depth of the cortical gray matter, rather than against the pial membrane. In this case one loses the "feeling" of the ball going along the pia, and thus in this circumstance, it is better to arbitrarily chose the depth of the transection.

8.7 Safe Limits of Resection

The posterior frontal premotor corticectomy can be carried out without concern of postoperative motor deficit, so long as the precentral motor cortex is not injured. This is especially true for the nondominant hemisphere. In the dominant hemisphere the removal of the SMA may be associated with a transient speech deficit, consisting of muteness. However, it is a transcortical motor aphasia. It usually lasts little more than 3 or 4 days but very occasionally can last as long as 2 or 3 weeks. A case in point will be noted here, not only because of the prolonged period of muteness but also because of the fact that the speech deficit occurred suddenly with a simple 1–2 mm discrete incision during the intraoperative course of the resection well above Broca's area in the parasagittal area. This young man was a R3 medical resident, who, following a grand mal seizure and the initiation of phenytoin, presented with intractable focal seizures characterized by alterations in speech or speech arrests that lasted up to an hour. The muteness he had suddenly during the operation remained while he was in hospital in which he remained for 10 days, as he was from another part of the country. During these 10 days we were all concerned about whether I had given him a permanent language deficit. He retained it for the best part of a week following discharge and 2 months later it was normal. The language experts felt that it had the characteristics of the transcortical motor aphasia. I accepted this diagnosis, but certainly I had never seen this last as it did with him.

The inferior Rolandic cortex can be removed with impunity, in either the nondominant or dominant hemisphere. This "inferior" cortex refers to that which is

Table 8.1 Distance between the Sylvian fissure and the thumb segment of the homunculus

Anatomical area	Mean distance above the Sylvian fissure (mm)	*n*	Range (mm)
Thumb segment of homunculus	28.8	26	18–45

inferior to the thumb area of the homunculus, i.e., those involving the face, larynx, pharynx, etc. As pointed out in the section on inferior Rolandic corticectomy (Sect. 8.4), there must not be encroachment upon the cortical thumb connectivity within the frontal stem in order to preclude an impairment of thumb movement. In the dominant hemisphere attention must additionally be directed to the very delicate removal of the cortex in the anterior and posterior borders, in the vicinity of the precentral and postcentral sulci, respectively, as the juxtaposed cortex is "eloquent"—Broca's and parietal speech cortex, respectively. The inferior Rolandic corticectomy frequently results in a transient dysarthria. However, it is worth reemphasizing the fact that once the incision is conducted at the juncture between head/neck and thumb on the Rolandic cortex, the remainder of this part of the procedure should be conducted as quickly as possible. Once this has been completed, in the absence of a deficit, then any deficit that subsequently develops will nearly *always* be self-limited, gradually disappearing, or markedly improving, within a few days postoperatively; the rate of this improvement or disappearance will be inversely related to the evident severity of the deficit (see Chap. 13).

Table 8.1 is simply a record of a number of measurable amounts of head and neck representations in the inferior Rolandic cortex. The range (18–45 mm) is not quite as great as that found by Penfield and Rasmussen, but it is still significant. The variation speaks to the effect that the use of local anesthesia for the conduct of the inferior Rolandic corticectomy is mandatory.

References

Brodmann K. Beiträge zur histologischen Lokalisation der Grosshirnrinde. I. Mitt, Der Rolandica. J Psychol Neurol. 1903;2:79–107.

Burns BD. Some properties of the cat's isolated cerebral cortex. J Physiol. 1949;110:9P (abstract).

Burns BD. Some properties of the cat's isolated cerebral cortex. J Physiol. 1950;111:50–68.

Burns BD. Some properties of isolated cerebral cortex in the unanaesthetized cat. J Physiol. 1951;112:156–75.

Colonnier ML. The structural design of the neocortex. In: Eccles JC, editor. Brain and conscious experience. New York: Springer; 1966. pp. 1–23.

Garey LJ. Description of individual brain maps. In: Garey JL, editor. Brodmann's 'Localization in the Cerebral Cortex'. London: Smith-Gordon and Company; 1994. pp. 107–74.

Girvin JP. Chapter 73. Complications of epilepsy surgery. In: Luders HO, editor. Epilepsy surgery. New York: Raven; 1991. pp. 653–60.

Lehman R, Andermann F, Olivier A, Tandon PN, Quesney LF, Rasmussen TB. Seizures with onset in the sensorimotor face area: clinical patterns and results of surgical treatment in 20 patients. Epilepsia. 1994;35:1117–24.

Morrell F. Multiple subpial transection for the surgical treatment of focal epilepsy. EEG Clin Neurophysiol. 1973;34:714 [abstract].

Morrell F, Whisler WW, Bleck TP. Multiple subpial transection: a new approach to the surgical treatment of focal epilepsy. J Neurosurg. 1989;70:231–9.
Penfield W. The cerebral cortex in man. I. The cerebral cortex and consciousness. Arch Neurol Psychiatr. 1938;40:417–42.
Penfield W, Jasper H. Epilepsy and the functional anatomy of the human brain. Boston: Little, Brown and Co; 1954. p. 896.
Penfield W, Rasmussen T. The cerebral cortex of man: a clinical study of localization of function. New York: Hafner Publishing Company; 1968. p. 248.
Penfield W, Rasmussen T. A clinical study of localization of function. In: Penfield W, Rasmussen T, eds. The cerebral cortex of man. New York: MacMillan; 1950. pp. 184–6.
Penfield W, Roberts L. Speech and brain-mechanisms. Princeton: Princeton University Press; 1959. p. 286.
Rasmussen T. Cortical resection in the treatment of focal epilepsy. In: Purpura DP, Penry JK, Walter RD, editors. Advances in neurology, vol. 8. New York: Raven; 1975a. pp. 139–54.
Rasmussen T. Surgery for epilepsy arising in regions other than the temporal and frontal lobes. In: Purpura DP, Penry JK, Walter RD, editors. Advances in neurology, vol. 8. New York: Raven; 1975b. p. 206–26.
Rasmussen T. Commentary: Extratemporal cortical excisions and hemispherectomy. In: Engel J, editor. Surgical Treatment of the Epilepsies. New York: Raven Press; 1987, pp. 417–24.
Whisler WW. Multiple subpial transection. Tech Neurosurg. 1995;1:40–4.
Wyler AR, Hermann BP, Somes G. Extent of medial temporal resection on outcome from anterior temporal lobectomy: a randomized prospective study. Neurosurgery. 1995;37:982–91.
Wyler AR. Multiple subpial transections. Chapter 88. In: Lüders HO, editor. Epilepsy Surgery, 2nd edition. New York: Raven Press; 2001. pp. 807–11.

9 Parietal Lobe Resections

9.1 Introduction

In this section the postcentral gyral cortex will not be considered, as it is more accurately included in the central, or Rolandic, cortex than the bulk of the parietal lobe cortex. Hence, the reader is referred to Chap. 8 regarding this cortex.

When one views the registries of epilepsy cases from many institutions, there is often a relative paucity of cases of parietal lobe epilepsy. While there is some variety in the percentage of parietal lobe epilepsy (PLE) cases, nevertheless many figures fall beneath the 10 % mark. I suspect that parietal lobe epilepsy is more common than is normally appreciated in these registries. One of the reasons for this is that this cortex cannot be considered "eloquent" in the way that it is defined and utilized in this book (see Sects. 3.1 and 4.1). Some refer to this as "association" cortex. Thus, it is not uncommon to have parietal foci in the mid- to posteroparietal cortex that comes to notice when the epileptic discharge spreads to juxtaposed cortices, which do represent eloquent cortex the stimulation of which exhibits clinically recognizable altered neurological function, e.g., visual, Rolandic, post-Sylvian temporo-occipitoparietal dominant cortex, etc. Under these circumstances clinical observations of the epileptic semiology lead to these epileptic foci being more likely attributed clinically to these eloquent cortices, than to the clinically silent (i.e., non-eloquent) association cortical foci in the parietal cortex, per se. This is exemplified in various parts of the literature. The statement "It has been long recognized that clinically similar seizures may arise from epileptic foci at different sites and that a focus at a particular site may give rise to a variety of seizure types by virtue of differing pathways of seizure spread" was the initial sentence of the very excellent paper devoted to a consideration of parietal and occipital lobe epilepsies by Sveinbjornsdottir and Duncan (1993). The publications of Williamson et al. (1992) and Salanova et al. (1995) are also good descriptions in dealing with PLE. The latter describes the patients with parietal lobe epilepsy who were investigated at the Montreal Neurological Institute over a 50-year period.

J.P. Girvin, *Operative Techniques in Epilepsy*,
DOI 10.1007/978-3-319-10921-3_9

The Montreal series of patients with parietal lobe epilepsy was similar to many epilepsy centres, in that a great number of their epileptic cases had primarily Rolandic semiology, either alone or with associated features such as "dizziness, cephalic sensation, conscious or unconscious contraversion, epigastric sensation, dysphasia, or automatism" (Rasmussen 1975b).

The medical students who were educated before the waning years of the twentieth century will remember learning that the parietal lobe cortex, posterior to the postcentral sulcus, was involved in numerous activities, such as dressing, distinguishing between right and left sides of the body, agnosia associated with the identification of fingers, etc. In large part the origin of these neurological deficits was attributed to the parietal cortex, posterior to the postcentral gyrus, by Critchley in his *The Parietal Lobes* (1955). However, it is now known that this is perhaps more the result of the destruction of the white matter underlying the mid- to posterior parietal cortex, as Rasmussen has shown that the removal of this cortex, per se, posterior to the postcentral sulcus, may infrequently be associated with mild, transient sensory deficits, but never associated with a permanent sensory neurological deficit (Corkin et al. 1970; Rasmussen 1975a, p. 298). That is to say, a pure "decortication" of this posterior parietal cortex results in no clinically demonstrable permanent defect. However, Mattingly et al. with the currently available much more sophisticated investigative technology have more recently demonstrated evidence of complex alterations in movements as determined by subtle unilateral neglect in patients with inferior parietal lobule (IPL) lesions (1998).

I will add to the immediate foregoing a paragraph in a letter that Dr. Rasmussen wrote to me in 1984: "In regard to the parietal cortical excisions, we have not seen the "parietal syndrome" from excisions in either the dominant or the non-dominant parietal lobe. I am sure this syndrome which is most clearly seen in patients with stroke is actually due to damage to projection fibers from the depths of the parietal lobe, and does not occur when the parietal lobe excisions are carried out the way they do for epilepsy. We have not seen this even when we have removed the posterior third of the non-dominant hemisphere up to the postcentral gyrus."

9.2 Superior Parietal Lobulectomy (SPLY)

9.2.1 Anatomy

The boundaries of the superior parietal lobule (SPL) are relatively well defined. The anterior boundary consists of the superior part of the postcentral sulcus dorsolaterally and the paracentral lobule medially, the medial extent is the subparietal sulcus, the lateral (inferior) boundary is the intraparietal sulcus, and the posterior boundary consists of the parieto-occipital sulcus medially and the arbitrary dorsolateral line between the superior aspect of the parieto-occipital sulcus superiorly and the "occipital notch" inferiorly. These features are illustrated in the dorsolateral (a) and medial (b) surfaces of a left cerebral hemisphere in Fig. 9.1.

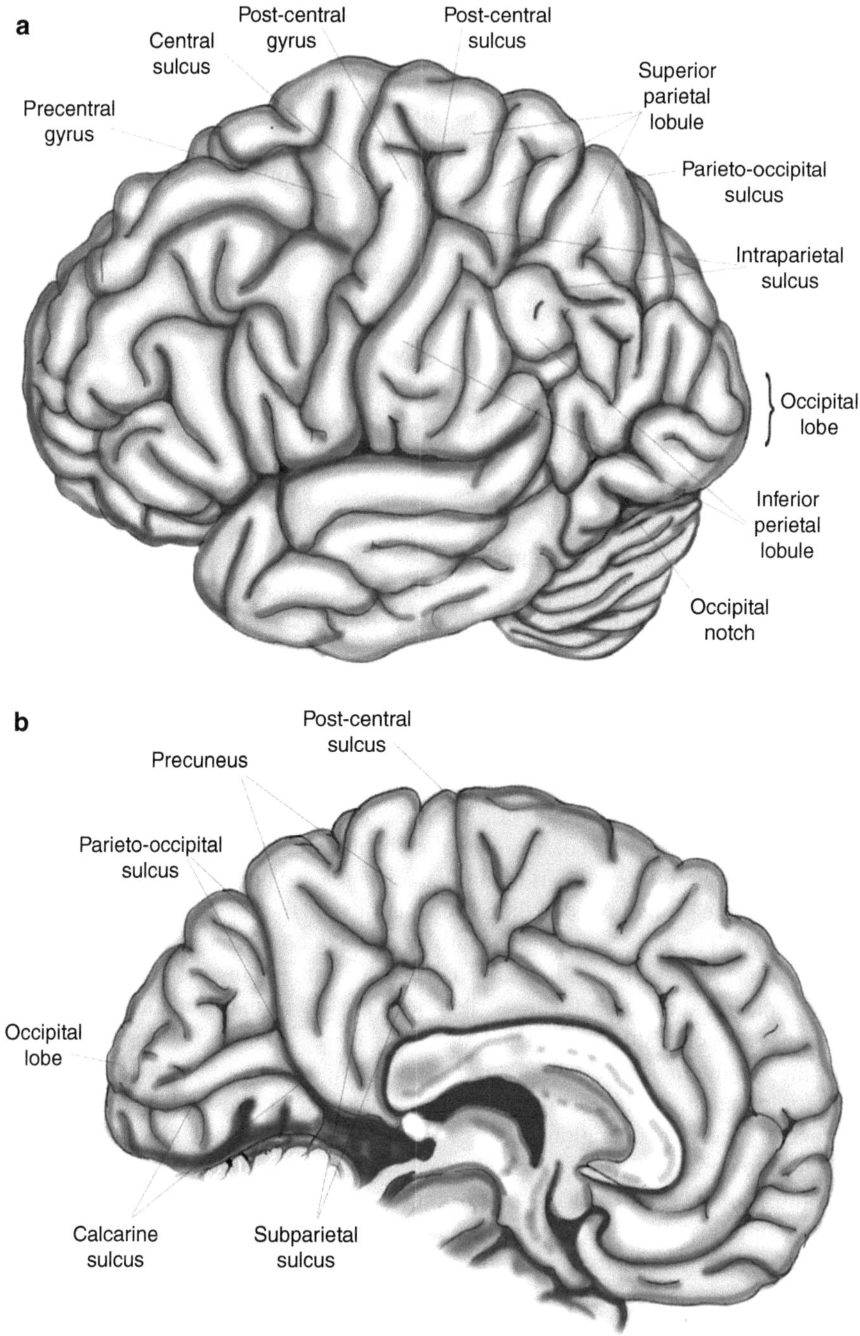

Fig. 9.1 The anatomy of the parietal lobe. It illustrates the dorsolateral (**a**) and medial (**b**) surfaces of a left cerebral hemisphere. The medial surface of the superior parietal lobule consists of primarily the precuneus. That part of the dorsolateral surface above the intraparietal sulcus simply takes the name "superior parietal lobule"

9.2.2 Surgery (Superior Parietal Lobulectomy)

The SPLY, both nondominant and dominant, is carried out with all the recommendations outlined in Chap. 5 with respect to corticectomies, particularly preserving the overlying *en passage* arterial vessels (Sect. 5.2) that do not terminate in the cortex being removed and the preservation of the subcortical white matter (Sects. 5.3 and 5.4) in the deeper parts of the lobulectomy.

Those resections, which include the cortex juxtaposed to the postcentral gyrus, are best conducted under local anesthesia, with good clinical monitoring and with all the precautions and the surgical strong points in precluding injuries to that cortex (see Sects. 5.5.3 and 7.2.2).

9.3 Inferior Parietal Lobulectomy (IPLY)

9.3.1 Anatomy

The inferior parietal lobule (IPL) is located over the dorsolateral surface of the hemisphere. Its boundaries are the postcentral sulcus anteriorly and the intraparietal sulcus superiorly. The inferior boundary consists of the posterior part of the Sylvian fissure and an arbitrary extension of a posterior line from its posterior extent to the posterior boundary, which consists of the segment of the often-called "dorsolateral line," a line that runs between the parieto-occipital sulcus superiorly and the "occipital notch" inferiorly. It also includes the undersurface of the parietal operculum posterior to the postcentral sulcus. These features are illustrated in Fig. 9.2.

The inferior part of the left IPL, anteroposteriorly, is composed of Wernicke's area (Brodmann's area 43) of the operculum behind the postcentral sulcus and then the supramarginal (inferior part of Brodmann's area 40) and angular gyri (area 39) posterior to the posterior end of the Sylvian fissure and the superior temporal sulcus, respectively. These areas are significantly neuronally connected to their juxtaposed areas of cortex involving auditory, visual, and somesthetic functions. This presumably is part of the reason for the striking complexity of their functions. All three areas have functions that are related to various aspects of speech. These complexities involve the understanding of speech, phonological and articulatory processing of words, semantic processing of language, reading, spelling, calculation, performance of reversible operations in space, digital recognition, etc. Injury to the areas can lead to typical Wernicke's speech problems, as well as to dyslexia and a variety of agnosias. The IPL is now one of the cortical regions that is being explored extensively with functional magnetic resonance imaging (fMRI).

The foregoing gives the reader some insight why inferior parietal lobe resections are so rarely conducted, especially in the dominant parietal lobe. My experience with electrocortical stimulation of the area is very sparse; what experience I had, if I recall accurately, was that which was usually associated with eloquent cortex and the stimulation of which seemed to have some disturbance of cognition, usually having to do with language. Many of the responses were not clearly dissimilar from

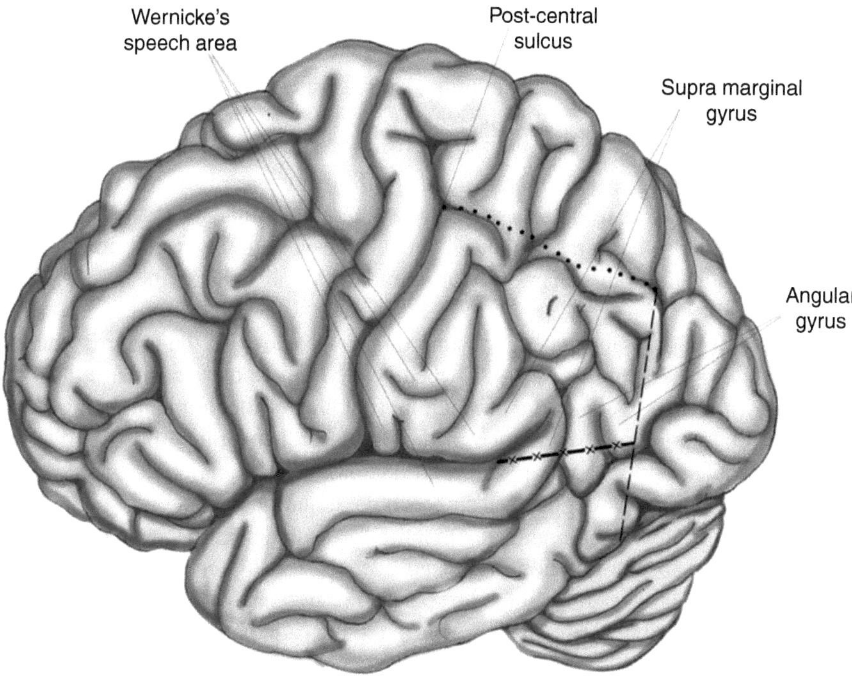

Fig. 9.2 Anatomy of the inferior parietal cortex. An illustration of the lateral surface of the left hemisphere, depicting the various anatomical boundaries and the cortical areas, which are located in the IPL (inferior parietal lobule). ×■ × ■ × ■ × ■ × arbitrary extension line from the posterior end of the Sylvian fissure (the inferior boundary of the posterior half of the IPL); — — — — the dorsolateral line, separating the parietal and occipital lobe; ●●●●●●●●● intraparietal sulcus (see text)

responses that one might have observed from stimulation of the two primary speech areas, e.g., Broca's and especially the temporal part of Wernicke's. With respect to surgical operations in this area, see the section pertaining to the posterior peri-Sylvian cortex (Sect. 9.3.4).

9.3.2 Nondominant (IPLY)

The nondominant IPLY is carried out much the same way as the SPLY noted in the foregoing. That is to say, the corticectomy is conducted as outlined for corticectomies in Chap. 5. As noted with the SPLY, it is important to preserve the overlying *en passage* arteries (Sect. 5.2) and mandatory to preserve the subcortical white matter (Sect. 5.4) in this corticectomy. Both of these aspects are more important in the IPLY, than the SPLY. Further, it is worth mentioning that in the IPLY, there are more vessels and some will be encountered emerging from the middle cerebral artery in the Sylvian fissure in the depths of transverse sulci of the parietal operculum.

9.3.3 Dominant (IPLY)

As might be intuitively noted, the significant areas of eloquent cortex in the inferior part of the IPL are the reason for the paucity of epileptic surgical resections of this area in the dominant hemisphere. These structures all consist of eloquent cortex and if they are normal, i.e., not injured in early life or displaced by space-occupying lesions, they cannot be resected. Further, any potential juxtaposed resections around these areas must be carried out under local anesthesia with the availability of functional mapping through electrocortical stimulation and good clinical monitoring during surgery.

Somewhat in this same category I am going to provide, for the reader's interest, a response of Dr. Rasmussen in 1984 when I asked him about a concern I had with a patient who had a lesion in the parietotemporal area of the dominant hemisphere: "The parietal-temporal speech zone in the dominant hemisphere poses a difficult surgical problem since there are no good anatomical landmarks, that identify the posterior and superior margins of the speech area, and one cannot rely on negative stimulation responses as guaranteeing that the cortex underneath the electrode is not concerned with speech functions. I looked over the last fifteen patients in whom I carried out cortical excisions in the left parietal region. In two of these, the amytal speech test proved that speech had transferred to the right hemisphere as result of an early lesion. In two thirds of the remainder, there was a temporary post-operative dysphasia similar in all respects that which sometimes follow anterior temporal lobectomy in the dominant hemisphere. The dysphasia cleared up in one to three weeks, following the same general time course as in anterior temporal lobe removals. In the remaining few cases, there was no dysphasia at all, although in two of them the excision approached the posterior margin of the parietal temporal opercular area more than I liked. In these cases, I suspect that the lesion responsible for the seizures had resulted in the parietal speech area being further anterior, or smaller than normal."

9.3.4 Posterior Peri-Sylvian (Temporoparieto-occipital) Corticectomy

I have labeled this as a separate category. The reason for this is purely personal and has to do with the fact that a number of lesions, including epileptic foci, exist in this area just posterior to the posterior end of the Sylvian fissure. I have chosen the term "posterior peri-Sylvian" because I feel that it more accurately localizes the area than the perhaps more commonly used "posterior parietal," "anterior occipital," "posterior temporoparietal," or "posterior temporoparieto-occipital." This is perhaps more germane to the dominant posterior peri-Sylvian region than the same region in the nondominant hemisphere. Hence, it involves much of the eloquent cortex of the IPL.

Anatomically it includes primarily the angular gyrus of the parietal lobe, the anterior middle gyrus of the occipital lobe, and the posterosuperior cortex of the temporal lobe. Thus, functionally it may be involved with some of the cognitive language complexity, vision, and part of the temporal speech area, respectively.

There is little need to mention much about this area in the nondominant lobe, other than to indicate that the most likely postoperative neurological deficit from a corticectomy in this area of the nondominant lobe would be a visual field defect. Thus, white matter and *en passage* arterial vessels must be attended to as noted in the foregoing. In the dominant lobe the same cautiousness and surgical technique require being used as noted in the foregoing discussion of the IPLY, with, of course, the added concern about the visual pathways.

I would like to give a brief review of a case of a 21-year-old female with an IFL lesion in the pre-MRI decade (1980), who had a 1-year history of seizures that began with episodes of difficulty speaking. She had both simple partial and complex partial seizures. She had some mild transient neurological deficits confined to her right hand. A CT scan disclosed a cystic/neoplastic lesion in the IPL, in the middle of what would be a typical anatomical Wernicke's speech area. At operation, in spite of a very thorough electrocortical stimulation of the area, there was difficulty in defining a clear-cut speech area and thus careful clinical monitoring was necessary in carrying out the removal of the tumor. The lesion was a ganglioglioma, which was removed with no adverse consequences. Her MRIs are normal and she has been seizure-free. I note this case to simply exemplify that lesions might be relatively easily removed from what is considered to be clearly eloquent cortex by operations carried out under local anesthesia, with electrocortical stimulatory mapping and particularly with ongoing clinical neurological examination during the resection. The prime reason for mentioning this case is that I have operated on a number of cases with lesions in this area, particularly arteriovenous malformations (AVMs) or, interestingly, gangliogliomas which were considered inoperable because of their locations, only to find, under local anesthesia and electrocortical stimulation, that the lesions could easily be removed without a postoperative neurological deficit. Preoperative *contralateral* intracarotid amytal tests (IAT) often aided in the preoperative investigation. (Ipsilateral IATs, in the case of significantly large AVMs, are usually of no value; however, perhaps the now current use of fMRI may be of value.) It goes without saying, but is still worth adding, that in such patients who have no, or very mild, neurological deficits preoperatively, there is often no evidence of speech around the lesion! Further, lesions that are present before birth or in the initial few years of infancy (e.g., up to 5–7) are often associated with the finding that speech has been "moved," often to the contralateral hemisphere in the same location or a few gyri away from the lesion; these include especially AVMs, hamartomas, and various benign cysts. It is difficult, in this respect, not to believe that the AVM, hamartoma, and ganglioglioma lesions may have had enough significance at birth or in the early years of infancy to bring about an alteration in the speech area (see Rasmussen and Milner 1975).

9.4 Safe Limits of Resection

9.4.1 Introduction

There is little more that can be added to the foregoing discussion regarding safe limits of surgical resection of the parietal lobe. However, I have added a "safe limits" section here primarily to describe two other relatively safe surgical pathways that exist within this anatomical region, allowing relative safe exposure to deeper lesions. One is the use of the superomedial part of the SPL, while the other is the use of the posterior end of the Sylvian fissure. Pilcher and Rusyniak consider the complications associated with the posterior and inferior parietal corticectomies (1993).

In the inferior lobulectomies (IPLYs), the subcortical white matter must be saved in order to reduce a potential postoperative lower quadrantic homonymous hemianopsia (Rasmussen 1975b).

9.4.2 Superomedial Parietal Surgical Pathway

I learned from Dr. T. Rasmussen many years ago that one of the safest areas of cortex that can be removed is that of the superomedial part of the SPL—as already noted in the foregoing, that area between the postcentral sulcus anteriorly and the occipital lobe posteriorly—consisting primarily of approximately a centimeter of the parasagittal dorsolateral cortex and the medial (precuneal) cortex. Keeping the subcortical white matter removal to a reasonable minimum and the *en passage* arteries intact, this approach can be utilized as a surgical pathway, with very little risk of postoperative neurological deficit, to reach the corpus callosum, especially the splenium, the pineal region, and the posterior lateral ventricular system. This is depicted in Fig. 9.3.

9.4.3 The Posterior Sylvian Fissure Pathway

Another pathway to deep structures is through the depth of the posterior Sylvian fissure. The appreciation of this potential pathway is obvious when one views a coronal cross section through the very posterior end of the fissure. Figure 9.4 is such a section. In this figure the very thin mantle of white matter between the ventricular surface of the trigone of the lateral ventricle and the depth of the posterior end of the Sylvian fissure is evident.

The surgery required for exposing this mantle requires a gentle and careful, but generous, surgical separation of the walls of the Sylvian fissure in its posterior extent. This separation needs no necessary surgical description, other than to indicate my bias that the arteries associated with the irrigation of one bank of the fissure are very unlikely to be involved with the other bank, even though the difficulty of the certainty of this eventuality may occur a number of times throughout such a dissection. The separation must be taken to the very depth of the fissure and, reemphasizing the

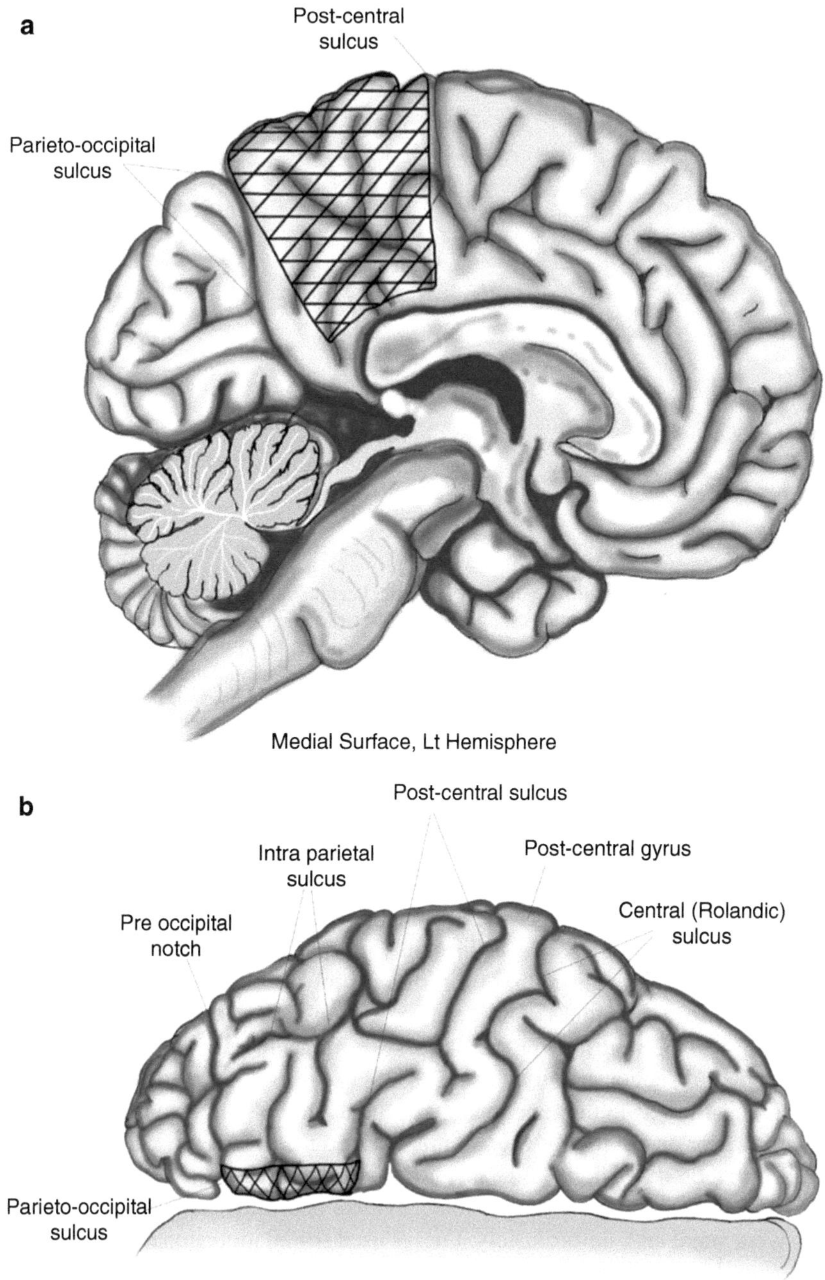

Fig. 9.3 Illustration of a "safe" transcortical pathway through the medial parasagittal parietal cortex. It illustrates a "safe" (surgically) area of excision in the medial parasagittal parietal cortex, behind the postcentral sulcus and anterior to the occipital (visual) cortex (parietooccipital sulcus) in the left hemisphere. It includes approximately 1 cm of the parasagittal dorsolateral surface (**a**) and the whole of the medial surface (**b**). The corticectomy is illustrated in the crosshatched areas (see text)

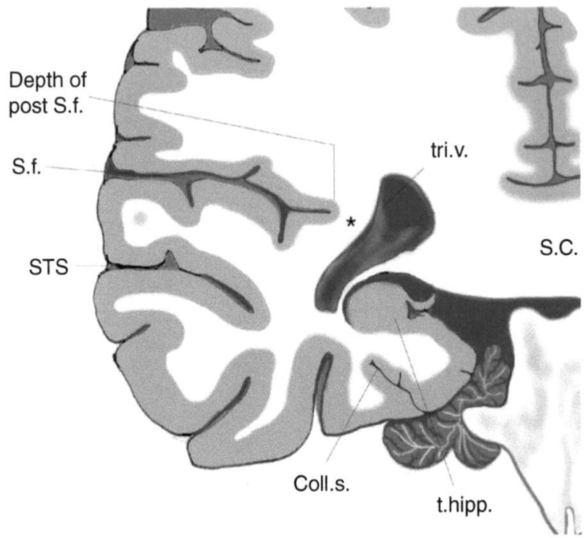

Fig. 9.4 A coronal section through the trigone of the lateral ventricle. A coronal section through the trigone of the lateral ventricle, which demonstrates the mantle of cerebral parenchyma that exists between the ependymal surface of the trigone and the depth of the posterior end of the Sylvian fissure. *coll.s.* collateral sulcus, *S.f.* Sylvian fissure, *s.c.* splenium of the corpus callosum, *STS* superior temporal sulcus, *t.hipp.* tail of the hippocampus, *tri.v.* trigone of the lateral ventricle, ∗ depicts the short line of the distance between the depth of the posterior Sylvian fissure and the trigone of the lateral ventricle

foregoing, there must be a significant separation more superficially in order to allow the room at the depth to carry out an instrumented surgery. Once having reached the bottom of it, the mantle can be incised with gentle suction and low current bipolar coagulation (much the same as will be seen utilized in the incision of the corpus callosum in the conduct of a corpus callosotomy in Chap. 11 (Sect. 11.2.4)).

The use of such a pathway has been significantly reduced by the sophistication of the stereotactic techniques of the last two decades. However, it can give relatively safe passage to the ventricle for those cases when that access is necessary and cannot be achieved stereotactically.

I am uncertain as to the functionality of the mantle of parenchyma in the depth of the posterior end of the Sylvian fissure, but I do feel that if this pathway were to be utilized, then it should be done under local anesthesia and neuroleptanalgesia. I have gained access in this manner without evident neurological deficit, but my incisions were small and, unfortunately, I never used stimulation along the bank of the fissure nor the mantle at its depth; rather I used clinical monitoring alone. If visual fibers were in this mantle, they can be recognized in the same way that visual cortex can be recognized, by stimulation of the surface and the production of phosphenes (see Chap. 10). These dots of light are much smaller when produced from stimulation of the visual cortical surface than when stimulating visual fiber pathways. If visual pathways exist in this cerebral mantle, then stimulation in the depth should reveal their presence by the production of phosphenes in response to the stimulation (see Sects. 4.6.4 and 10.2.1).

References

Corkin S, Milner B, Rasmussen T. Somatosensory thresholds – contrasting effects of post-central gyrus and posterior parietal-lobe excision. Arch Neurol. 1970;23:41–58.

Critchley M. The parietal lobes. London: Edward Arnold; 1955.

Mattingly JB, Husain M, Rorden C, Kennard C, Driver J. Motor role of unman inferior parietal lobe revealed in unilateral neglect patients. Nature. 1998;392:179–82.

Pilcher WH, Rusyniak WG. Complications of epilepsy surgery. Neurosurg Clin N Am. 1993;4:311–25.

Rasmussen T. Cortical resection in the treatment of focal epilepsy. In: Purpura DP, Penry JK, Walter RD, editors. Advances in neurology, vol. 8. New York: Raven; 1975a. p. 139–54.

Rasmussen T. Surgery for epilepsy arising in regions other than the temporal and frontal lobes. In: Purpura DP, Penry JK, Walter RD, editors. Advances in neurology, vol. 8. New York: Raven; 1975b. p. 206–26.

Rasmussen T. [9.1, 9.3.3*, 9.4.2]

Rasmussen T, Milner B. Clinical and surgical studies of the cerebral speech areas in man. In: Zulch KJ, Creutzfeldt O, Galbraith GC, editors. Cerebral localization: an Otfrid Foerster symposium. New York: Springer; 1975. p. 238–57.

Salanova V, Andermann F, Rasmussen T, Olivier A, Quesney LF. Tumoural parietal lobe epilepsy: clinical manifestations and outcome in 34 patients treated between 1934 and 1988. Brain. 1995;118:1289–304.

Sveinbjornsdottir KS, Duncan JS. Parietal and occipital lobe epilepsy: a review. Epilepsia. 1993;34:493–521.

Williamson PD, Boon PA, Thadani VM, Darcey TM, Spencer DD, Spencer SS, Novelly RA, Mattson RH. Parietal lobe epilepsy: diagnostic considerations and results of surgery. Ann Neurol. 1992;31:193–201.

Occipital Lobe Resections

10

10.1 Introduction

10.1.1 Anatomy

The occipital lobe, the smallest of the cerebral lobes, has three surfaces—dorsolateral, medial, and inferior. Because of the curvilinear aspect of the junction of the posterior falx cerebri and the tentorium cerebelli, the junction of the medial and inferior surfaces of the occipital lobe is somewhat ill defined. Histologically, the lobe is comprised primarily of the three cytoarchitectonic areas, 17, 18, and 19 of Brodmann.

The dorsolateral surface is that cortex posterior to the "occipital line" which extends from the superior extent of the parieto-occipital sulcus superiorly to the "occipital notch" inferiorly; the notch is approximately 4 cm anterior to the occipital pole at the junction of the dorsolateral and inferior surfaces (see Fig. 10.1a). The medial surface is that cortex posterior to the parieto-occipital sulcus superiorly and anterior limb of the calcarine sulcus, which ends just beneath the splenium of the corpus callosum (see Fig. 10.1b). The inferior surface is less well delineated; it includes the posterior part of the temporal lobe, extending behind an arbitrary line between the occipital notch and the isthmus of the cingulate gyrus. Thus, it includes, from lateral to medial, respectively, the posterior part of the inferior temporal gyrus, posterior part of the fusiform (occipitotemporal) gyrus, and the lingual gyrus.

The dorsolateral surface is defined by some as consisting of three, superior, middle, and inferior, occipital gyri. Others fail to acknowledge such a distinction of three gyri, which is my position. In my view it consists of a number of gyri and shallow sulci, which have little, if any, predictability. The cortex of the medial surface that is posterior to the parieto-occipital sulcus and superior to the posterior limb of the calcarine sulcus is the cuneus. That below the sulcus consists primarily of the lingual gyrus. The inferior surface may have gyral names that vary somewhat, depending upon the neuroanatomical text. Thus, these may variously be referred to as the posterior parts of the lingual, temporo-occipital, parahippocampal, and even some of the inferior temporal gyri. These features are illustrated in Fig. 10.1.

J.P. Girvin, *Operative Techniques in Epilepsy*,
DOI 10.1007/978-3-319-10921-3_10

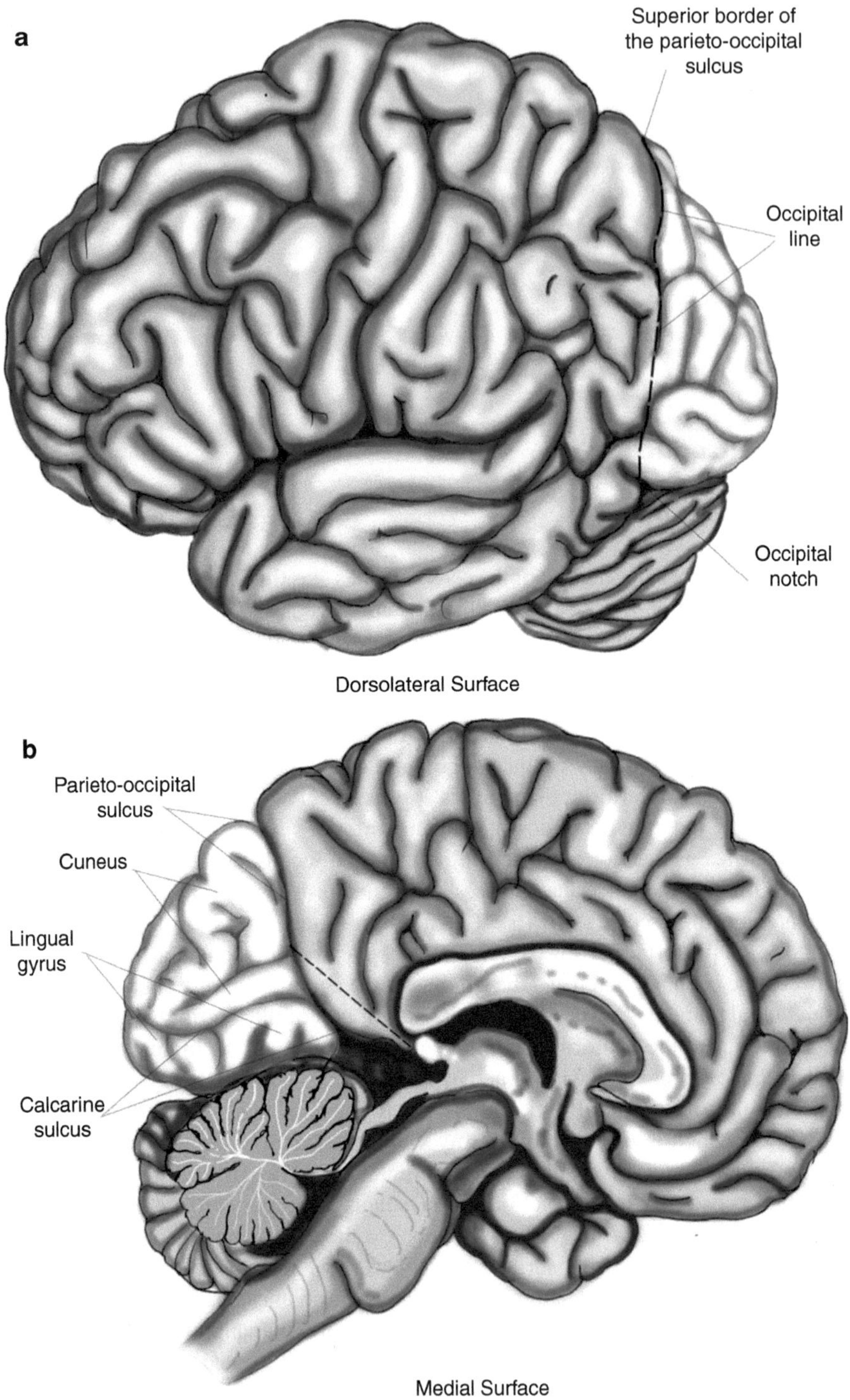

Fig. 10.1 Anatomy of the occipital lobe. An illustration of the anatomical features of the three surfaces of the occipital lobe of the left hemisphere: (**a**) dorsolateral, (**b**) medial, and (**c**) inferior (see text)

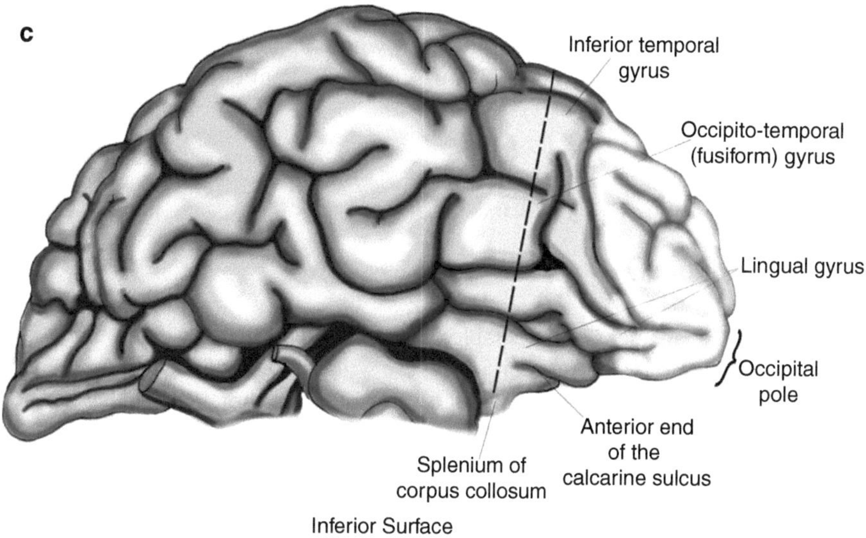

Fig. 10.1 (continued)

10.1.2 Physiology

The occipital cortex has an array of connectivity with other areas of the cerebrum like other lobes, but it has a very closely associated connectivity with the posterior temporal lobe. This association is significantly reflected in the semiology of the occipital and the posterior temporal seizures.

The semiology of occipital lobe seizures exhibits a remarkable variety, perhaps to a greater extent than other lobes. Its connectivity is such that epileptic foci in the parietal and temporal lobes may disclose characteristics of the semiology that clinically they are initially attributed to those lobes. The reverse is just as likely, i.e., foci in the occipital lobe spreading to the eloquent cortex in other cortical areas, leading to the clinical view that the epileptic foci are in those areas. The majority of seizures arising in the occipital cortex have some remnants of altered vision—altered vision that is usually in the contralateral visual field. These may be alterations in brightness, color, size of objects, appearance of various hallucinations, etc.

The significant connectivity to the posterior temporal lobe results in the primary semiology of the occipital lobe foci to be very characteristic of the results of electrocortical stimulation of the occipital cortex. Such stimulation results in so-called "elementary" aspects of vision, which never consists of the elements of normal human vision. Moving from the occipital pole to the posterior temporal cortex, the quality of human vision becomes increasing normal. The results of stimulation of the occipital cortex produce, in the contralateral visual field, elements of light with sizes from a pinpoint to huge balls, figures of unrecognizable flashes/dots/balls/stars/etc., color, and the absence of depth. Hallucinations that could be recognized as normal, i.e., brightness, color, figures, speech, depth, etc., are the typical semeiotic hallucinatory or relatively normal pictorial data from stimulation of posterior temporal foci. These may exhibit normal pictorial humans, color, depth, auditory output, etc., which appear in both halves of the visual fields (see Penfield and Rasmussen 1952; Penfield and Jasper 1954; Brindley 1973).

10.2 Surgical Management

10.2.1 Introduction

The surgical management of intractable occipital epilepsy includes both the lobectomy as well as various corticectomies. These will be briefly described, as there is little that is absolutely specifically associated with the occipital cortex that has not already been covered. The most important aspect of the surgical management depends upon the visual status of the patient and whether or not a visual field defect is something that has been agreed upon (by the patient and surgeon) as an acceptable postoperative deficit. If the latter is not acceptable, then the patient is best operated upon under local anesthesia and neuroleptanalgesia. In Chap. 4 (Sect. 4.6.4), stimulation of the visual cortex was discussed. Punctate stimulation, identifying the visual cortex, is primarily located on the medial surface of the occipital lobe and not uncommonly over a very narrow medial strip of the dorsolateral cortex bordering on the midline. Between this and clinical monitoring during the surgery, there should not be significant concern about the surgery leading to an unanticipated postoperative visual field deficit. The only circumstance in which there is no concern about producing a homonymous hemianopia is in the case of a functional hemispherectomy (see Chap. 12), especially those caused by fetal or early infant infarcts.

From Chap. 4, the reader will realize that punctate stimulation of the visual cortex results in the production of small dots of light, called phosphenes, which, with the eyes held stationary, are immobile in the contralateral visual field. Through this methodology, the visual cortex subserving the contralateral visual field can be reasonably well defined. (Only "reasonably well" in that two-thirds of the visual cortex is "buried," as shown by Stensaas et al. in 1974, and hence is not able to be accessed by surface stimulation.) The clinical monitoring can be easily undertaken by using a large visual field chart on a stand, turned through 90° and placed comfortably in front of the patient's "window" in the surgical drapes. This can then be used at any time to carry out a visual field examination or to have the patient identify exactly where in the visual field a phosphene is seen, in response to ongoing electrocortical stimulation.

10.2.2 Lobectomy

The operative intervention in the case of occipital lobe epilepsy will vary according to a number of variables, which will not be covered fully here. Providing the patient has a permanent homonymous hemianopia or that the seizures are of such disability that the patient is willing to sacrifice a half of the visual field, then a full occipital lobectomy may be carried out. There are times that a lobectomy ends up being the surgery of choice when corticectomies that have initially been conducted, avoiding the visual cortex, have failed to control the epileptic disorder.

If the resection is truly confined to the occipital lobe, then there may be little difference between the consideration of a nondominant and a dominant intervention. My choice would still be to use local anesthesia and neuroleptanalgesia when conducting the dorsolateral resection in order to make certain that some function of the angular gyrus is not being removed.

10.2.3 Corticectomy

The occipital corticectomies are primarily confined to the inferior and dorsolateral surfaces. The closer these are to the inferolateral junction between the two surfaces, the less risk there is with respect to the production of a visual field defect from a resection. If the visual area, bordering on the corticectomy, is to be a boundary of the corticectomy, then the operation should be conducted under local anesthesia so that electrocortical stimulation can be carried out initially in order to determine the perimeter of the visual cortex the stimulation of which gives rise to phosphenes (Sect. 4.6.4, and the foregoing Sect. 10.2.1). This is true also for the dorsolateral corticectomy that may border on the IPL in the dominant hemisphere.

Realizing the relative benignity of an upper quadrantic visual field defect, this gives the surgeon some extra license in the size of the corticectomy. That is to say, if the electrocortical stimulation demonstrates that part of the epileptic focus involves the visual cortex associated only with the cortex associated with contralateral upper quadrantic vision, then it may be removed without the concern of the much more significant visual impairment from inferior quadrantic vision. Surgically, the corticectomy is carried out in keeping with all the recommendations noted in Chap. 5.

References

Brindley GS. Sensory effects of electrical stimulation of the visual and paravisual cortex in man. In: Jung J, editor. Handbook of sensory physiology, volume VII/3B, Central Processing of Visual Information. New York: Springer-Verlag; 1973. p. 583–94.

Penfield W, Jasper H. Epilepsy and the functional anatomy of the human brain. Boston: Little, Brown and Co.; 1954. p. 896.

Penfield W, Rasmussen T. The cerebral cortex of man. New York: Macmillan; 1952. p. 135–47, 165–6.

Stensaas SS, Eddington DK, Dobelle WH. The topography and variability of the primary visual cortex in man. J Neurosurg. 1974;40:747–55.

Corpus Callosotomy (CCY) 11

11.1 General Observations Regarding the Corpus Callosum (CC)

11.1.1 Introduction

Corpus callosotomy (CCY) is not a resective epilepsy operation, but rather comes under the heading of "interruption of conducting pathways," which is another group of operations that are utilized in special cases of epilepsy. I am covering it here very briefly, as it is a commonly utilized epilepsy operation; further, it does form part of the functional hemispherectomy (fHSPY), which will be discussed in the next chapter.

11.1.2 Embryology

The development of the corpus callosum (CC) begins during the fifth week of fetal life (39 days) with the formation of the primitive lamina terminalis, which thickens to form the commissural plate. Failure of development of this plate results in a lack of the necessary guide for the CC crossing fibers and, hence, a probable agenesis. Glial cells coalesce to form a bridge-like structure, which serves as a guide for the callosal fibers crossing the longitudinal cerebral fissure to reach their target positions in the contralateral hemisphere. The interhemispheric projection of the first axons is preceded by microcystic degeneration in the commissural plate and physiological death of astrocytes. The lack of degeneration of the plate leaves a glial barrier that will interfere with the crossing corpus callosal fibers and, hence, an abnormal, or lack of, development of the CC. The earliest callosal axons appear at ~74 days in the human embryo, the genu and the splenium are recognized at 84 days, and the adult morphology is achieved by 115 days.

Neurons giving rise to commissural fibers from the neocortex are located in the supra-granular layers of the cortex, mainly layer III, and terminate in the vicinity of layer IV of the homotopic area in the opposite hemisphere. There is a paucity of

J.P. Girvin, *Operative Techniques in Epilepsy*,
DOI 10.1007/978-3-319-10921-3_11

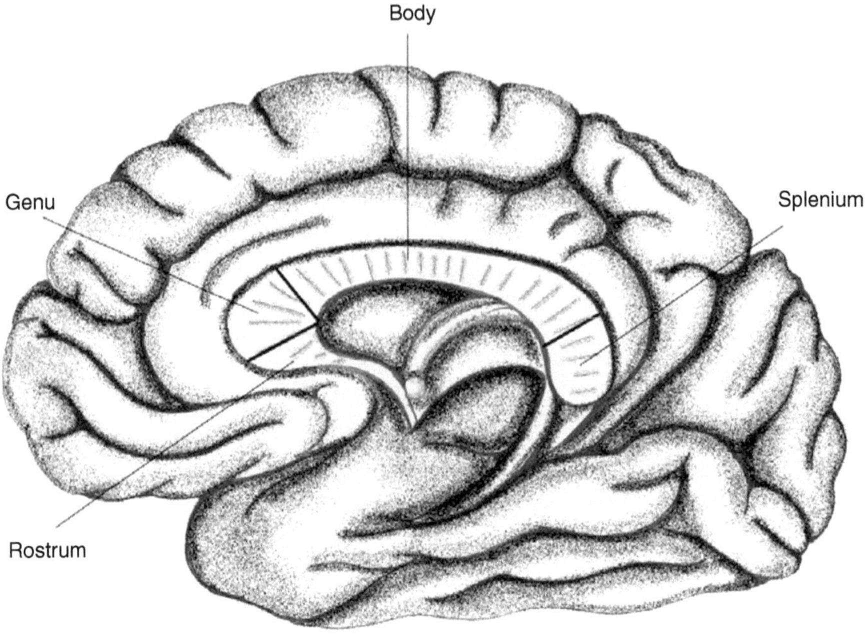

Fig. 11.1 Medial aspect of the right hemisphere, exhibiting the four anatomical divisions of the corpus callosum.

fibers representing the distal portions of the limbs and most of visual area 17 (except near the border with area 18), as compared to most other neocortical areas.

11.1.3 Anatomy

The CC is the largest of the three hemispheric commissures. It primarily connects homotopic areas of the two hemispheres with one another. It develops in concert with the neocortex. In humans, it consists of ~200 million fibers. It consists of four relatively easily identifiable parts: rostrum, genu, body, and splenium, anteroposteriorly (see Fig. 11.1). The CC is something of the order of 10 cm in length, with its anterior end (genu) ~4 cm behind the frontal pole and the posterior end (splenium) ~6 cm anterior to the occipital pole.

11.1.4 The Corpus Callosum and Epilepsy

Given that there is no neuronal cortex or neuronal networks in the CC, what is the rationale for a so-called corpus callosotomy? Experimental animal investigations have shown that (1) bilaterally synchronous discharges augment seizures with bilateral motor manifestations; (2) the CC can be shown to be a major pathway for seizure propagation, as noted in the well-described electroencephalographic "secondary bilateral synchrony" (with a transcallosal conduction time of ~5–15 ms); and (3) a CC section decreases or abolishes synchronous epileptiform discharges. Erickson showed in monkeys that electrically produced seizures in one hemisphere spread to the other, but that corpus callosotomy abolished the interhemispheric spread (1940). These types of observations have led to the view that the CC is heavily involved in the transmission of facilitation—particularly in the context of bihemispheric epileptogenicity. However, the experimental literature leaves little doubt but that there are alternate pathways, besides the CC, that provide the neuronal substrate for the appearance of bihemispheric synchrony.

Van Wagenen and Herren experimented with a corpus callosotomy (CCY) in a few human patients after a long practice history of observations in which the spontaneous destruction of transcallosal tissue by naturally occurring phenomena, e.g., stroke, tumors, etc., led to a significant reduction of seizures (1940). Their operations had a number of outcomes, but certainly the authors were convinced that there was a general reduction in seizures. Others followed who conducted also the incision of multiple interhemispheric commissures in addition to the CC, e.g., anterior commissure and hippocampal commissure (Bogen et al. 1965, 1969; Luessenhop 1970; Luessenhop et al. 1970; Wilson et al. 1975). However, surgery of multiple commissures caused significant concern about postoperative morbidity. Wilson and colleagues initially experimented with incising all three cerebral commissures (Wilson et al. 1975) but eventually felt that CCY alone was the most appropriate and safest, from the point of view of neurological and neuropsychological outcomes (Wilson et al. 1978, 1982). A review of the changes to the procedure over the middle of the twentieth century can be found in excellent reviews by Spencer et al. (1987) and Maxwell et al. (1987).

11.2 Corpus Callosotomy (CCY)

11.2.1 Indications

The indications for the conduct of a CCY are much less rigid than in most of the resective operations that have been discussed to this point. The group of indications might be looked upon by the uninitiated as a *potpourri* of intractable epileptic disorders. The indications are less generally accepted and vary considerably from one center to another. Indications include (1) seizures with absence of resectable epileptic foci; (2) cases of multiple seizure types, especially if the most troublesome consists of "drop attacks"; and (3) frontal epileptic foci with rapid secondary bilateral synchrony.

In the article by Maxwell et al. there is a very good account of the historical evolution of the CCY over the twentieth century after the pioneering work of Van Wagenen and Herren (1940). Their discussion is replete with the variety of

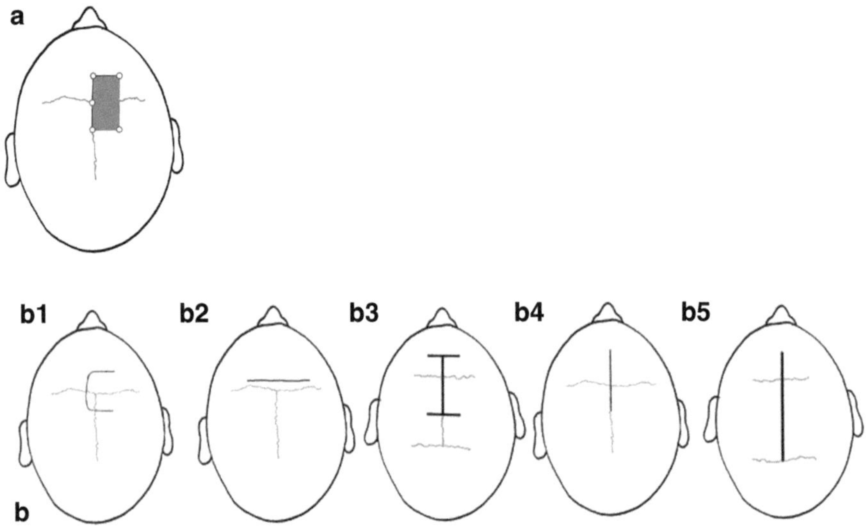

Fig. 11.2 The scalp incisions used for conducting a corpus callosotomy (CCY). An illustration of the various incisions that have been used in the scalp in order to provide the craniotomy opening for access to the corpus callosum for the conduct of a CCY. (**a**) Demonstrates an outline of the approximate craniotomy that is required in order to gain this access. (**b**) Illustrates the choice of scalp incisions, which have been used to provide adequate access to the craniotomy site. Subfigures (**B1**–**B5**) (see text)

supportive measures of the procedure used at the University of Minnesota. Certainly there is marked contrast between what I will describe below and what they utilized. For example, I have never used preoperative steroids or intraoperative antibiotics or mannitol nor found it necessary to consider dividing the sagittal sinus. I would agree that if the ventricular (ependymal) surface can be left intact, it is probably preferable, but if the surgeon feels that this might compromise the completeness of the incision in a particular part of the CC, then I have no concern about recommending being more radical, at the expense of placing rents in the integrity of the ventricular surface, which I have never felt resulted in *any* complications.

11.2.2 Craniotomy

The common craniotomy, per se, is demonstrated in Fig. 11.2a; this is a narrow ~2–3 cm wide (mediolateral) parasagittal opening into the nondominant frontal lobe, approximately centered, in an anteroposterior direction, over the coronal suture. Figure 11.2b demonstrates the common scalp incisions that have been noted in the literature in order to gain access to the amount of bone requiring exposure for the craniotomy. Figure B1 depicts a typical parasagittal craniotomy incision, which is perhaps one of the commonest incisions used. Figure B2 discloses a transverse incision, near or just anterior and parallel to the coronal suture. I have included figure B3 simply because I used this incision for a number of years. It works perfectly well but it is unnecessarily more difficult in its production and certainly much more in its closure at the end of the CCY. Figure B4 is an anterior midline incision and one that was commonly used for the first phase of the CCY, by those carrying out the CCY in two phases (Wilson et al. 1982; Maxwell et al. 1987). The Dartmouth group chose to use two transverse incisions and 5 cm trephinations, one just anterior to the coronal suture and a second more posteriorly located (Roberts 1985; Roberts and Siegel 2001). My own preference is shown in figure B5, which is a simple generous length of a midline incision running from just behind the hairline of the forehead back to the lambda area. This incision is very easily extended anteriorly and/or posteriorly if more surgical "room" is required medially, laterally, or anteroposteriorly. Further, the clearly delineated tissue planes provide for a very easy surgical closure.

The reason for my preference for the longer incision shown in figure B5 is that I have always carried out a more radical callosotomy than what seemed to have become the standard at the time, which was a so-called *anterior two-thirds* callosotomy, i.e., an incision estimated as involving approximately the anterior two-thirds of the CC. A depiction of this CCY is illustrated in Fig. 11.3a. The following text will outline my preference for a more radical CCY, as illustrated in Fig. 11.3b.

11.2.3 Surgical Access to the CC

As noted earlier, the mediolateral extent of the craniotomy need not be more than ~2 cm. The length of it will depend to some extent upon the proposed length of the callosotomy. As noted in the foregoing, my own preference would be to err on the side of too much length, rather than too little. Very small length craniotomies can lead to difficulties in situations where there happens to be large parasagittal veins, which the surgeon may wish to leave intact, but which create significant difficulties in securing easy access and visualization of the whole length of the proposed CCY. The medial two or three burr holes may be placed according to the surgeon's individual preference. I personally like to place them *over* the superior sagittal sinus (SSS), and then with good curettes and one of the periosteal dissectors, the separation of the SSS from the cranial bone is achieved. The bone is incised with a Gigli saw such that the bevel of the incision in the bone results in its outer edge being on the opposite side of the sinus to the craniotomy opening, e.g., usually the left. This allows easy removal of the inner layer of bone, i.e., the inner portion of the bevel, over the sinus through the use of curettes and/or rongeurs. This in turn partially mobilizes the sinus, which leads to less awkwardness of retraction. Even the few millimeters that one may gain through clearing the sinus of its adherence to the underside of bone may greatly facilitate the final exposure of the CC.

The dura is opened as in any parasagittal craniotomy and retracted. Exploration of the superior aspect of the hemisphere will then lead to the identification of any

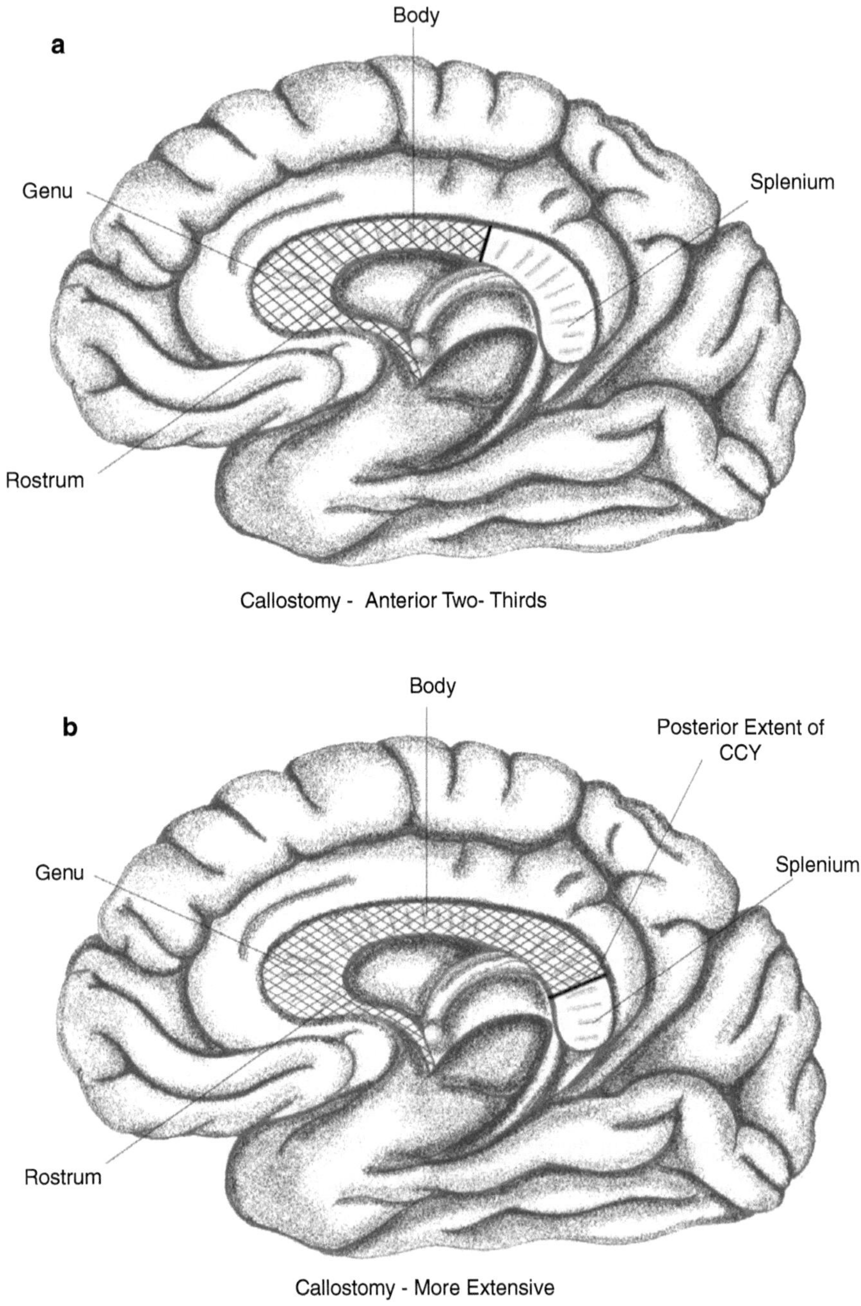

Fig. 11.3 (**a**) A typical sagittal depiction of an "anterior two thirds CCY." (**b**) A typical sagittal depiction of a more extensive CCY, i.e., the posterior extent reaches the anterior part of the splenium (see text). cross-hatching (xxx) exhibits the extent of the callosotomy

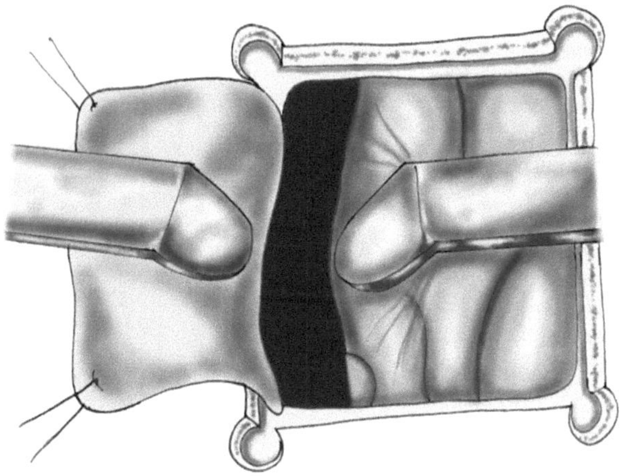

Fig. 11.4 Interhemispheric exposure of the superficial aspect of the surgical pathway to the corpus callosum. Illustration of the use of two retractors, facilitating the visualization of the deeper part of the exposure. As indicated in the text, the retractor against the falx and superior sagittal sinus may expand the opening by only a millimeter or two, but even this may be enough to significantly improve the visualization once the CC is reached. The second retractor is placed against the medial aspect of the hemisphere

veins that may be traversing the proposed pathway between the retracted falx cerebri and the medial aspect of the hemisphere, as shown in Fig. 11.4. This discloses the initiation of the separation of the medial hemisphere from the midline. Notice that a retractor is also used against the superior sagittal sinus; once this is mobilized, even a small amount of it can be moved; even a 1–2 mm movement may pay significant dividends in visualization when the CC is reached in the depth. The final satisfactory visualization is gradually achieved through the gentle advance of the retractors in small steps.

The most aggravating, exasperating, and labor-intensive aspect of securing the pathway is encountered when there is significant adherence between the leptomeninges of the medial aspects of the hemispheres, which is most likely to occur below the inferior extent of the falx. In cases where the adherence is severe and the surgical exposure reluctantly involves entrance into the subpial areas of each medial hemispheric surface, then it is important to make certain that in the final exposure, the arteries that have been encountered under those circumstances are kept to their respective sides under the retractors. Dealing with this same adherence in the conduct of a medial frontal corticectomy, which is quite a different problem, is discussed at some length in Chap. 7 (Sect. 7.2.3).

Once again, the importance of the gentleness and small steps in moving the retractors inferiorly, as the dissection is conducted inferiorly, cannot be overemphasized. The CC is recognized by the two obvious pericallosal arteries lying on top of it (Fig. 11.4) and its strikingly white color; the brightness of the white CC is greater than the medial hemispheric cortex.

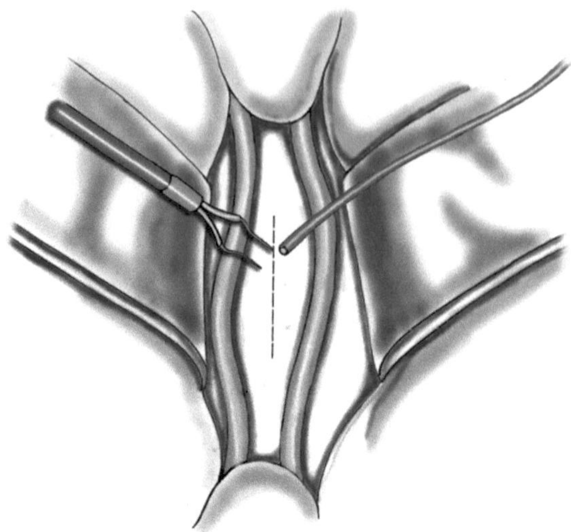

Fig. 11.5 Interhemispheric exposure of the corpus callosum. Illustrates the corpus callosum at the *bottom* of the exposure as a result of the satisfactory retraction of the medial cortex of both hemispheres. Not commonly, one, or even both, pericallosal arteries may be included in the retraction. The *broken line* is where the start of the callosotomy is initiated (see text)

11.2.4 Incision of the CC

Once the CC and the two arteries are visualized, the latter can be gently separated and held separated by the retractors. They can also be held apart with either the suction cannula with a small cottonoid patty and/or the blades of the coagulating forceps, depending upon which one is not at the moment being used to incise the CC. I am not *absolutely* certain that branches of the pericallosal arteries never cross from one hemisphere to the other, yet I do believe this to be nearly always, if not always, the case (Fig. 11.5).

The incision can then be made with the combination of the coagulating forceps, mild irrigation, and suction. The suction is the primary instrument used for making the incision, but the forceps ensure ongoing meticulous hemostasis, which minimizes the likelihood of a significant amount of blood getting into the ventricular system. A large cottonoid patty can be a valuable aid in bringing about satisfactory mild compression of the sides of the incision when required, but it should be left only for short periods (1–3 min), then irrigated with saline solution, removed, and replaced with a fresh patty, as emphasized earlier (Sect. 2.1.5), until clear abolition of any bleeding has been achieved. The incision is taken down to the ventricular surface; it is very unusual, in my experience, to carry out a CCY without significantly making rents in this surface, e.g., thus creating potential passages for blood entering the ventricular system. It is best to carry out the CC incision over the whole of whatever part of the body of the CC is easily visualized at this point. That is to say, it should be taken as far posteriorly and anteriorly as possible at this stage of the surgery, and cottonoid patties, usually the large patties with attached strings (one of my very uncommon uses of cottonoid patties at the end of attached strings! see Sect. 2.1.5), can be left in the extents of the incision. The latter is simply taking as much advantage as possible when there is a satisfactory placement of retractors. If part of a potential CC incision is not carried out under that circumstance, then there is a likelihood of having to make their same placements once again further on in the surgery. Thus, both time and potential retractor injury are lessened.

Once visualization of the more anterior part of the CC is required, the operating table can be altered such that the head is lowered. Between this and the anterior advancement of the tips of the retractors, the remainder of the genu and most of the rostrum can be followed between the pericallosal arteries, which also serve to help in the identification of the rostrum, as its curving position becomes more inferior and posterior. Once this incision is completed, the table orientation is reversed, such that the posterior aspect of the head is lower than the anterior aspect, thus increasing the ease of visualization of the more posterior part of the CC. The incision is now carried posteriorly until there is clearly an increase in the size of the CC, indicating that the smaller incision through the body of the CC has now been gradually replaced by the obviously larger size of the anterior splenium (see Fig. 11.3a). Once this has been reached, the CCY has been completed. I have never observed anything to make me feel that this more radical CCY, than the popular "anterior two-thirds callosotomy," is any less safe.

At this juncture, if required, a combination of cottonoid patties, bipolar coagulation, irrigating fluid, and suction can be utilized to achieve a satisfactory bloodless completion of the CC incision.

11.2.5 Surgical Closure

The closure is simply that of the preference of the individual surgeon. As with most epilepsy operations, I fill the closed dura with irrigation fluid at body temperature under slightly increased pressure and close the bone with silk and the scalp with deep sutures in the periosteum/galea and a simple, running 3–0 nylon suture in the skin.

11.2.6 Potential Postoperative Complications

Besides general neurosurgical complications, there are some that are primarily related to the CCY, per se. Perhaps the commonest is clinically evident partial or complete mutism, which is seen after retraction of the dominant frontal cortex, thought to be the result of excessive retractor pressure, applied over the supplementary motor area. It has the language characteristics of transcortical motor dysphasia. It is a transient impairment and commonly lasts only a few days and rarely is there any evidence of it remaining after a week.

Memory impairment can be seen after incisional splitting of the posterior part of the body of the CC. It is postulated to be the result from the CC incision interrupting the hippocampal commissure(s), which are juxtaposed to the underside of the posterior CC.

Disconnection syndromes, through impaired interhemispheric transfer of visual, tactile, or auditory information, and somewhat bizarre syndromes have been reported, interpreted as independent/conflicting behaviors between the two hemispheres, and finally impairment of speech is now accepted as a potential complication that may occur in the case of "crossed dominance," i.e., when language representation is in the contralateral hemisphere to that of hand dominance (see also Pilcher and Rusyniak 1993).

References

Bogen JE, Fisher ED, Vogel PJ. Cerebral commissurotomy. A second case report. JAMA. 1965;194:1328–9.

Bogen JE, Sperry RW, Vogel PH. Addendum: commissural section and propagation of seizures. In: Jasper HH, Ward Jr AA, Pope A, editors. Basic mechanisms of the epilepsies. Boston: Little, Brown and Co; 1969. p. 439–40.

Erickson TE. Spread of epileptic discharge: an experimental study of the after-discharge induced by electrical stimulation of the cerebral cortex. Arch Neurol Psychiat. 1940;43:429–52.

Luessenhop AJ. Interhemispheric commissurotomy: (the split brain operation) as an alternate to hemispherectomy for control of intractable seizures. Am Surg. 1970;36:265–8.

Luessenhop AJ, dela Cruz TC, Fenichel GM. Surgical disconnection of the cerebral hemispheres for intractable seizures: results in infancy and childhood. JAMA. 1970;213:1630–6.

Maxwell RE, Gates JR, Gumnit RJ. Corpus callosotomy at the university of Minnesota. In: Engel J, editor. Surgical treatment of the epilepsies. New York: Raven; 1987. p. 659–66.

Pilcher WH, Rusyniak WG. Complications of epilepsy surgery. Neurosurg Clin N Am. 1993;4:311–25.

Roberts DW. Corpus callosotomy: surgical technique. In: Reeves AG, editor. Epilepsy and the corpus callosum. New York: Plenum Press; 1985. p. 259–67.

Roberts DW, Siegel AM. Corpus callosotomy. In: Lüders HO, Comair YG, editors. Epilepsy surgery. 2nd ed. Philadelphia: Lippincott Williams & Wilkins. 2001; p. 747–56.

Spencer SS, Gates JR, Reeves AR, Spencer DD, Maxwell RE, Roberts D. Corpus callosum section. In: Engel J, editor. Surgical treatment of the epilepsies. New York: Raven; 1987. p. 425–44.

Van Wagenen WP, Herren RY. Surgical division of commissural pathways in the corpus callosum: relation to spread of an epileptic attack. Arch Neurol Psychiat. 1940;44:740–59.

Wilson DH, Culver C, Waddington M, Gazzaniga M. Disconnection of the cerebral hemispheres: an alternative to hemispherectomy for the control of intractable seizures. Neurology. 1975;25:1149–53.

Wilson DH, Reeves A, Gazzaniga G. Division of the corpus callosum for uncontrollable epilepsy. Neurology. 1978;28:649–53.

Wilson DH, Reeves AG, Gazzaniga G. "Cerebral" commissurotomy for intractable generalized epilepsy: series two. Neurology. 1982;32:687–97.

Hemispherectomy 12

12.1 Anatomical (aHSPY)

12.1.1 History

The history of the operation of surgical anatomical hemispherectomy (aHSPY) is an interesting one. Its initial use consisted of the surgical management of two different clinical conditions: (1) cerebral gliomas and (2) intractable seizures in children with infantile hemiplegia. The rationale for both was the anatomical removal of most of the involved abnormal hemisphere, leaving only the forebrain gray matter. There have been brief reviews of the history of hemispherectomies, the current types, and the reasons for their variations (e.g., Almeida et al. 2006; Binder and Schramm 2006).

12.1.2 Anatomical Hemispherectomy (aHSPY) for Gliomas

The treatment of cerebral gliomas can be found in the literature in a plethora of papers. The use of aHSPY began in the early part of the twentieth century when the then current surgery for glioblastoma multiforme (GBM) was so very disappointing. The notion developed that perhaps the removal of the whole of the diseased hemisphere would be likely to remove *all* of the associated peripheral parenchyma, which was considered to be the source of the continued growth of the tumor postoperatively. On the basis of the then understanding of the natural history of the GBM, it was initially considered that an aHSPY would cure the tumor. This was attempted by many of the well-known surgeons of the day (Dandy 1928, 1933; L'Hermitte 1928; Zollinger 1935; Bell and Karnosh 1949; Hillier 1954; Gardner 1953; Gardner et al. 1955; Austin and Grant 1955). The view that an anatomical hemispherectomy (aHSPY) might be a curative surgical management of glioblastoma multiforme was settled by the middle part of the century. The postoperative quality of life in these patients was very, very poor, by nearly any standard, but perhaps more importantly,

J.P. Girvin, *Operative Techniques in Epilepsy*,
DOI 10.1007/978-3-319-10921-3_12

the gliomas were not cured. Thus, the use of the aHSPY simply prolonged very low-quality lives of the patients and hence was discarded. However, the one aspect of the operations, which was of some importance, was that it was clearly evident that patients could survive this radical procedure, certainly more radical than any previous neurological surgery. In any hemispherectomy, it is true that ". . . the more pronounced the neurological defect, the more advantageous will be the operation" (Goodall 1957). There is no argument with the fact that those with an already poor quality of life because of neurological deficits from the GBM, per se, would not suffer as much as those who were neurologically intact preoperatively, but also the fact remained that the GBM was not cured and the quality of life, irrespective of the preoperativc state, was far worse postoperatively.

12.1.3 The Use of the aHSPY in Infantile Hemiplegia and Epilepsy

The treatment of intractable seizures of children with infantile hemiplegia and epilepsy was a different story and stood in marked contrast to that for gliomas. The initial attempt at its use in this condition was by Dr. Kenneth McKenzie in Toronto (1938; see also Williams and Scott 1939). Its success led to its widespread use in the ensuing years (Krynauw 1950; Cairns 1951; Polani 1952; McKissock 1953, 1954; Meyers 1958). The most exciting report was that of Krynauw in South Africa. He carried out aHSPYs on 12 patients, between the ages of 8 months and 21 years. They all had the syndrome of infantile hemiplegia, intractable hemispheric seizures, and mental changes. His operation consisted of the anatomical removal of the hemisphere with the exception of "the thalamus and the caudate nucleus and its tail." There was one immediate postoperative death. The operation, beginning with McKenzie, was often called "hemidecortication" (Meyers 1958; Carmichael 1966), which in some ways is a more accurate anatomical description of the procedure. The pathology of the removed hemispheric components was a *potpourri* of abnormalities with no single pervasive morphological identified abnormality. Krynauw's patients had transient increased motor impairments. However, eventually the motor abilities were improved, if anything. There was a profound cortical sensory impairment, which never completely resolved. There was a contralateral hemianopia, if it had not existed preoperatively, with macular sparing, which was of no clinical consequence.

12.1.4 Postoperative Courses

The popularity of the operation for epilepsy was really attributed to the outcomes of the patients. In all the patients, the seizures were abolished, without the use of anticonvulsant medication. In all, there were profound improvements in behavioral abnormalities, e.g., temper tantrums, improved cognitive function, improved motor function, and improvement in what were referred to as "personality" traits. The latter were so striking that there were some who considered that the aHSPY should be conducted for this abnormality alone! Thus, by the middle of the twentieth century, there was general consensus that the operation of aHSPY was the most beneficial operation for epilepsy, when the patients presented with intractable seizures based on cerebral hemiatrophy and infantile hemiplegia. Unlike the poor postoperative cognition of the tumor patients having undergone an anatomic hemispherectomy, those with seizures and infantile hemiplegia were the reverse in that there was nearly *always* significant cognitive improvement (McFie 1961; Smith and Sugar 1975). This was the consensus by neuropsychologists who commented upon it in the literature.

Most disappointingly, the foregoing excitement about the beneficial outcomes of the operation did not last long, for it was about the same time when there began to appear in the literature the odd article describing peculiar complications in the longer postoperative courses of some patients. The original article by Noetzel in 1940 was followed by other articles, which ushered in the evidence of delayed complications that led to the demise of the operation of anatomical HSPY (McKissock 1953; Cabieses et al. 1957; Laine et al. 1964; Oppenheimer and Griffith 1966; Griffith 1967; Falconer and Wilson 1969; Wilson 1970a, b).

The initially described complications were not uniform, and there was no standard acceptance as to why the complications occurred. However, gradually it became evident that the common complications included subdural appearance of a membrane or more than one membrane, fluid in the resective cavity that was xanthochromic or bloody, granular ependymitis, and often hydrocephalus (Noetzel 1940; Adams 1983). The latter could be managed, but the former failed any reasonable management. It soon became a recognizable hemorrhagic syndrome that eventually was simply designated a "delayed" intracranial hemorrhage. Its actual location was not easily identified nor absolute. It was labeled by some as "subdural" (Oppenheimer and Griffith 1966; Falconer and Wilson 1969; Wilson 1970a, b), and there was nearly always associated evidence of hemosiderin in the brain and spinal cord (Falconer and Wilson 1969; Wilson 1970b). This hemorrhagic complication became associated with a number of names with various designations, but eventually the term "superficial cerebral hemosiderosis" (SCH) probably became the one used most commonly (Rasmussen 1973, 1975, 1983; Rasmussen and Andermann 1983).

No source of bleeding was found to which one might attach a specific physiological etiology nor was there any recognition suggesting a potential prophylaxis or certain satisfactory treatment of the complication. The notion arose that it was the large area left by the hemispherectomy that somehow gave rise to the bleeding, which led to various suggestions as to how the cavity might be reduced in volume. Oppenheimer and Griffith were the first to suggest managements of the complications; these included the disconnection of a part of the hemisphere, but leaving it in place, thus reducing the cavity size (1966), which was echoed by Wilson (1970b). Another suggestion was to simply use a corpus callosotomy as a replacement for hemispherectomy (Wilson et al. 1975). Rasmussen reviewed the MNI results of both aHSPYs as well as multi-lobar resections for the management of intractable epilepsy. Approximately a third of the former developed the SCH syndrome, but none of the latter developed the hemorrhagic complication (1973, 1983). He and his colleagues considered that "this syndrome results after anatomically complete hemispherectomy from lack of adequate support of the remaining hemisphere within the skull and its consequent vulnerability to minimal jolts to the head or brief physiological increases in intracranial pressure (e.g., coughing, sneezing) leading to repeated leakage of red blood cells into the intracranial cavity" (Tinuper et al. 1988).

In order to reduce or abolish the SCH syndrome, Rasmussen, in 1968, began carrying out operations associated with leaving in place (and connected) at the least epileptogenic 25–33 % of the hemisphere in patients with infantile hemiplegia, an operation that he referred to as a "subtotal hemispherectomy." However, the seizure outcomes in these patients were less efficacious (45 % vs 59 %), but as expected, the SCH syndrome was not observed (Rasmussen 1983). This "cost of a significant lessening of the effectiveness of the cortical excision" in the subtotal hemispherectomies led Rasmussen to further revise the operation by "disconnecting the remaining segment of the bad hemisphere from the rest of the brain by sectioning the white matter down to the medial pial surface," which involved "the remaining frontal or occipital pole ..... separated from the corpus callosum and the upper brain stem, resulting in a functional complete but anatomical subtotal hemispherectomy" (Rasmussen 1983; Tuniper et al. 1988; Villemure and Rasmussen 1990). The latter, or a modification of it, is what eventually developed and came to be called a "functional hemispherectomy" (fHSPY). This fHSPY was joined by a more recent, less invasive, technique, which has been labeled a "hemispherotomy," in which nearly the whole of the disconnected hemisphere is left intact (Delalande et al. 1992, 2001). This will be discussed briefly in Sect. 12.3.

Thus, in summary, as clinical experience accumulated, it became evident that this late hemorrhagic complication occurred many years (a minimum of 3–4 years and up to 20+ years) postoperatively after an aHSPY, that it involved approximately 25–33 % of the aHSPYs carried out, and that 50 % of those who developed the complication died. Thus, in the final analysis, one out of every seven or eight cases undergoing an aHSPY died some years later by complications attributable to the operative procedure, which had been conducted many years earlier! As a result, shortly after the middle of the twentieth century, the use of the aHSPY as an operative procedure for the surgical management of epilepsy gradually came to an end.

12.2 Functional (fHSPY)

12.2.1 Introduction

There have been many examples of fHSPYs with slightly different alterations in methodology. Independently, I have used the same technical fHSPY, as described in this section, since the 1970s (see Girvin and Baessa 2006). It is not dissimilar to the final revision of what was used at the Montreal Neurological Institute by Villemure and Rasmussen and their colleagues (1993). It has been a very satisfactory procedure in my hands, and, as a result, I have thus seen no reason to change it, on the basis of what I interpret to be minor suggestions of alterations in the literature. The reader may be interested in reviewing many of these modifications, which have appeared in the literature since the turn of the century (Schramm 2002; Binder and Schramm 2006; Almeida et al. 2006). I will not comment on these fHSPYs, as I truly believe that it is what a surgeon develops on his/her own, or learned during residency, that best determines the best procedure for him/her. The article of Binder and Schramm outlines the advantages that they feel exist in their "transsylvian functional hemispherectomy" as compared with the Rasmussen version. I could quite honestly make a similar comparison of the advantages of the one I will describe in the following narrative, compared with Binder's and Schramm's method, but I do not feel that it is terribly useful. In considering the many different techniques that may emerge from a given surgical operation, one should be aware of Cushing's very relevant statement in Keen's *Surgery: Its Principles and Practice*, "Many of the views to be expressed are purely personal ones and are given with the full knowledge that the instruments and operative details found satisfactory to one individual may be entirely unsuited to the operative requirements of others" (1910, p.261). For those in academic institutions with neurosurgery residency programs, these operations provide significantly rewarding learning experiences for residents!

My fHSPY consists of the removal of the temporal lobe and the lower part of the Rolandic cortex, but leaving the remaining disconnected hemisphere (frontal and posterior parietal and occipital lobes and the superior Rolandic cortex) in place, with no mortality, a paucity of morbidity, and nearly always with the abolition of seizures or greater than a 90 % reduction in seizures. A significant portion of the patients is off anticonvulsant medication and free of seizures. It is a safe procedure and easily performed. I have arbitrarily divided the technical procedure into a continuum of five relatively individually isolated surgical steps, which I have labeled: (1) radical temporal lobectomy (TLY), (2) central (Rolandic) corticectomy, (3) corpus callosotomy, (4) posterior medial and orbitofrontal incision, and (5) anteroposteromedial parietal incision.

12.2.2 Indications

The indications for an fHSPY are varied. That for which it was originally indicated in the management of intractable epilepsy related particularly to infantile hemiplegia and it remains the most appropriate procedure for treatment of this condition and one of the most efficacious surgical managements of intractable epilepsy. However, it also has become a very satisfactory operation for certain patients with Rasmussen's encephalitis, hemi-megalencephaly, and a variety of other less common diseases, e.g., some cases of Sturge-Weber disease, porencephalic cysts, etc. King et al. were the first to consider the use of hemispherectomy in the surgical management of hemimegalencephaly (1985). The reader who is interested in the complexities of hemimegalencephaly is referred to more comprehensive reviews in the literature (Dekaban and Sakuragawa 1977; DeMyer 1999; Di Rocco and Iannelli 2000).

12.2.3 General Surgical Considerations

One feature of the surgical conduct of either type of hemispherectomy is the difference between the cases with large ventricles as compared to those in which ventriculomegaly is not present. This difference is *not* minor by any means. The surgery of the latter takes much longer. In those with large ventricles (infantile hemiplegia with typical hemispheric atrophy, some porencephalic cases, and occasional Rasmussen's encephalitis), the whole operation can be easily carried out within 2–3 h. However, those with small ventricles, or anatomically distorted small ventricles, which may especially be seen in hemimegalencephaly with significantly distorted anatomy, can take up to 5–6 h or even more infrequently. In these latter cases it takes more time to incise the much thicker mantles of parenchyma, more time to sort out distorted anatomy, more time to easily find and follow the small ventricles, more time to achieve satisfactory hemostasis, and more time to retract parenchyma. Any one of these potential eventualities can head the list of added labor-intensive features in the conduct of fHSPYs in which there are small and distorted ventricles and/or postoperative complications, especially in infants below the age of 9 months (see DiRocco and Iannelli 2000).

Another aspect of the fHSPY, which is different from general neurosurgery, is that the vascular supply to the disconnected parts of the hemisphere that are being left in place, i.e., the posterior parietal, occipital, and frontal lobes, should be preserved. This is another aspect of the fHSPY, which is more tedious in the group of cases with small ventricles and larger volumes of parenchyma. Adams indicated the importance of good hemostasis in this operative procedure, noting that it should be "immaculate" (1983)!

12.2.4 Scalp Incision

The preferred scalp incision is not dissimilar to that used for the aTLY, as noted and illustrated in Chap. 6 (Sect. 6.2.2). It does not need to be any larger than the interrupted line in Fig. 12.1a that is the same as that for an aTLY demonstrated in Fig. 6.1, *if* the operation is for disorders in which there is significant hydrocephalus, e.g., infantile hemiplegia. However, if it is for one of the conditions with small ventricles and large amounts of parenchyma, then it needs to be somewhat more posterior and superior, reaching approximately the temporo-occipital junction in the former and within 2–3 cm of the midline in the latter, as illustrated by the solid line in Fig. 12.1a. This is more easily understood by referring to Figs. 12.1b, c. B illustrates the case of the very large ventricles, which characterize the cases of infantile hemiplegia. The lateral ventricle is not only extremely enlarged, but the anterior extent of the large trigone is more anteriorly situated because of the atrophy of the parenchyma of the temporal lobe, the insula, and the forebrain nuclei, i.e., thalamus and hypothalamus. C illustrates the usual (normal) position of the trigone as a result of the normal or above normal amount of parenchyma, both cortical and in the gray matter nuclei of the forebrain. Thus, the scalp incision must be carried more posteriorly and medially in order to easily achieve the second (see Sect. 12.2.5) and third (see Sect. 12.2.6) steps, respectively, of the fHSPY described in the following sections.

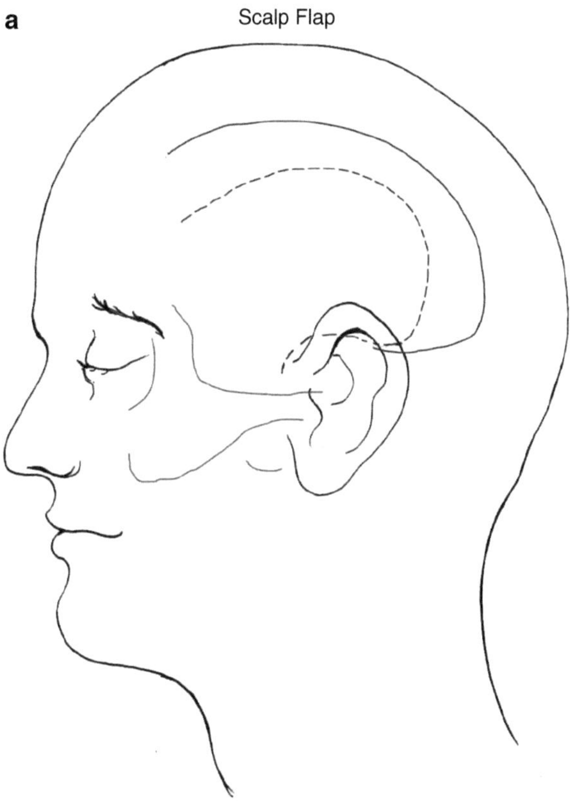

Fig. 12.1 Scalp incision for a functional hemispherectomy (fHSPY). (**a**) Illustration of the typical scalp incision for an aTLY, which is also perfectly satisfactory for an fHSPY in the case of infantile hemiplegia (*interrupted line*). The larger incision of the same shape (*solid line*) is the recommended incision for the fHSPY associated with conditions that have a normal, or greater than normal, amount of parenchyma and normal-sized or distorted small ventricles. The different-sized scalp incisions are depicted in figures (**b**), which shows the large ventricle and atrophied forebrain gray matter (thalamus and hypothalamus) that typifies that of the infantile hemiplegic hemisphere, and (**c**), which demonstrates the very small ventricles typically seen in some cases of Rasmussen's encephalitis, hemimegalencephaly, and Sturge-Weber disease. The *arrows* demonstrate the posterior extents (e.g., the posterior resection lines) of the TLYs, which must be reached in the two examples in order to gain comfortable access to the trigone of the lateral ventricle. The cross-hatched area depicts the size of the forebrain gray matter nuclei (see text)

Fig. 12.1 (continued)

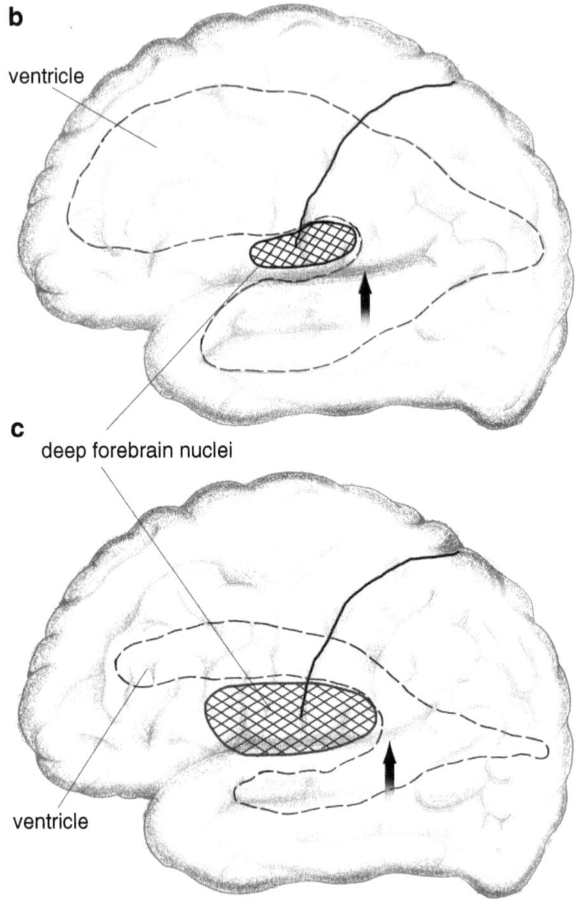

12.2.5 Radical Temporal Lobectomy (TLY)

This is a radical extension of the aTLY in that it is not "anterior" to any extent. It is a true radical complete temporal lobectomy (TLY), extending back to the trigone of the lateral ventricle, e.g., near the junction of the temporal and occipital lobes. Its surgical technique is the same as that outlined earlier for the aTLY (Sect. 6.2). The major difference is its extent, with the posterior resection (PRL) line being at the coronal cross section of the posterior trigone of the lateral ventricle; thus, its posterosuperior extent will be very close to, at, or even behind the posterior extent of the Sylvian fissure. This is illustrated in Fig. 12.2a. This is the initial stage of the fHSPY, and the very posterior removal greatly facilitates the other two steps that isolate the posterior part of the hemisphere, which will end up being disconnected from any remaining functioning cortex. The posterior cerebral artery (PCA) must be preserved, as it will be irrigating the cerebral parenchyma that will be disconnected, but otherwise left intact. This also applies to any significantly sized middle cerebral arterial (MCA) branches that cross the posterior resection line, which take the label of *en passage* arteries. Other than these points, this step is simply a more radical removal of the temporal lobe cortex than the aTLY, but its surgery is roughly the same. In those with marked atrophy, e.g., infantile hemiplegia, the TLY is much easier and less time consuming than the small ventricle/large amount of parenchyma disorders, e.g., especially megalencephaly. Figure 12.2b illustrates the surgical bed of the temporal lobectomy.

a

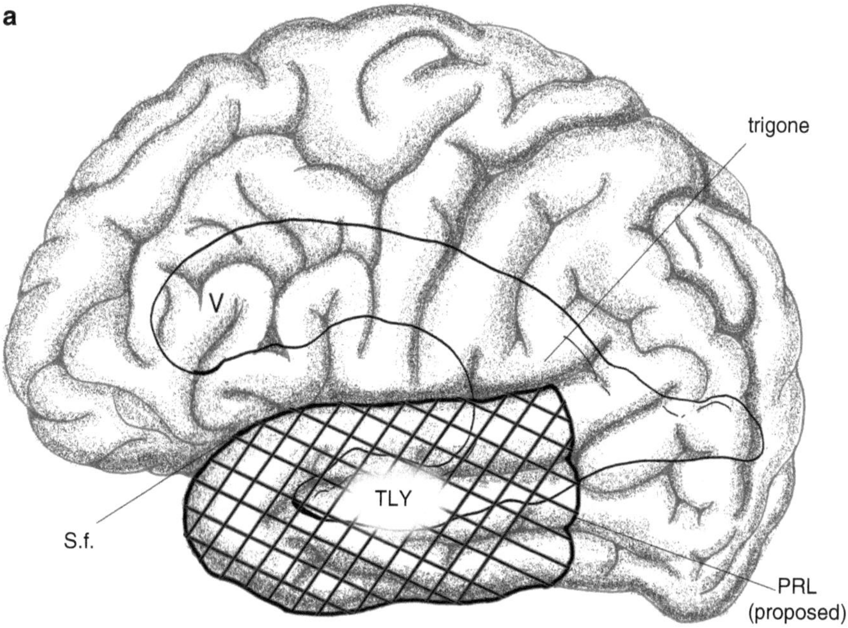

Fig. 12.2 First step of the fHSPY—radical temporal lobectomy (TLY). Illustration of the radical TLY—the initial step of the fHSPY. (**a**) The temporal lobe to be removed; as noted earlier, the posterior resection line (PRL) of this TLY will *always* reach a point that allows easy entry into the trigone of the lateral ventricle (after the lobectomy). (**b**) Diagrammatic representation of the surgical bed of the TLY. *br. stem* brain stem, *Cr.N.3* oculomotor nerve, *en.p.art.* "en passage" artery, *falx* falx cerebri, *floor* floor of the middle fossa, *fr.op.* frontal operculum, *inf. ins.* inferior insula, *lept.* leptomeninges, *med.TLlept.* medial temporal lobe leptomeninges, *PCA* posterior cerebral artery, *p.op.* parietal operculum, *PRL* posterior resection line of the TLY, *S.f.* Sylvian fissure, *t.stem.* temporal stem, *tent.c* free edge of the tentorium cerebelli, *trigone* trigone of the lateral ventricle, *TL* temporal lobe, *TLY* temporal lobectomy (radical), *V* ventricle (Redrawn, with permission, from Girvin and Baeesa (2006))

b

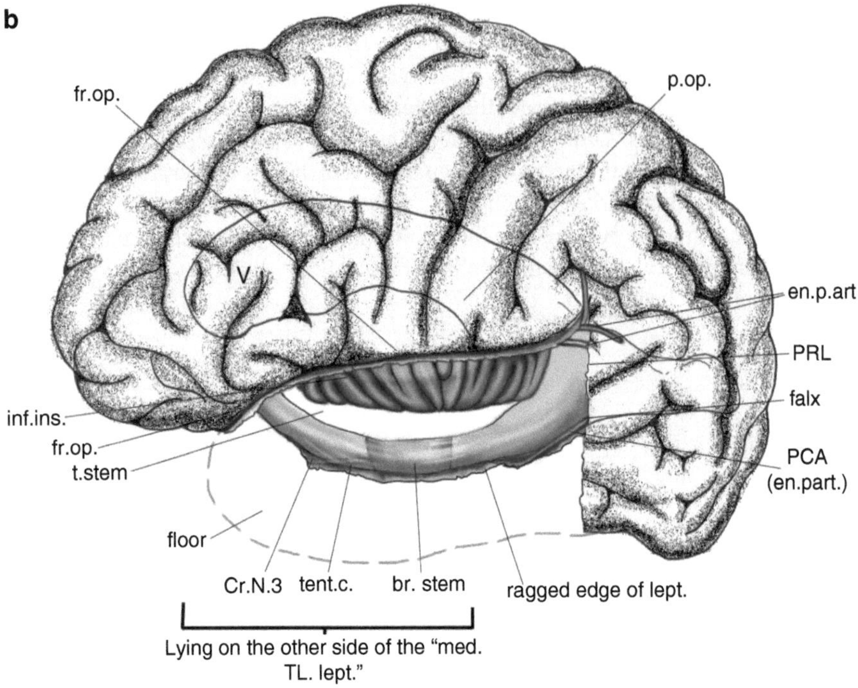

Fig. 12.2 (continued)

12.2.6 Central (Rolandic) Corticectomy

This "central corticectomy" or "Rolandic window" is the second stage of the fHSPY; it provides full access to the lateral ventricle, which is required for step three, which consists of the corpus callosotomy. Figure 12.3a outline its boundaries: (1) *inferior*, Sylvian fissure; (2) *posterior*, the extension superiorly of the posterior resection line (PRL) of the TLY; (3) *anterior*, mid-frontal, dorsolateral incision at roughly a coronal level of the sphenoid wing; and (4) *superior*, sufficient horizontal cortical and subcortical incision to achieve access to the roof of the body of the lateral ventricle, through which the corpus callosotomy will be conducted.

The surgery of a corticectomy is outlined in Chap. 5. However, this corticectomy, for the fHSPY, does not require as much attention to the preservation of the subcortical white matter (Sects. 5.3 and 5.4), the periphery of the corticectomy (Sect. 5.5), or even the preservation of overlying vessels (Sect. 5.2), which were discussed in Chap. 5. However, with respect to the latter, it becomes a matter of judgment, as the surgeon proceeds, whether there is relatively clear evidence that some vessels, which emerge from the Sylvian fissure, do irrigate the cortex that is being left intact. The superior border of the Rolandic corticectomy is near the junction of the anterior and middle cerebral arteries, which makes the likelihood of significant *en passage* vessels very small. However, if such is judged to be the case, then they should be saved intact, which may require the steps in their preservation (Sect. 5.2).

The corticectomy is initiated at the Sylvian fissure with the frontal operculum being removed subpially, as described and illustrated in the conduct of the inferior Rolandic corticectomy in Chap. 8 (Sect. 8.4.2). The operculum is removed subpially in exactly the same way as the superior temporal gyrus is removed in the initiation of an aTLY (Sect. 6.2.4). In the aTLY, the inferior insular cortex is exposed (viewed through the double layer of leptomeninges), while the removal of the frontoparietal operculum exposes in the same way the superior insular cortex. Starting with this boundary has the advantage of removing the major portion of the vascular

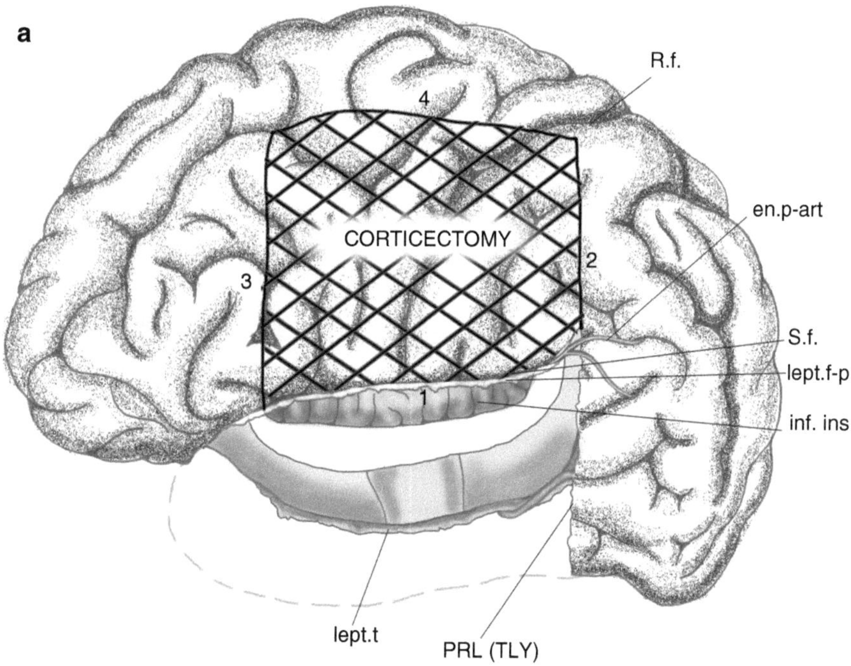

Fig. 12.3 Second step in the fHSPY—the Rolandic corticectomy. Illustrations of the second step of the fHSPY—the "Rolandic corticectomy" (or the "central" window). It is the most important step in most ways, as it paves the way for the corpus callosotomy and the following disconnection of the posterior parieto-occipital lobes posteriorly and the frontal lobe anteriorly. (**a**) Illustration of the location of the corticectomy in the central aspect of the dorsolateral surface of the (*left*) hemisphere (#s 1–4 outline the periphery of the corticectomy; see text). (**b**) A coronal section through the level of the thalamus; the *large arrow* indicates a satisfactory position of the SRL (superior resection line). (**c**) Illustration of the anatomy (same illustration as in **a**) of the surgical bed after the corticectomy. (**d**) The same coronal section as (**b**), after the corticectomy. *1* (*IRL*) inferior resection line, *2* (*PRL*) posterior resection line, *3* (*ARL*) anterior resection line (corticectomy), *4* (*SRL*) superior resection line, *b.MCA* branch(es) of the middle cerebral artery, *en.p.art.* "en passage" artery, *falx* falx cerebri (bottom edge), *fr.op.* frontal operculum, *inf.ins.* inferior insula, *ins.* insula, *j.* junction of the inferolateral and orbitofrontal cortices (also junction of the lateral and inferior surfaces of the frontal lobe and junction of the inferior and anterior boundaries of the corticectomy), *lept.f-p* (or *lept.f*) the fragments of the leptomeninges of the frontoparietal operculum, remaining following the Rolandic corticectomy, *lept.t.* fragments of the medial temporal leptomeninges, remaining after the TLY, *p.op.* parietal operculum, *R.f.* Rolandic (central) fissure, *S.f.* Sylvian (lateral) fissure, *SRL* superior resection line (also: ----), *tent* tentorium cerebelli, *Th.* thalamus, *TLY* temporal lobectomy, *V* lateral ventricle

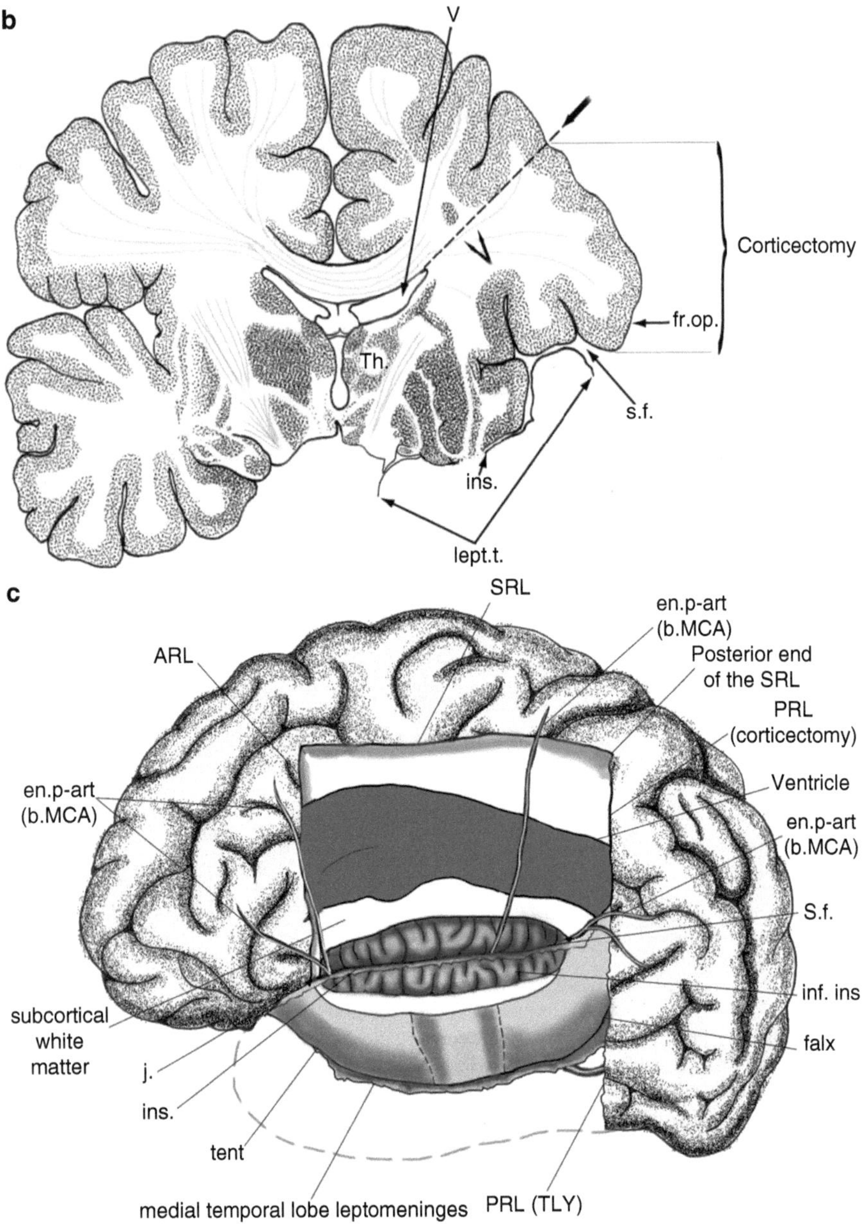

Fig. 12.3 (continued)

d

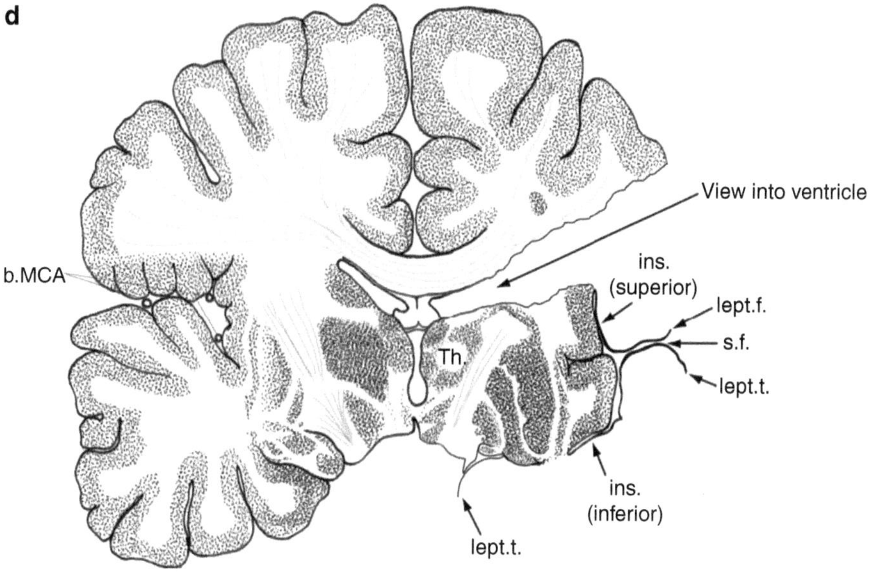

Fig. 12.3 (continued)

supply to the cortex being removed; this precludes having to do it twice, which would be the case to some degree should one chose to initiate the corticectomy at the superior boundary. The subpial removal is carried through the Rolandic operculum and then superiorly over the insula until the leptomeningeal investment of the operculum ends at the superior border of the insula, e.g., as conducted in the inferior Rolandic corticectomy. In an anteroposterior direction, this boundary will extend through the operculum posteriorly until the superior aspect of the PRL of the TLY is reached. Anteriorly, it will be carried to where an approximate coronal section would be through the posterior aspect of the orbitofrontal cortex and the sphenoid wing of the temporal bone, which will be anterior to the insula. This point will also be the inferior extent of what will become the anterior border of the corticectomy. If there are sufficiently large vessels emerging superiorly from the Sylvian fissure that clearly irrigate the frontal cortex that will be left behind after the corticectomy is completed, then they should be considered *en passage* arterial vessels and saved. *En passage* arteries are much more likely being either posterior, irrigating the posterior parietal lobe, or anterior, irrigating the frontal lobe, than superior. There are often variable numbers of middle cerebral arterial branches flowing deeply off the leptomeninges of the insular cortex that will be in this category.

The corticectomy should be primarily the cortex, once it extends superior to the insula. The base of the resection will be subcortical white matter (see Fig. 12.3c), which will protect the nuclei of the forebrain that are beneath it and should be left intact. The posterior boundary of the corticectomy is simply a superior extension of the PRL of the TLY. This will be carried out through the cortical mantle, i.e., the cortex and subcortical white matter, between the dorsolateral surface and the lateral wall of the ventricle. Its superior extent must be at, or slightly higher, than the roof of the body of the lateral ventricle, which is easily recognized as the incision is extended more and more superiorly, as illustrated in Fig. 12.3c, i.e., the subcortical white matter between the ventricle and the SRL. Figure 12.3b is a coronal section that illustrates the superior extent of the posterior resection line (large arrow), which will provide satisfactory visualization of the body of the lateral ventricle (V). Figure 12.3c also reminds the reader that any arterial vessels, which are considered to be *en passage* vessels, should be saved. The main difficulty in this corticectomy when the ventricle is normal, distorted, or smaller than normal is its identification. This fails to be troublesome if the PRL is established initially or preferably after the inferior resection line has been established at the Sylvian fissure, since its beginning, at the top of the TLY PRL, is in the trigone of the lateral ventricle. Thus, the PRL of the Rolandic corticectomy is simply carried superiorly until the roof of the ventricle is reached. Finally, Fig. 12.3d illustrates the clear visualization of the lateral ventricle, and it can be easily appreciated how the corpus callosotomy may be carried out.

In the case of a large ventricle (e.g., infantile hemiplegia), there is never a problem in finding the ventricle, both because of its size and the thinness of the mantle of the cortex and white matter overlying it. In the case of the small ventricle, it is more difficult. As noted in the foregoing paragraph, if the choice is to incise the superior boundary before the posterior boundary, then it can lead to significant difficulty in identifying the ventricle, especially in the case of hemimegalencephaly, as often in this case, the surgeon is relegated to a position of having to guess where the ventricle should be located beneath the incision. Under this circumstance, the surgeon has to deepen the superior incision, guessing that the ventricle will be in the depths of the chosen incision. If this strategy is chosen, it is far safer to err on the side of the incision being too superior rather than too inferior in which the thalamus might be entered. However, as stated in the foregoing, the posterior boundary can be easily carried out prior to the superior boundary and taken superiorly to the roof of the lateral ventricle from which the incision of the superior boundary can very easily and confidently be conducted satisfactorily.

Once the roof of the ventricle is reached by the extension of the PRL, then the superior resection line (SRL) can be initiated slightly superior to it (see Fig. 12.3b) and carried anteriorly, somewhat above but using the roof to determine the SRL. The latter is carried anteriorly until there is clear evidence of an increase in the (rostrocaudal, e.g., from above down) size of the ventricle having been reached, which is the usual indication that the posterior extent of the frontal horn of the lateral ventricle has been reached. The incision is then turned downward, and the anterior resection line (ARL) is completed by carrying the incision inferiorly to the anterior extent of the inferior resection line, which has already been completed. As noted earlier, this will be near the anterior extent of the Sylvian fissure, approximately above the sphenoid wing of the temporal bone, anterior to the insula, and at the junction of the lateral and orbitofrontal cortices. There are nearly always some middle cerebral arterial branches, which will be preserved as they emerge from the fissure to irrigate parts of the dorsolateral and lateral orbital frontal cortex.

The final part of the corticectomy, most prominently in those cases of the small ventricle fHSPYs, is resecting the cortex of the Rolandic window. This requires removal of the gray matter (cortex) while leaving a generous amount of the underlying white matter between the inferior boundary, which, with the inferior frontal operculum removed, will have been elevated above the Sylvian fissure and the superior boundary. This figure also demonstrates that the white matter incision is always in a superior direction from the superior insular border, which avoids the possibility of entering the thalamus. Once this has been achieved, the whole of the ventricle can be more easily visualized, as depicted in Fig. 12.3c, d. Any difficulty in the visualization can be reduced by removal of more of the white matter bordering on the ventricle.

12.2.7 Corpus Callosotomy (CCY)

A corpus callosotomy is now conducted from *within* the ventricle. This can only be achieved satisfactorily by identifying the anatomical features that will allow confidence in the placement of the incision in the appropriate part of the corpus callosum (CC). What are the features? They include the interhemispheric fissure, the pericallosal arteries, and the recognition of the white matter that has the characteristics of the CC, e.g., its intense white colored fibers, as compared to the cortex, and its thinness and bundled morphology. It helps to see both pericallosal arteries, but the most important is being certain that the ipsilateral artery is recognized as such. This can be done through the roof of the ventricle, erring if there is concern, by initiating the exploration too ipsilaterally. This may seem unnecessary, but one way of getting into trouble is if the initial surgery crosses the midline and produces injury contralaterally, but believing that it is on the ipsilateral side of the interhemispheric fissure. I truly do not think the strategy needs to be defended—a position that is very strongly held by those who have suffered the kind of troubles just noted!

Figure 12.4a depicts an enlarged focal illustration of the surgical pathway entrance into the body of the lateral ventricle, which was shown in Fig. 12.3d. In this illustration are shown the interhemispheric fissure, the two pericallosal arteries, the corpus callosum, and the midline septum separating the bodies of the two lateral ventricles. The surgeon must choose the anatomical feature that will provide a safe CCY from the anterior tip of the rostrum back to the posterior border of the splenium. From experience, my preference, which is a strong preference, is to incise the CC, identify the *ipsilateral* pericallosal artery, and follow the pericallosal artery throughout the extent of the CC. This is a very easy method of carrying out the CCY, even in the absence of a protective element surrounding the artery, such as a leptomeningeal barrier. As the posterior part of the CCY is reached, the artery may be small, may disappear, or may be replaced by a small posterior pericallosal artery, but none of these changes is very important in altering the ease of completing the CCY. By far and away, the most difficulty in this step is the absolutely certain identification of the CC in the most appropriate place that allows the accurate identification of the anatomy above it, e.g., the pericallosal arteries in particular.

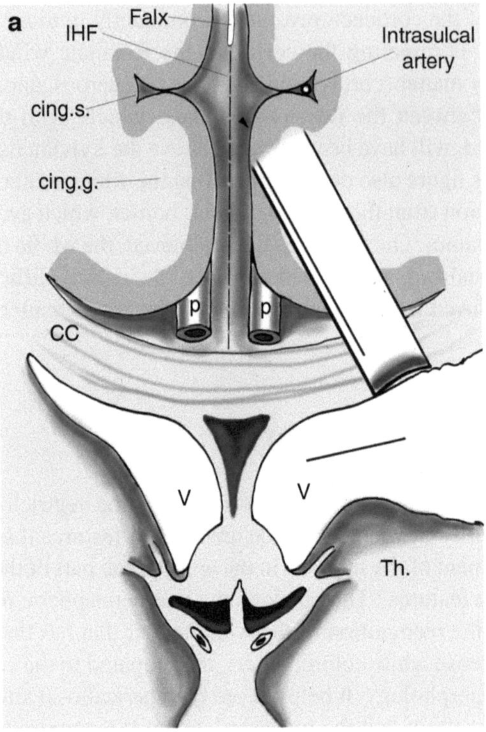

Fig. 12.4 Third step in the fHSPY—corpus callosotomy from within the lateral ventricle. This illustrates the various strategies and potential difficulties associated with the anatomical recognition of the ipsilateral pericallosal artery, along which the corpus callosotomy is carried out. (**a**) A coronal section, through the "window" into the body of the lateral ventricle, which results from the Rolandic corticectomy. (**b**) A demonstration of incisions (*arrows*) in the CC that should not be made, e.g., they are too medial: the result?—an initiation of the incision near the midline that then angles across the CC and ends up in the contralateral hemisphere parenchyma and/or lateral ventricle (see text). (**c**) An enlarged incision in the CC that shows the two pericallosal arteries. (**d**) An illustration of a method of identifying the midline anatomy by initiating the incision ipsilaterally, well lateral to the midline, entering the ipsilateral cingulate gyrus, and then removing its parenchyma over to the medial leptomeningeal investment; (**e**) a depiction of the cingulate cortex having been removed inferiorly by intrinsic subpial resection after which the pericallosal artery can be visualized (see *arrow*) through the remaining leptomeninges (see text). (**f**) An illustration of what the final exposure of the ipsilateral pericallosal artery should look like; it also reflects what would be seen in any coronal section, e.g., a diagram of the CCY being carried out from the rostrum to the splenium, following the pericallosal artery. *CC* corpus callosum, *CCi* CC incision, *cing.g.* cingulate gyrus, *cing.s.* cingulate sulcus, *falx* inferior edge of falx cerebri, *IHF* interhemispheric fissure, *med.lept.* medial (hemispheric) leptomeninges, *p* pericallosal artery, *Th* thalamus, *V* ventricle (body), *X* unacceptable paths initiating a corpus callosotomy (from within the ventricle)

Fig. 12.4 (continued)

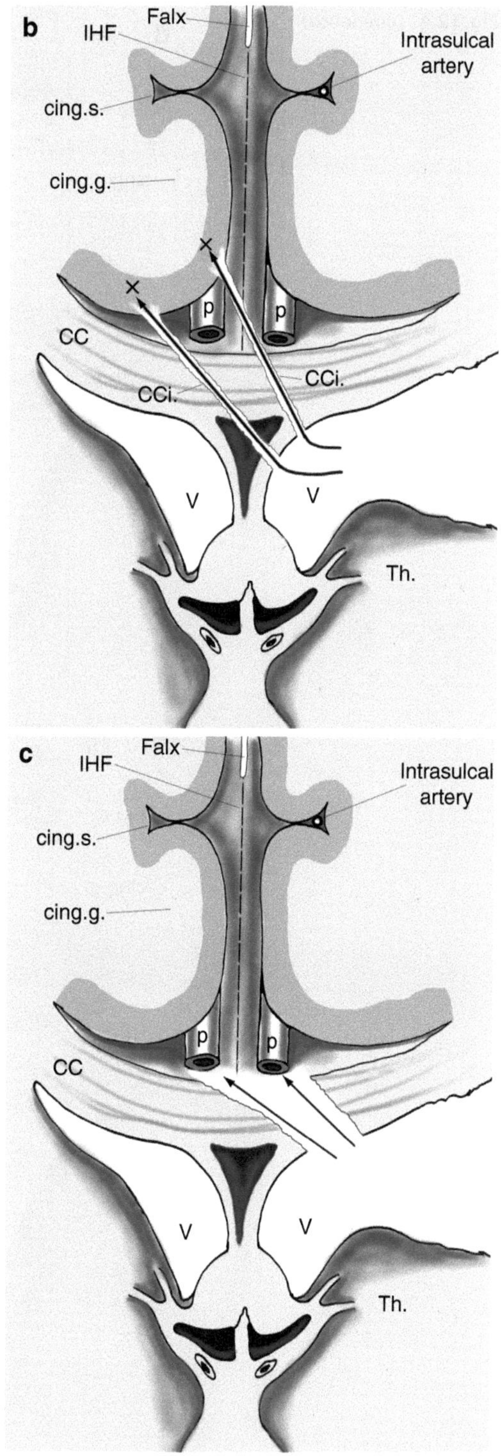

Fig. 12.4 (continued)

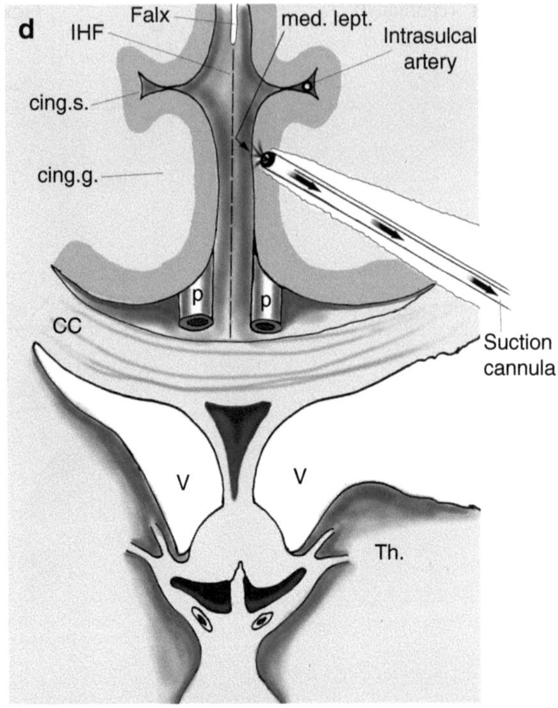

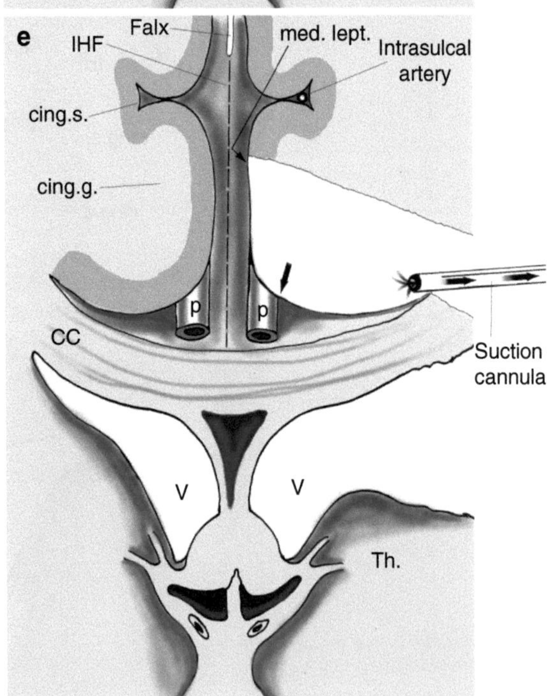

Fig. 12.4 (continued)

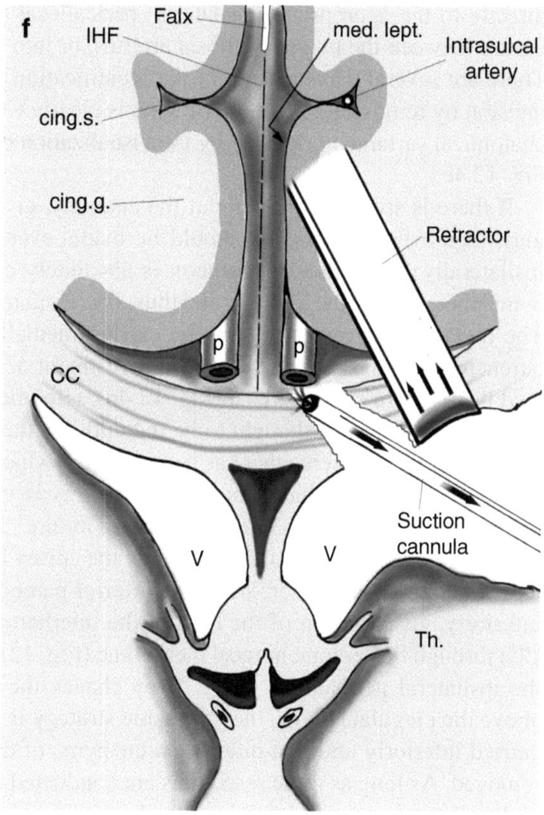

Figure 12.4b depicts what should *not* be done, i.e., crossing the midline and entering the contralateral hemisphere, usually the cingulate gyrus, or identifying the contralateral pericallosal as the ipsilateral artery. A single pericallosal artery should *never* be identified and considered to be the ipsilateral artery. Rather, both pericallosal arteries should be identified. When this is achieved, then the CCY through the CC lateral to the ipsilateral artery is straightforward and can be safely achieved in the absence of entering the contralateral hemispheric ventricle and/or parenchyma. The latter is usually the result of initiating the incision too medial, through the roof of the ventricle, resulting not in a perpendicular incision through the CC that is difficult to achieve with certainty, but rather an angled incision that enters the contralateral side of the midline. There is nothing wrong with this occurring *IF* the surgeon recognizes the potential error, halts the process, and starts over again.

The preferred strategy is to slowly and gently initiate the incision well ipsilateral to what is considered the midline on the undersurface of the CC. This may lead directly to the appropriate (ipsilateral) pericallosal artery, to the interhemispheric fissure between the two pericallosal arteries, or into the ipsilateral cingulate gyrus. There are several ways to help in the identification of the anatomy. Enlarging the incision by removing *only* more of what is clearly CC may be sufficient to provide anatomical certainty, primarily by the visualization of the two arteries, as shown in Fig. 12.4c.

If there is still confusion about the anatomy, given the foregoing noted strategies, then a further incision should be made, even more proximally (e.g., more ipsilaterally), such that the surgeon is absolutely certain to be on the ipsilateral hemisphere side of the midline, and thus, the (ipsilateral) cingulate gyrus is entered. The incision can very gradually be carried medially in the gyrus, removing the parenchyma until the leptomeningeal investment of the medial aspect of the operated hemisphere is recognized (Fig. 12.4d). (Be mindful that if the resection continues beyond what is thought to be the midline, then it must be considered that it is the contralateral gyrus that has been entered, which, of course, has no leptomeningeal membrane in that direction.) Once this is visualized, the surgeon can be confident of being at the interhemispheric fissure. The inferior white matter then can be removed, while at the same time, the cortex is removed subpially using the leptomeninges as a barrier. When the inferior parenchyma of the gyrus is removed inferiorly, visualization of the base of the interhemispheric fissure (the top of the CC) through the leptomeningeal membrane (Fig. 12.4e) allows the identification of the ipsilateral pericallosal artery. If by chance the latter type incision is carried above the cingulate gyrus, then the same strategy is utilized, i.e., subpial resection carried inferiorly until the inferior parenchyma of the gyrus over the CC has been removed. As long as these resections are conducted on the ipsilateral side and subpially, there is *no* risk of injury to the arteries, e.g., calloso-marginal or other branches (Fig. 12.5).

Irrespective of how the exposure of the ipsilateral pericallosal artery has been achieved, enlargement of the incision antero-posteriorly along the artery will now easily allow the minimal superior retraction of the tissue lateral to it (see Fig. 12.5), which facilitates the visualization required for completion of the CCY. Once this is initiated, the CCY can be easily and quickly achieved by the suction cannula and bipolar forceps. This is illustrated in the coronal section of Fig. 12.4f and in a sagittal plane in Fig. 12.5. In the latter, a small segment of the CCY is illustrated. That segment is shown as a result of retraction of the ventricular roof lateral to the incision, which of course includes a portion of the CC, thus exposing both the pericallosal artery and the incised CC edge. As the CCY is moved forward, the size of the artery helps make it easier to follow the path of the incision. Moving posteriorly the artery gradually becomes smaller, but usually a small posterior pericallosal artery is present that can be followed satisfactorily to the posterior end of the splenium. Anteriorly the curvilinear incision can be followed over and around the genu and down inferiorly along the majority of the rostrum.

After the CCY, the only remaining parenchyma that requires disconnection is that of the medial and inferior frontal cortices and a small part of the medial parietal cortex.

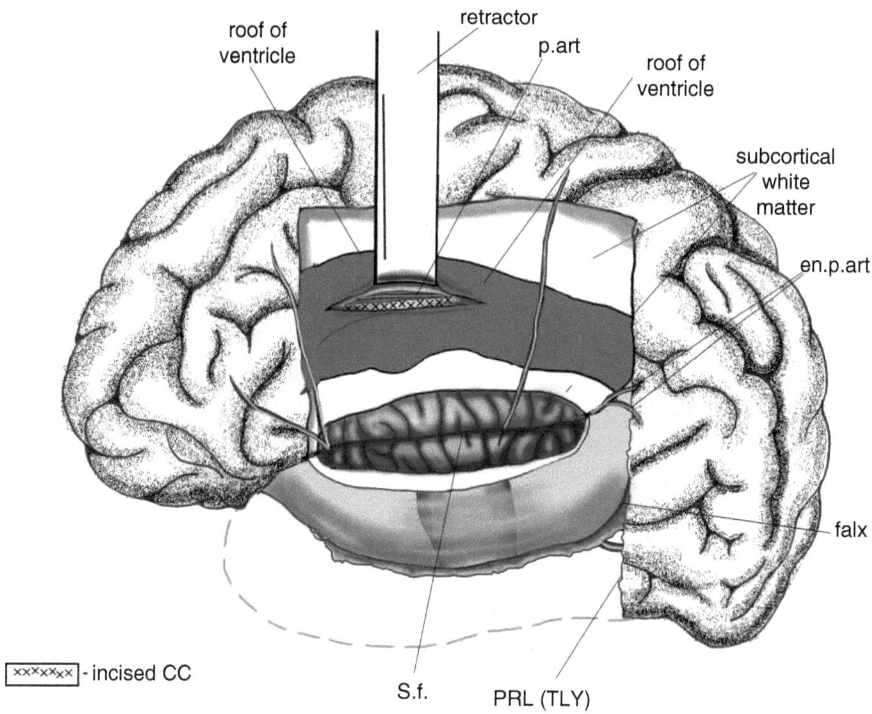

Fig. 12.5 Sagittal section illustrating the CCY from within the ventricle. This is the same figure as Fig. 12.3c with some modification. It is a sagittal section of the resection bed of the Rolandic corticectomy, demonstrating most particularly the opening into the body of the lateral ventricle. It shows a fragment of the CCY beneath the retractor blade, which is retracting the ventricular roof; a segment of the CC has been incised (crosshatched) following the pericallosal artery that can be seen in the background. *en.p.art.* en passage artery, *CC* corpus callosum, *falx* inferior falx cerebri, near its base at its junction with the tentorium cerebelli, *p.art.* pericallosal artery, *PRL* posterior resection line of the temporal lobectomy

12.2.8 The Posteroinferior Frontal Incision

This incision can be made as the last (step 5) or next to the last (step 4) incision required to complete the fHSPY. These are the last incisions leading to the disconnection of the frontal lobe and are located in the small segment of the inferomedial cortex, inferior to the anterior incision end of the CCY (see Fig. 12.6a), and the posterior orbitofrontal cortex, from the anteroinferior junction of the boundaries of the Rolandic corticectomy to the medial cortex (Fig. 12.6b). The figure illustrates these incisions as dotted lines over the medial surface (a) and the inferior orbital surface (b). Both incisions are conducted completely subpially from within, i.e., without incising the leptomeninges, as extended continuities of parenchymal incisions from the earlier steps of the surgery. Thus, since they are conducted subpially, any arterial vessels irrigating the disconnected frontal parenchyma will remain intact.

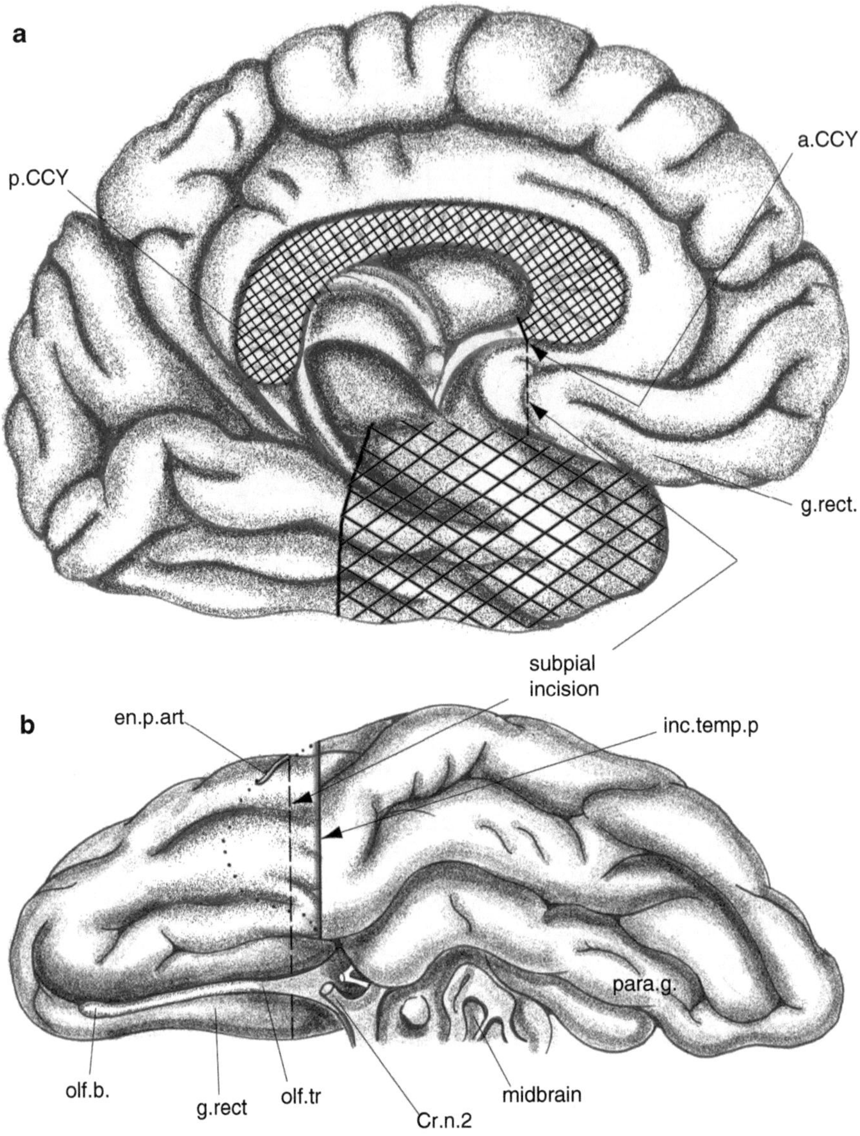

Fig. 12.6 Illustrations of the disconnections required to complete the fHSPY. Illustration of the disconnections that are required in order to complete the isolation of the frontal lobe parenchyma that is being left in place, as part of the fHSPY. The disconnecting incisions of a left frontal lobe are shown on the outside of the medial (**a**) and inferior (**b**) surfaces and the *interrupted lines* mark the paths of the subpial disconnecting incisions. However, the leptomeninges and arterial vessels and the olfactory bulb and tract exterior to the leptomeninges are left completely intact, as the incisions are conducted subpially, i.e., from inside the leptomeninges (see text). *a.CCY* anterior extent of the corpus callosotomy, *Cr.N.2* optic nerve, *en.p.art.* en passage artery, *g.rect.* gyrus rectus, *inc. temp.p.* the incision used to remove the temporal pole (for this illustration), *olf.b* olfactory bulb, *olf. tr.* olfactory tract, *p.CCY* posterior extent of the corpus callosotomy, *para.g.* parahippocampal gyrus (for the ease of the illustration, the temporal lobe remains true, the crosshatching in the (**a**) figure simply depicting the prior removal of the TL and the completion of the CCY) (Redrawn, with permission, from Girvin and Baeesa (2006))

The medial incision is initiated at the anterior end of the CCY incision (Fig. 12.6a) and carried inferiorly, by subpial resection, across the cortex and the underlying white matter. It will end at the leptomeninges of the inferior surface, which will be over the posterior part of the olfactory tract. In this resection, the branches of the pericallosal artery will be outside of the protective leptomeningeal membrane. The disconnection is then completed by completing a posterior orbitofrontal subpial incision, which laterally begins at the anteroinferior point of the Rolandic corticectomy and is carried medially until the medial hemispheric leptomeninges are reached at the point where the medial incision had ended, e.g., over the posterior part of the olfactory tract (Fig. 12.6b). Again, in this latter part of the frontal lobe isolation, there will be arteries that will be preserved by virtue of being outside the leptomeninges.

In large part, this incision is outlined in Chap. 7 (Sect. 7.2.4), but in the latter case, the eventual achievement is an orbitofrontal corticectomy with removal of the cortex and some of the underlying white matter. In the disconnection associated with the fHSPY, the only "removal" is that of the subpial incision line, with removal of just enough parenchyma to provide sufficient visualization to ensure that the incision does isolate the cortex and *all* the underlying frontal white matter.

12.2.9 Anteromedial Parietal Incision

This can be done as either step 4 or step 5 in the hemispherectomy. It involves the final disconnection of the remaining parietal and occipital lobes of the operated hemisphere. This is a short incision extending inferiorly from the posterior (splenial) end of the CCY down to the postero-superomedial extent of the PRL (posterior resection line) of the radical TLY. The latter point will be in the parahippocampal gyrus of the temporal lobe. This is most easily carried out by following the anterior curvilinear aspect of the falx cerebri, starting inferiorly in the superior aspect of the posterior resection line of the radical TLY. This tissue, depending upon the neuroanatomical textbook that is reviewed, may variously be referred to as the medial occipitotemporal, parahippocampal, fusiform, or even the posterior lingual gyrus. I have always referred to it as the "isthmus of the cingulate gyrus." Irrespective of what it is called, it is anatomically the continuity between the cingulate and parahippocampal gyri, which occurs at the very posterior end and undersurface of the splenium of the corpus callosum. It is also in this small area where the most anterior part of the calcarine cortex is located. This is illustrated in Fig. 12.7.

Figure 12.7 is a surface view of the medial aspect of the hemisphere. An interrupted line on the surface marks this disconnecting incision between the posterior end of the CCY in the splenium and the postero-superomedial extent of the radical TLY. As with the foregoing step, there is no incision through the leptomeninges. Rather, these and the underlying arterial vessels remain intact; the only incision is made subpially through the cortex and its underlying white matter. Once again the surgical technique is to conduct the incision through the medial wall of the ventricle and the small parenchymal mantle of the isthmus until the medial leptomeningeal investment of the isthmus is recognized. Reference to the base of the falx is illustrated in Figs. 12.7c and 12.5 near or at its junction with the tentorium cerebelli. The curvilinear aspect of the falx is then followed superiorly. As the splenium is

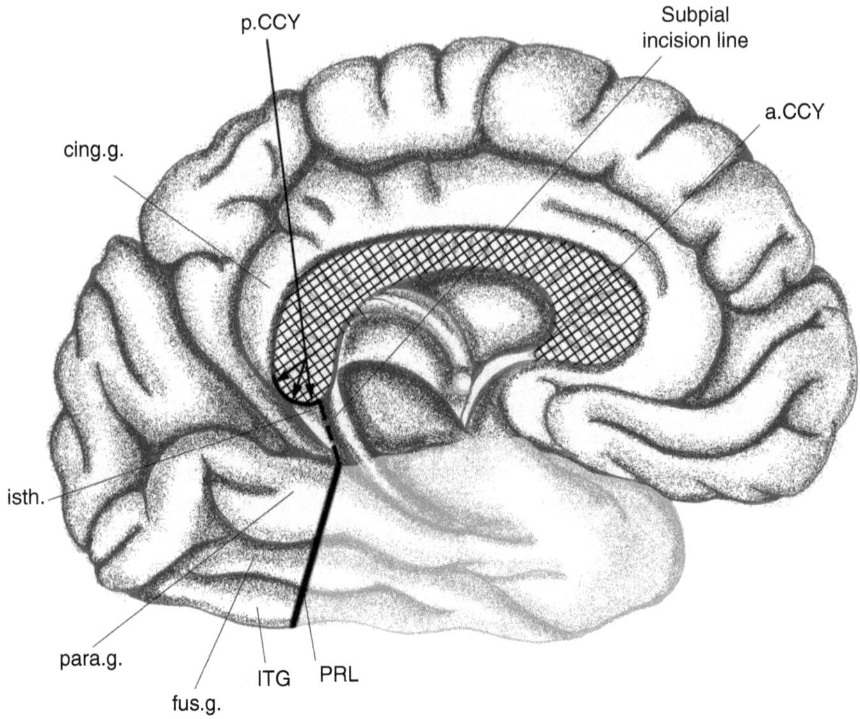

Fig. 12.7 The final medial disconnection in the fHSPY. This illustrates the medial surface of the hemisphere. The *broken line* is the pathway of the subpial incision that is required to isolate the posterior parenchyma of the hemisphere that is being left intact. It extends from the posterior extent of the splenium, i.e., the posterior extent of the CCY, to the antero-superomedial aspect of the PRL (posterior resection line) of the TLY. The CCY is illustrated by crosshatching and the TLY by dark/light shading. *a.CCY* anterior extent of the corpus callosotomy, *cing.g.* cingulate gyrus, *fus.g.* fusiform gyrus, *isth.* isthmus of the cingulate gyrus, *ITG* inferior temporal gyrus, *para.g.* parahippocampal gyrus, *p.CCY* the posterior extent of the corpus callosotomy, *PRL* posterior resection line of the radical TLY (Redrawn, with permission, from Girvin and Baeesa (2006))

approached, the falx is more posteriorly located than the proposed incision, as it extends behind and then above the splenium. Thus, the leptomeningeal investment alone, e.g., without the advantage of the fibrous protective element of the underlying falx, must be followed more cautiously over the last few millimeters to reach the splenium, without passing through the ipsilateral leptomeninges and injuring the contralateral hemispheric cortex. That is to say, as one approaches the splenium, the incision will eventually be anterior to the falx, but carefully identifying and keeping intact the medial leptomeningeal investment of this last bit of the cortex being removed should allow a satisfactory subpial resection and incision ending up in continuity with the posterior extent of the splenial incision of the CCY.

12.2.10 Is the Insular Cortex Removed in a Hemispherectomy?

Villemure and Rasmussen noted the Montreal method of functional hemispherectomy, which was similar to most functional hemispherectomies in keeping with Dr. Rasmussen's suggestion and course of action (Rasmussen 1973, 1983, 1987; Rasmussen and Andermann 1983; Villemure and Rasmussen 1990; Villemure et al. 1993). Since the middle of 1990s, Villemure has, as have many neurosurgeons, altered the methodology of his hemispherectomy to hemispherotomy from a peri-insular approach, which he viewed as bringing about a hemispherectomy with the removal of the smallest amount of parenchyma (Villemure and Mascott 1993, 1995). More recently he has entitled his now three-step functional hemispherectomy a "peri-insular hemispherotomy" (PIH). It is not that different from what I have outlined in the foregoing. However, on the basis of the increasing acceptance of seizures observed in the insular cortex, he has included disconnection of the insular cortex. I would recommend the reader to review his very excellent outlined PIH methodology in a more recent article (Villemure and Daniel 2006).

To return to the question of this section, "Is the insular cortex removed in a hemispherectomy?," there is controversy with respect to the answer to this question! Villemure and colleagues in 1989 reviewed a significant equal number of hemispherectomies in which the insular cortex was removed and in which it was not removed with the conclusion that their "Our data suggest that the insular cortex does not necessarily have to be removed in hemispherectomy." Freeman et al. concluded that in the case of Rasmussen's syndrome, it was mandatory to remove the insula (1994). At about this same time, Villemure and Mascott indicated, "The insula may or not need to be excised" (1993). However, in Villemure's most recent paper, regarding insular cortex removal, he noted that given his own experience and that of Freeman and of Cats et al (2007), "the presence of residual cortex correlated positively with persistent postoperative seizures" (Villemure and Daniel 2009). Thus, the current evidence would suggest that the insular cortex should be removed or isolated in a hemispherectomy.

12.3 Hemispherotomy

The technique of hemispherotomy was introduced by Delalande et al. as a method that achieved the disconnection of the whole hemisphere without a significant associated cortical resection as the basis of the fHSPY (1992, 2001). In Dr. Delalande's hands, this is more satisfactory than an fHSPY. As I noted earlier, there are many ways of disconnecting (i.e., isolating), but leaving in place, parts of the hemisphere, and the surgeon needs to simply choose the one with which he/she feels most comfortable.

References

Adams CBT. Hemispherectomy – a modification. J Neurol Neurosurg Psychiatry. 1983;46:617–9.
Almeida AN, Marino R, Aguiar PH, Teixeira MJ. Hemispherectomy: a schematic review of the current techniques. Neurosurg Rev. 2006;29:97–102.
Austin GM, Grant FC. Physiologic observations following total hemispherectomy in man. Surgery. 1955;38:239–58.
Bell E, Karnosh LJ. Cerebral hemispherectomy. Report of a case ten years after operation. J Neurosurg. 1949;6:285–93.
Binder DK, Schramm J. Transsylvian functional hemispherectomy. Childs Nerv Syst. 2006;22:960–6.
Cabieses F, Jeri R, Landa R. Fatal brain-stem shift following hemispherectomy. J Neurosurg. 1957;14:74–91.
Cairns H. Hemispherectomy in the treatment of infantile hemiplegia: with a psychological supplement, by M. A Davidson. Lancet. 1951;2:411–5.
Carmichael EA. The current status of hemispherectomy for infantile hemiplegia. Clin Proc Child Hosp (Wash). 1966;22:285–93.
Cats EA, Kho KH, Van Nieuwenhuizen O, Van Veelen CW, Gosselaar PH, Van Rijen PC. Seizure freedom after functional hemispherectomy and a possible role for the insular cortex: the Dutch experience. J Neurosurg. 2007;107 Suppl 4:275–80.
Cushing H. Chapter XXXVI. Surgery of the head. In: Keen WW, editor. Surgery: its principles and practice, vol. III. Philadelphia: W.B. Saunders Company; 1910. p. 261.
Dandy WE. Removal of right cerebral hemisphere for certain tumors with hemiplegia: preliminary report. JAMA. 1928;90:823–5.
Dandy WE. Physiological studies following extirpation of the right cerebral hemisphere in man. Bull Johns Hopkins Hosp. 1933;53:31–51.
Dekaban A, Sakuragawa N. Megalencephaly. In: Vinken PJ, Bryyn GW, Myrianthopoulos NC, editors. Handbook of Clinical Neurology, Congenital Malformations of the Brain and Skull, Chapter 25. Elsevier: North-Holland Biomedical Press; 1977. p. 647–60.
Delalande O, Pinard JM, Basdevant C, Gauthe M, Plouin P, Dulac O. Hemispherotomy: a new procedure for central disconnection. Epilepsia. 1992;33 Suppl 3:99–100. Abstract.
Delalande O, Fohlen M, Jalin C, Pinard JM. From hemispherectomy to hemispherotomy. In: Lüders HO, Comair YG, editors. Epilepsy surgery. 2nd ed. Philadelphia: Lippincott Williams & Wilkins; 2001. p. 741–6.
DeMyer W. Chapter 18. Microcephaly, micrencephaly, megalocephaly, and megalencephaly. In: Swaiman KF, Ashwal S, editors. Pediatric neurology: principles and practice. 3rd ed. St. Louis: Mosby; 1999. p. 301–11.
Di Rocco C, Iannelli A. Hemimegalencephaly and intractable epilepsy: complications of hemispherectomy and their correlations with the surgical technique. A report on 15 cases. Pediatr Neurosurg. 2000;33:198–207.
Falconer MA, Wilson PJE. Complications related to delayed hemorrhage after hemispherectomy. J Neurosurg. 1969;30:413–26.
Freeman JM, Arroyo S, Vining EPG, Breiter SN, Barker PB, Pardo CA, Carson BS, Zuckerberg AL. Insular seizures: a study in Sutton's Law. Epilepsia. 1994;35 Suppl 8:49. Abstr.
Gardner WJ. Removal of cerebral hemisphere for glioma. Proc 5th Int Cong Neurol, Lisbon. 1953;4:307–13.
Gardner WJ, Karnosh LJ, McClure CC, Gardner AK. Residual function following hemispherectomy for tumour and for infantile hemiplegia. Brain. 1955;78:487–502.
Girvin JP, Baeesa SS. Functional hemispherectomy for the treatment of intractable seizures. Neurosciences. 2006;11:72–7.
Goodall RJ. Cerebral hemispherectomy: present status and clinical indications. Neurology. 1957;7:151–62.
Griffith HB. Cerebral hemispherectomy for infantile hemiplegia in the light of the late results. Ann R Coll Surg. 1967;41:183–201.

Hillier WF. Total left cerebral hemispherectomy for malignant glioma. Neurology. 1954;4:718–21.

King M, Stephanson JBP, Ziervogel M, Doyle D, Galbraith S. Hemimegalencephaly—a case for hemispherectomy? Neuropediatrics. 1985;16:46–55.

Krynauw RA. Infantile hemiplegia treated by removing one cerebral hemisphere. J Neurol Neursurg Psychiatry. 1950;13:243–67.

L'Hermitte J. L'ablation complète de l'hémisphère droit dans les cas de rumeur cérébrale localisée compliquée d'hémiplégie: la décérébration suprathalamique unilateréale chez l'homme. Encéphale. 1928;23:314–23.

Laine E, Pruvot P, Osson D. Résultats éloignés de l'hémisphérectomie dans les d'hémiatrophie cérébrales infantile génératrice d'épilepsie. Neurochirugie. 1964;10:507–22.

McFie J. The effects of hemispherectomy on intellectual functioning in cases of infantile hemiplegia. J Neurol Neurosurg Psychiatry. 1961;24:240–9.

McKenzie KG. The present status of a patient who had the right cerebral hemisphere removed. JAMA. 1938;111:168–83.

McKissock W. Infantile hemiplegia. Proc R Soc Med. 1953;46:431–4.

McKissock W. The operative technique for cerebral hemispherectomy in the treatment of infantile hemiplegia. Zentbl Neurochir. 1954;14:42–8.

Meyers R. Recent advances in the neurosurgery of cerebral palsy. In: Illingworth RS, editor. Recent advances in cerebral palsy. London: Churchill; 1958. p. 330–86.

Noetzel H. Diffusion von Blutfarbstoff in der inneren Randzone und äusseren Oberfläche des Zentralnervensystems bei subarachnoidaler Blutung. Arch Psychiatry NervKrankh. 1940;111:129–38.

Oppenheimer DR, Griffith HB. Persistent intracranial bleeding as a complication of hemispherectomy. J Neurol Neurosurg Psychiatry. 1966;29:229–40.

Polani PE. Encephalo-trigeminal angiomatosis (Sturge-Weber syndrome) treated by removal of the affected cerebral hemisphere. Proc R Soc Med. 1952;45:860–2.

Rasmussen T. Postoperative superficial hemosiderosis of the brain, its diagnosis, treatment and prevention. Trans Am Neurol Assoc. 1973;98:133–7.

Rasmussen T. Surgery for epilepsy arising in regions other than the temporal and frontal lobes. In: Purpura DP, Penry JK, Walter RD, editors. Advances in neurology, vol. 8. New York: Raven; 1975. p. 206–26.

Rasmussen T. Hemispherectomy for seizures revisited. Can J Neurol Sci. 1983;10:71–8.

Rasmussen T. Commentary: extratemporal cortical excisions and hemispherectomy. In: Engel J, editor. Surgical treatment of the epilepsies. New York: Raven Press. 1987. p. 417–24.

Rasmussen T, Andermann F. Hemispherectomy for seizures revisited. Can J Neurol Sci. 1983;10:71–8.

Schramm J. Hemispherectomy techniques. Neurosurg Clin N Am. 2002;13:113–34.

Smith A, Sugar O. Development of above normal language and intelligence 21 years after left hemispherectomy. Neurology. 1975;25:813–8.

Tinuper P, Andermann F, Villemure JG, Rasmussen TB, Quesney LF. Functional hemispherectomy for treatment of epilepsy associated with hemiplegia: rationale, indications, results, and comparison with callosotomy. Ann Neurol. 1988;24:27–34.

Villemure JG, Daniel RT. Peri-insular hemispherotomy. Childs Nerv Syst. 2006;22:967–81.

Villemure J-G, Mascott CR. Hemispherotomy: the periinsular approach. Technical aspects. Epilepsia. 1993;34 Suppl 6:48. Abstract.

Villemure JG, Mascott CR. Peri-insular hemispherotomy: surgical principles and anatomy. Neurosurgery. 1995;37:975–81.

Villemure JG, Rasmussen T. Functional hemispherectomy: methodology. J Epilepsy. 1990;3(Suppl):177–82.

Villemure JG, Mascott CR, Anderman F, Rasmussen T. Is removal of the insular cortex in hemispherectomy necessary? Epilepsia. 1989;30:721. Abstr.

Villemure JG, Adams CBT, Hoffman HJ, Peacock WJ. Hemispherectomy. In: Engel J, editor. Surgical treatment of the epilepsies. 2nd ed. New York: Raven; 1993. p. 511–8.

Villemure JG, Daniel RT. Hemispherectomy. In: Lozano AM, Gildenberg PL, Tasker R, editors. Textbook of stereotactic and functional neurosurgery. 2nd ed. Springer-Verlag, Berlin/ Heidelberg; 2009. p. 2741–60.

Williams DJ, Scott JW. The functional responses of the sympathetic nervous system of man following hemidecortication. J Neurol Neurosurg Psychiat. 1939;2:313–22.

Wilson PJE. Cerebral hemispherectomy for infantile hemiplegia. A report of 50 cases. Brain. 1970a;93:147–80.

Wilson PJE. More 'second thoughts' on hemispherectomy in infantile hemiplegia. Dev Med Child Neurol. 1970b;12:799–800.

Wilson DH, Culver C, Waddington M, Gazzaniga M. Disconnection of the cerebral hemispheres: an alternative to hemispherectomy for the control of intractable seizures. Neurology. 1975;25:1149–53.

Zollinger R. Removal of left cerebral hemisphere. Report of a case. Arch Neurol Psychiatry. 1935;34:48–63.

13 Postoperative Course

13.1 Introduction

The postoperative course of resective epilepsy operations is usually relatively predictable, similar to any uncomplicated neurosurgical operative intervention with respect to any etiology, e.g., surgery involving vascular, neoplastic, and traumatic lesions. That is to say, resection of epileptic foci of seizures may be associated with a small incidence of postoperative complications such as infection, hemorrhage, and general anesthetic complications. These need no specific attention in a discussion here. Rather the most important considerations of complications arising from epilepsy surgery are those related to the outcomes with respect to postoperative seizure control, on the one hand, and the question of any altered neurological function resulting from the operative procedure, on the other hand.

13.2 Causes of Postoperative Neurological Deficits

13.2.1 Neuroparalytic Edema

It was perhaps Penfield and his colleagues who initially discussed in some detail the issue of postoperative neurological deficits following resective surgery for the management of intractable epilepsy. Their observations were undertaken in the early half of the twentieth century, long before the introduction of the quality imaging that might have added significant certainty to what was empirically considered to be the etiology of such deficits. The term "neuroparalytic edema" was coined by Penfield and was thought to be a significant cause of the deficits; it was considered to be an edematous swelling of cerebral parenchyma in the vicinity of the cortical excisions and was usually transient (1958). Penfield felt that it was at least partially related to the duration of the operative exposure of the cortex. He considered that the clinical symptomatology consisted of headache, paresis, focal ("neighborhood") seizures, dysphasia, etc. These were usually transient, reaching their peak during

J.P. Girvin, *Operative Techniques in Epilepsy*,
DOI 10.1007/978-3-319-10921-3_13

the initial 5 days and then gradually declining. There have been a number of discussions related to the possible explanations of Dr. Penfield's "neuroparalytic edema," but none has been accepted as a consensus. It is not now considered, if indeed it occurs, as a complication!

13.2.2 Aseptic Meningitis

Penfield also described aseptic meningitis as a separate postoperative difficulty (Finlayson and Penfield 1941; Penfield 1958). It was a term used by Rasmussen as well. It consists of headache, stiff neck, and elevated body temperature. Its etiology was considered to be the result of blood in the cerebral ventricle, and it was felt that "ventricular closure" decreased its likelihood. The CSF examination at the time was amber in color and exhibited a leukocytosis, which was lower than what might have been expected with meningitis. Similar to Sect. 13.2.1, the term doesn't really have the criteria to consider it a complication.

13.2.3 Intraoperative Mechanical (Surgical) Retraction

It is well known that mechanical retraction of cerebral cortex can transiently abolish whatever physiological function is associated with the retracted tissue. It has also been well known that excessive retraction, lasting for significant periods of time may not only transiently alter its function, but indeed may lead to permanent loss of function or even visually obvious destruction (bruising) of cortical tissue. Albin, a neuroanesthesiologist, and his colleagues conducted a number of studies on both human patients and experimental animals and demonstrated that pressures of greater than 30 mmHg applied to the brains of dogs for 60 min led to reductions in the somatosensory evoked potentials (SSEPs), even distant to the cortex that was actually being compressed (Albin et al. 1977, 1980; Albin and Bunegin 2003; Bennett et al. 1977a, b). Pressures that become "excessive" were those greater than 30 mmHg for these lengths of time—excessive in that they led to neurological deficits that lasted longer than 3 days and permanent histological neuronal loss in the compressed cortex. These effects were exaggerated if the cerebral blood flow to the animals was reduced significantly. RosenØrn and Diemer carried out similar studies with similar conclusions on rats (1982). Therefore, as mentioned earlier (Sects. 2.2.4 and 8.4.1), any retraction that is forceful should be applied to parenchyma that is being removed, not to that which is being left. (The surgery of an fHSPY is the only instance, in my view, in which traction may be applied to parenchyma that is being left, without much concern.)

13.2.4 Interruption in Blood Supply

This complication really needs no specific discussion here. It is obvious that arterial irrigation to cerebral parenchyma that is not being resected should be left healthy and most certainly with its blood supply intact. Any loss of this irrigation results in the loss or alteration of normal function, and if it is "eloquent" cortex, the loss of function will be associated with a postoperative neurological impairment. This begs a reiteration of the importance of recognizing the role of *en passage* arteries once again and the necessity of their preservation (Sect. 5.2). If it involves the non-eloquent cortex, it may lead to the origin of epileptogenic foci, as Penfield warned in 1958.

13.2.5 Hemorrhage

Postoperative hemorrhage is not as common a clinical problem in epilepsy surgery as it is in general neurosurgery. If the epileptic surgery is truly resective, then there is space for minor hemorrhage to occur which is of little clinical significance. For example, the majority of resective epileptic surgery leaves behind a significant "empty space"—a space into which small self-limited postoperative hemorrhages may occur without any clinical evidence of such. On the other hand, that same hemorrhage in many general neurosurgical operations where there is no resection may well give rise to clinical symptomatology—symptomatology that may even be sufficiently significant to require a second operative procedure to remove the hemorrhage.

I noted the foregoing, not only for indicating the relatively minor postoperative hemorrhages that may be considered benign but also to follow up to indicate the clinical difference that may occur in the case of postoperative hemorrhages that are not self-limited. I have always remembered a patient who had a perfectly normal postoperative course for 36–48 h after a routine uneventful aTLY, who, in the period between the second and third postoperative days, began to exhibit a little bit of intermittent drowsiness, then some intermittent confusion, and finally some contralateral paresis. My initial thought was that this was simply more-than-usual edema; however, a CT clearly disclosed a temporal lobe resection cavity filled with blood and a midline displaced by a few millimeters. Thus, on the fourth day postoperative, the patient had her second operation! I mention this case, because we were taught, and we teach, that postoperative hemorrhage is usually found in the very early postoperative course, e.g., hours, or a day or so, following the completion of surgery. This is true, but in the case of significant resections, it is not only more likely to occur further (later) into the postoperative course, but also there is a rather more slowly developing clinical evidence of its presence. To summarize, the clinical evidence of a developing hemorrhage following significantly sized epileptic surgical resections is much more likely to be less acute than in operations that are unassociated with resections of cerebral parenchyma.

The hemorrhage that I just described in the foregoing is the only such hemorrhage I have witnessed. Why might this be? I am uncertain as to why. Certainly a very obsessive compulsion of making certain that *every* possible small area of *any* oozing of blood has been dealt with (of course, coagulation with very low current!) is likely the reason, but as I noted in Chap. 3 (Sect. 3.6.8), I have been of the impression that the insertion of fluid into the closed (dural) cavity under pressure after the dura is closed might perhaps help in avoiding such hemorrhage. Whether this impression has any truth to it remains unknown!

13.2.6 Damage to the Eloquent Cortex in the Depths of the Sulci

The importance of being aware of potential eloquent cortex within the depths of the sulci was discussed in Chaps. 4 (Sect. 4.5.2) and 5 (Sects. 5.5.3 and 5.4). This deficit will ordinarily be recognized during the course of the surgery, if it is carried out under local anesthesia. This is discussed in more detail elsewhere (Girvin 1991).

13.2.7 Seizure Activity

The most common resections likely to be often associated with seizures postoperatively are those following Rolandic or peri-Rolandic resections. It is always important to warn patients and their caregivers about the very high incidence of immediate postoperative seizures in these cases. It is perfectly reasonable to add that these types of so-called "neighborhood" seizures, to use Dr. Rasmussen's labeling of such seizures, do not herald the onset of permanent seizures, but rather they are more commonly the result of a transient physiological alteration in the cortex at the periphery of the resection and they should largely disappear after a few days, usually not greater than a week or so.

13.2.8 Neuropsychological Deficits

As noted earlier there were reports in the latter quarter of the last century, indicating that cognitive deficits were likely to occur following dominant aTLYs (Ojemann and Dodrill 1985, 1987; Ivnik et al. 1987). This was a reflection of the increasing quality of the psychometric subtests used in neuropsychological assessment. In large part it was Brenda Milner from Cambridge and the Montreal Neurological Institute who was the founder of modern-day neuropsychology as a result of her many, many research observations that gave so much to the discipline, beginning in the middle of the twentieth century.

Having noted the foregoing, I would be remiss in not indicating the tremendously increased sophistication of neuropsychological assessments, which have gradually appeared over the last 50 years. I do not believe that a thorough review is pertinent in this monograph, but I also believe that the reader should be aware of two or three of such reviews. I have already mentioned the very good longitudinal review of Helmstaedter et al. in 2003 and the very thoughtful recent 2011 meta-analysis of postoperative neuropsychological outcomes by Sherman et al. (see Sect. 6.7.4).

13.3 Clinical Course of Postoperative Neurological Deficits

13.3.1 Introduction

What is the time course of postoperative deficits? These are not very dissimilar to any postictal deficits, irrespective of the etiology of the ictus, e.g., trauma, stroke, epilepsy seizure, surgery, etc. That is to say, the same principles apply to all of these situations in which relatively sudden deficits in neurological function are produced. In the examples noted in which the ictus is a spontaneous clinical event, the term "postictal recovery" is commonly utilized to describe the time course of recovery of the resulting neurological deficit, which is attributable to the seizure. By definition this is primarily associated with insults to the "eloquent" cortex.

Such ictuses may be nonstructural, e.g., purely functional, i.e., physiological, such as epileptic seizures, which involve the "eloquent" cortex. That is to say, such seizures *transiently* compromise the *function* of that cortex. The mechanism of that compromise is not definitively understood, but it is understood that the compromise is nearly always physiological and thereby is transient, and thus reversible, i.e., it is self-limited. However, some ictuses may result in structural damage, e.g., trauma, stroke, tumor, neurosurgical operations, etc. While some of the deficits produced by such ictuses may be transient and self-limited, a significant percentage of these are not reversible, but rather permanent to some degree.

Irrespective of whether ictal deficits are transient or permanent, the typical recovery is not linear. The nonlinearity is rather more logarithmic. For example, whatever the rapidity or the slowness of the recovery, there is greater recovery in a given time period shortly after the ictus than in a similar time period later during the course of the recovery. Such a recovery, if it is complete, may be so within minutes, hours, days, weeks, or months. Thus, such a deficit may be considered "transient." For those deficits that never recover completely, e.g., a residuum of the deficit remains "permanent," there is reasonable consensus that whatever recovery might take place will do so within about 18–24 months. In such cases, probably something of the order of 50 % of the recovery will have occurred in the initial few weeks or a very few months. The result of such a partial recovery is that the significant majority of it will have occurred within roughly 3–6 months of the insult.

Finally, I should mention an important rule of thumb that I have held to be true with respect to postoperative deficits: "If there is no deficit when an operative procedure is completed, then there will be no permanent deficit, irrespective of what might be the post-operative clinical course!" The reader will be correct in guessing that this statement applies particularly to operations carried out under local anesthesia, as the most worrisome deficits are those that occur very rapidly following surgery under local anesthesia and those which are present after surgery under general anesthesia in which the surgeon is, of course, uncertain as to whether they were present at the completion of surgery on cerebral parenchyma or not.

13.3.2 The Time Course of Deficits Following Operative Procedures

Figure 13.1 (redrawn from Girvin 1991) allows a discussion of some of the features of the clinical course of postoperative neurological deficits. While these three curves may be representative of deficits caused by a number of causes, e.g., strong retraction, altered vascular irrigation, edema in the resection area, etc., nevertheless, the majority emerge from surgical encroachment on eloquent cortex. Thus, it will be the proximities of these encroachments to the eloquent cortex that will be used to describe the various postoperative courses. Under these specific circumstances, one

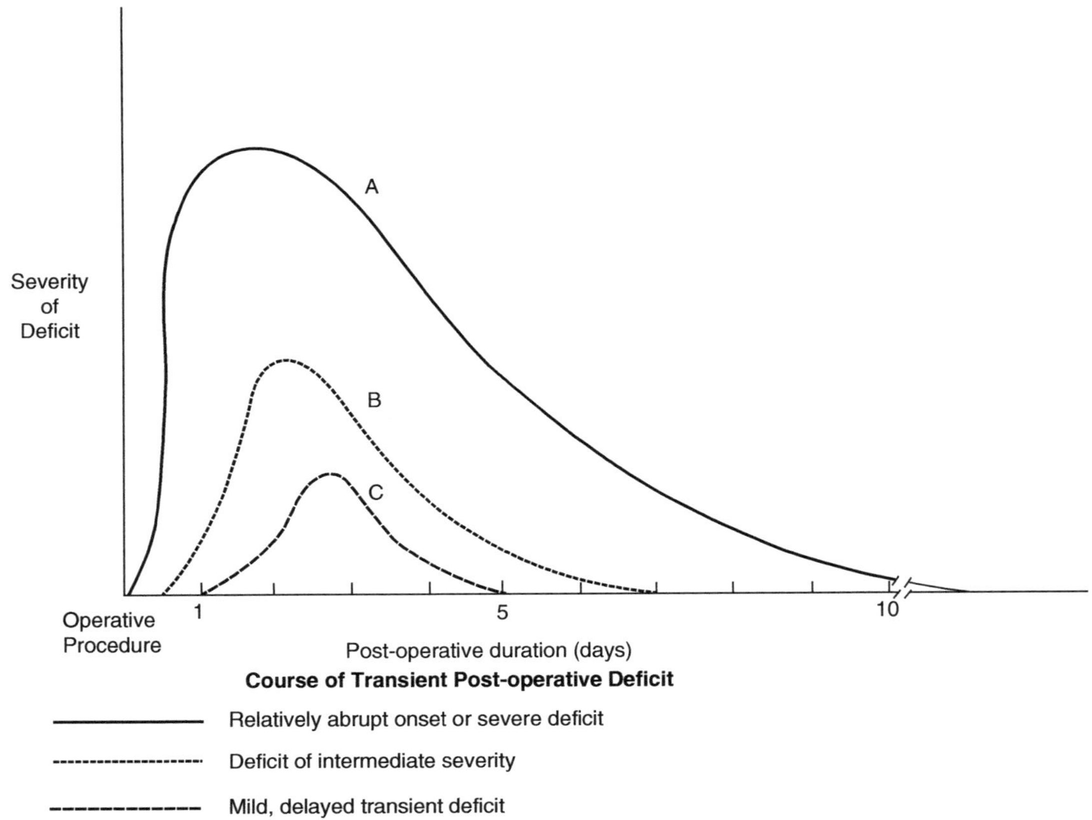

Fig. 13.1 Illustration of potential transient time courses of postoperative neurological deficits, as a result of the surgery. This illustrates a group of curves depicting the time courses and severity of postoperative transient neurological deficits (Redrawn, with permission, from Girvin (1991))

can provide a number of relatively accurate statements with regard to the three curves. For example, the nearer the resection is to the eloquent cortex, the more quickly will a deficit manifest itself, as illustrated in curve A, which has its onset during or immediately after the termination of the resection (see *x* axis), and its altitude (see *y* axis) indicates the greatest deficit of the three curves. Curve B may then presume to have been a resection further away from the eloquent cortex than the case in A, and curve C would imply resection even further away from the eloquent cortex than that which gave rise to curve B. Also, the later the deficit emerges after surgery, the less severe the deficit is. From the examination of these three curves, some tentative conclusions may be made. The closer the resection has been to the eloquent cortex, (1) the sooner the deficit will become evident (*x* axis), (2) the more rapidly the deficit will occur (the rise time of the curve is more rapid), (3) the greater the deficit (the height of the peak on the *y* axis) will be, and (4) the longer it will take for the deficit to resolve (the length of time of its evidence, as noted on the *x* axis).

Within limits the foregoing gives a reasonable insight into the general considerations of neurological deficits resulting from epileptic surgical procedures. Once again, I remind the reader that if there is not a deficit when the surgical resection has been completed, then there is nearly never the appearance of a permanent deficit. Thus, these curves are the results of data that has been retrieved from operations conducted under local anesthesia and neuroleptanalgesia and had no deficit at the completion of the surgical resections.

References

Albin MS, Bunegin L. The insidiousness of brain retractor pressure: another "smoking gun"? Anesth Analg. 2003;96(1):306–7.

Albin MS, Bunegin L, Bennett MH, Dujovny M, Jannetta PJ. Clinical and experimental brain retraction pressure monitoring. Acta Neurol Scand Suppl. 1977;64:522–3.

Albin MS, Bunegin L, Helsel P, et al. Intracranial pressure and regional cerebral blood flow responses to experimental brain retraction pressure. In: Shulman K, Marmaru A, Miller S, editors. Intracranial pressure IV. Proceedings of the 5th International Symposium on Intracranial Pressure. Heidelberg: Springer; 1980. p. 131–4.

Bennett MH, Albin MS, Bunegin L, Dujovny M, Hellstrom H, Jannetta PJ. Evoked potential changes during brain retraction in dogs. Stroke. 1977a;8:487–92.

Bennett MH, Bunegin L, Albin MS, et al. Evoked potential correlates of graded brain retraction pressure. Stroke. 1977b;8:487–92.

Finlayson AI, Penfield W. Acute postoperative aseptic leptomeningitis. Review of cases and discussion of pathogenesis. Arch Neurol Psychiatry. 1941;46:250–76.

Girvin JP. Chapter 73. Complications of epilepsy surgery. In: Luders HO, editor. Epilepsy surgery. New York: Raven; 1991. p. 653–60.

Helmstaedter C, Kurthen M, Lux S, Reuber M, Elger CE. Chronic epilepsy and cognition: a longitudinal study in temporal lobe epilepsy. Ann Neurol. 2003;54:425–32.

Ivnik RJ, Sharbrough FW, Laws ER. Effects of anterior temporal lobectomy on cognitive function. J Clin Psychol. 1987;43:128–37.

Ojemann GA, Dodrill CB. Verbal memory deficits after left temporal lobectomy for epilepsy. Mechanism and intraoperative prediction. J Neurosurg. 1985;62:101–7.

Ojemann GA, Dodrill C. Intraoperative techniques for reducing language and memory deficits with left temporal lobectomy. Adv Epileptology. 1987;16:327–30.

Penfield W. Pitfalls and success in surgical treatment of focal epilepsy. Br Med J. 1958;1:669–72.

Rosenørn J, Diemer NH. Reduction of regional cerebral blood flow during brain retraction pressure in the rat. J Neurosurg. 1982;56:826–9.

Sherman EMS, Wiebe S, Fay-McClymont B, Tellez-Zenteno J, Metcalfe A, Hernandez-Ronquillo L, et al. Neuropsychological outcomes after epilepsy surgery: systematic review and pooled estimates. Epilepsia. 2011;52:857–69.

Glossary

Cortex

"Buried" ("hidden") Cortex that is not on what is called the "surface" cortex; rather it is beneath the surface, in sulci and/or fissures, thus increasing the complexity of stimulating the cortex from the surface and requiring surgery for its exposure.

"Dispensable" or "silent" Cortex that can be removed and/or stimulated without evidence of an alteration in clinical function. Penfield used both terms "silent area" and "dispensable cortex" [see Penfield and Rasmussen 1969, p. 201].

Eloquent Cortex, the stimulation of which results in an identifiable clinical response and the surgical resection of which results in an identifiable clinical deficit, e.g., speech, motor movements, sensory perceptions, visual responses, etc.

Non-eloquent Cortex, the electrical stimulation or injury of which does not result in a clinically observable response or deficit (however, this should not be construed as a cortex which can necessarily be described as having no neurological function, in that very large areas of injury to the non-eloquent cortex may contribute to deficits) [also see Penfield and Rasmussen 1969].

Diprivan (*DI*-iso*PR*opyl *IV AN*esthetic), propofol, a short-acting, non-barbiturate sedative drug, introduced in 1986.

"En passage" blood vessels Usually refers to vessels that are simply passing by, over, or through parenchyma being removed but providing vascular irrigation to parenchyma other than that upon which surgery is being undertaken.

Frontal stem The content of afferent and efferent connectivity in the subcortical white matter of the eloquent frontal lobe cortex, primarily with respect to the Rolandic cortex; it is the frontal lobe counterpart of a similar label in the temporal lobe.

Skeletonize A term which means "reducing to a skeleton"; it is used in surgery to isolate a portion of an *en passage* vessel, by coagulating and incising its connections (e.g., its branches that irrigate parenchyma, which is being removed), thereby having skeletonized that portion of the parent vessel, which is left intact so that its irrigation of parenchyma that is also left intact remains normal.

J.P. Girvin, *Operative Techniques in Epilepsy*,
DOI 10.1007/978-3-319-10921-3

Stimulation

Bifocal A more accurate term for "bipolar" stimulation.

Unifocal A more accurate term for "unipolar" stimulation.

Temporal stem That broad bundle (sometimes called the *tapetum*) of subcortical white matter that carries the connectivity of the anterior temporal lobe cortex to other areas of the lobe or elsewhere in the cerebrum.

Bibliography

Adams CBT. Hemispherectomy – a modification. J Neurol Neurosurg Psychiatry. 1983;46:617–9 [12.1.4, 12.2.3].

Agnew WF, Yuen GH, Pudenz RH, Bullara LA. Electrical stimulation of the brain. IV. Ultrastructural studies. Surg Neurol. 1975;5:438–48 [4.2.3].

Agnew WF, Yuen TGH, Pudenz RH. Neuropathological effects of intracerebral platinum salt injections. J Neuropathol Exp Neurol. 1977;36:533–46 [4.2.3].

Agnew WF, Yuen TGF, McCreery DB. Morphologic changes after prolonged electrical stimulation of the cat's cortex at defined charge densities. Exp Neurol. 1983;79:397–411 [4.2.3].

Albin MS, Bunegin L. The insidiousness of brain retractor pressure: another "smoking gun"? Anesth Analg. 2003;96(1):306–7 [13.2.3].

Albin MS, Bunegin L, Bennett MH, Dujovny M, Jannetta PJ. Clinical and experimental brain retraction pressure monitoring. Acta Neurol Scand Suppl. 1977;64:522–3 [13.2.3].

Albin MS, Bunegin L, Helsel P, et al. Intracranial pressure and regional cerebral blood flow responses to experimental brain retraction pressure. In: Shulman K, Marmaru A, Miller S, et al, editors. Intracranial pressure IV. Proceedings of the 5th international symposium on intracranial pressure. Heidelberg: Springer; 1980. p. 131–4 [13.2.3].

Alexander W. The treatment of epilepsy by ligature of the vertebral arteries. Brain. 1883;5:170–87 [1.1].

Almeida AN, Marino R, Aguiar PH, Teixeira MJ. Hemispherectomy: a schematic review of the current techniques. Neurosurg Rev. 2006;29:97–102 [12.1.1, 12.2.1].

Austin GM, Grant FC. Physiologic observations following total hemispherectomy in man. Surgery. 1955;38:239–58 [12.1.2].

Bailey P, Gibbs FA. The surgical treatment of psychomotor epilepsy. JAMA. 1951;145:365–70 [1.2, 6.1].

Bailey P, Green JR, Amador L, Gibbs FA. Treatment of psychomotor states by anterior temporal lobectomy. A report of progress. Res Publ Assoc Res Nerv Ment Dis. 1935;31:341–6 [1.2].

Bates JAV. The surgery of epilepsy. In: Williams D, editor. Modern trends in neurology, vol. 3. Washington: Butterworths; 1962. p. 125–37 [1.2].

Bell E, Karnosh LJ. Cerebral hemispherectomy. Report of a case ten years after operation. J Neurosurg. 1949;6:285–93 [12.1.2].

Bennett MH, Albin MS, Bunegin L, Dujovny M, Hellstrom H, Jannetta PJ. Evoked potential changes during brain retraction in dogs. Stroke. 1977a;8:487–92 [13.2.3].

Bennett MH, Bunegin L, Albin MS, et al. Evoked potential correlates of graded brain retraction pressure. Stroke. 1977b;8:487–92 [13.2.3].

Billings JS. The surgical treatment of epilepsy. Cincinnati Lancet Observ. 1861;4:334–41 [1.1].

Binder DK, Schramm J. Transsylvian functional hemispherectomy. Childs Nerv Syst. 2006;22:960–6 [12.1.1, 12.2.1].

Blümcke I, Wiestler OD. Gangliogliomas: an intriguing tumor entity associated with focal epilepsies. J Neuropathol Exp Neurol. 2002;61:575–84 [5.7].

Blume WT, Jones DC, Pathak P. Properties of after-discharges from cortical electrical stimulation in focal epilepsies. Clin Neurophysiol. 2004;115:982–9 [4.3.5].

J.P. Girvin, *Operative Techniques in Epilepsy*,
DOI 10.1007/978-3-319-10921-3

Bogen JE, Fisher ED, Vogel PJ. Cerebral commissurotomy. A second case report. JAMA. 1965;194:1328–9 [11.1.4].
Bogen JE, Sperry RW, Vogel PH. Addendum: commissural section and propagation of seizures. In: Basic mechanisms of the epilepsies. Boston: Little, Brown and Co; 1969. p. 439–40 [11.1.4].
Branch C, Milner B, Rasmussen T. Intracarotid sodium Amytal for the lateralization of cerebral speech dominance: observations on 123 patients. J Neurosurg. 1964;21:399–405 [4.6.1.3. 4.7].
Brindley GS. Sensory effects of electrical stimulation of the visual and paravisual cortex in man. In: Jung J, editor. Handbook of sensory physiology, vol. VII/3B, Central processing of visual information; New York: Springer-Verlag; 1973. pp. 583–94 [4.6.4, 10.1.2].
Brindley GS, Lewin WD. The sensations produced by electrical stimulation of the visual cortex. J Physiol. 1968;196:479–93 [4.6.4].
Broca P. Sur la siège de la faculté du language articulé. Bull Soc Anat Paris. 1861;6(2 Série):355 [4.6.1.1].
Brodmann K. Beiträge zur histologischen Lokalisation der Grosshirnrinde. I. Mitt, Der Rolandica. J Psychol Neurol. 1903;2:79–107 [8.1.1].
Brodmann K. In: Barth JA, editor. Vergleichende Lokalisationslehre der Grosshirnrinde in ihren Prinzipien dargestellt auf Grund des Zellenbaues. Leipzig; 1909 (reprinted 1925, XII). p. 324 [8.1.1].
Brown TG, Sherrington CS. On the instability of a cortical point. Proc Roy Soc. 1912;85:250–77 [4.6.2].
Bubnoff N, Heidenhain R. Ueber Erregungs- und Hemmungs-orgänge innerhalb der motorischen Hirncentren. Arch ges Physiol. 1881;26:137–200. (English trans: von Bonin, McCulloch WS. In: Bucy PC, editor. The precentral motor cortex. Urbana: University of Illinois Press. Chapter VII, p. 173–210) [4.3.4].
Burns BD. Some properties of the cat's isolated cerebral cortex. J Physiol. 1949;110:9P (abstract) [8.6.2].
Burns BD. Some properties of the cat's isolated cerebral cortex. J Physiol. 1950;111:50–68 [8.6.2].
Burns BD. Some properties of isolated cerebral cortex in the unanesthetized cat. J Physiol. 1951;112:156–75 [3.1, 8.6.2].
Cabieses F, Jeri R, Landa R. Fatal brain-stem shift following hemispherectomy. J Neurosurg. 1957;14:74–91 [12.1.4].
Cairns H. Hemispherectomy in the treatment of infantile hemiplegia: with a psychological supplement, by M. A. Davidson. Lancet. 1951;2:411–5 [12.1.3].
Carmichael EA. The current status of hemispherectomy for infantile hemiplegia. Clin Proc Child Hosp (Wash). 1966;22:285–93 [12.1.3].
Cats EA, Kho KH, Van Nieuwenhuizen O, Van Veelen CW, Gosselaar PH, Van Rijen PC. Seizure freedom after functional hemispherectomy and a possible role for the insular cortex: the Dutch experience. J Neurosurg. 2007;107 Suppl 4:275–80 [12.2.10*].
Colonnier ML. The structural design of the neocortex. In: Eccles JC, editor. Brain and conscious experience. New York: Springer; 1966. p. 1–23 [8.1.1-2, 8.6.1].
Comair YG. The transsylvian functional hemispherectomy: patient selection and results. In: Lüders HO, Comair YG, editors. Epilepsy surgery. 2nd ed. Philadelphia: Lippincott Williams & Wilkins; 2001. pp. 702–3 [6.4].
Corkin S, Milner B, Rasmussen T. Somatosensory thresholds – contrasting effects of post-central gyrus and posterior parietal-lobe excision. Arch Neurol. 1970;23:41–58 [5.4, 9.1].
Critchley M. The parietal lobes. London: Edward Arnold; 1955 [5.4, 9.1].
Cushing H. A note upon the faradic stimulation of the postcentral gyrus in conscious patients. Brain. 1909;32:44–53 [1.2].
Cushing H. Chapter XXXVI. Surgery of the head. In: Keen WW, editor. Surgery: its principles and practice, vol. III. Philadelphia: W.B. Saunders Company; 1910. p. 17–276 [4.6.2, 12.2.1].
Cutter IS, Benjamin W. Dudley and the surgical relief of traumatic epilepsy. Int Abstr Surg. 1930;50:189–94 [1.1].
Dandy WE. Removal of right cerebral hemisphere for certain tumors with hemiplegia: preliminary report. JAMA. 1928;90:823–5 [12.1.2].

Dandy WE. Physiological studies following extirpation of the right cerebral hemisphere in man. Bull Johns Hopkins Hosp. 1933;53:31–51 [12.1.2].

Dekaban A, Sakuragawa N. Chapter 25. Megalencephaly. In: Vinken PJ, Bryyn GW, Myrianthopoulos NC, editors. Handbook of clinical neurology, congenital malformations of the brain and skull. Elsevier: North-Holland Biomedical Press; 1977. pp. 647–60 [12.2.2].

Delalande O, Pinard JM, Basdevant C, Gauthe M, Plouin P, Dulac O. Hemispherotomy: a new procedure for central disconnection. Epilepsia. 1992;33 Suppl 3:99–100. Abstract. [12.1.4, 12.3].

Delalande O, Fohlen M, Jalin C, Pinard JM. From hemispherectomy to hemispherotomy. In: Lüders HO, Comair YG, editors. Epilepsy surgery. 2nd ed. Philadelphia: Lippincott Williams & Wilkins; 2001. p. 741–6 [12.1.4, 12.3].

DeMyer W. Chapter 18. Microcephaly, micrencephaly, megalocephaly, and megalencephaly. In: Swaiman KF, Ashwal S, editors. Pediatric neurology: principles and practice. 3rd ed. St. Louis: Mosby; 1999. p. 301–11 [12.2.2].

Di Rocco C, Iannelli A. Hemimegalencephaly and intractable epilepsy: complications of hemispherectomy and their correlations with the surgical technique. A report on 15 cases. Pediatr Neurosurg. 2000;33:198–207 [12.2.2, 12.2.3].

Dobelle WH, Mladejovsky M. Phosphenes produced by electrical stimulation of human occipital cortex, and their application to the development of a prosthesis for the blind. J Physiol. 1974;243:553–76 [4.3.6].

Dobelle WH, Mladejovsky MG, Girvin JP. Artificial vision for the blind: electrical stimulation of visual cortex offers hope for a functional prosthesis. Science. 1974;183:440–4 [4.3.6, 4.6.4].

Dobelle WH, Turkel J, Henderson DC, Evans JR. Mapping the representation of the visual field by electrical stimulation of human visual cortex. Am J Ophthalmol. 1979;88:727–35 [4.6.4].

Drake C. Personal communication [2.1.5].

Dudley BW. Observations on injuries of the head. Transylvania J Med. 1828;1:9–40 [1.1].

Dymond AM, Kaechle LE, Jurist JM, Crandall PH. Brain tissue reaction to some chronically implanted metals. J Neurosurg. 1970;33:574–80 [4.2.3].

Erickson TE. Spread of epileptic discharge: an experimental study of the after-discharge induced by electrical stimulation of the cerebral cortex. Arch Neurol Psychiatry. 1940;43:429–52 [4.3.5, 11.1.4].

Evans JP. A study of the sensory defects resulting from excision of cerebral substance in humans. Public Assoc Res Nerv Ment Dis. 1935;15:331–70 [5.4].

Falconer MA, Wilson PJE. Complications related to delayed hemorrhage after hemispherectomy. J Neurosurg. 1969;30:413–26 [12.1.4].

Feindel W. The nervi tentorii and intracranial pain. Anat Rec. 1954;118:298. Abstract. [3.5.4, 3.5.5.3].

Feindel W. Memory and speech function in the temporal lobe in man. In: Brazier MA, editor. Brain function, vol. 2. 1964. p. 277–98 [6.6].

Feindel W. Electrical stimulation of the brain during surgery for epilepsy—historical highlights. Int Anesthesiol Clin. 1986;24:75–87 [1.2].

Feindel W, Rasmussen T. Temporal lobectomy with amygdalectomy and minimal hippocampal resection: review of 100 cases. Can J Neurol Sci. 1991;18:603–5 [6.1].

Feindel W, Penfield W, McNaughton F. The tentorial nerves and localization of intracranial pain in man. Neurology. 1960;10:555–63 [3.5.4, 3.5.4.2, 3.5.5.2].

Feindel W, Leblanc R, Nogueira DE, Almeida A. Epilepsy surgery: historical highlights 1909–2009. Epilepsia. 2009;50(S3):131–51 [1.2].

Ferrier CH, Aronica E, Leijten SS, Spliet WGM, van Huffelen AC, van Rijen PC, Binnie CD. Electrocorticographic discharge patterns in glioneuronal tumors and focal cortical dysplasia. Epilepsia. 2006;47:1477–86 [5.7].

Finlayson AI, Penfield W. Acute postoperative aseptic leptomeningitis. Review of cases and discussion of pathogenesis. Arch Neurol Psychiatry. 1941;46:250–76 [13.2.2].

Foerster O. Zur Pathogenese und Chirurgischen Behandlung der Epilepsia. Zentralbl Chir. 1925;52:531–49 [1.2].

Foerster O. Zur operativen Behandlung der Epilspsie. Dtsch Z Nervenheilkd. 1926;89:137–47 [1.2, 4.1].
Foerster O. Sur Pathogenese und chirurgischen Behandlung der Epilepsie. Zentralbl Chir. 1929a;52:531–49 [1.2, 4.1, 4.6.4].
Foerster O. Beiträge zur Pathophysiologie der Sehbahn und der Schsphäre. J Psychol Neurol Lpz. 1929b;39:463–85 [1.2, 4.1].
Foerster O. Uber die bedeutung und reichweite des lokalisation-sprinzips im nervensystem. Verh Dtsch Ges Inn Med. 1934;46:117–211 [1.2].
Foerster O. Sensible corticale Felder. In: Bumke O, Foerster O, editors. Handbuch der Neurologie, vol. 6. Berlin: Springer; 1936a. p. 1–448 [1.2, 4.1].
Foerster O. The motor cortex in man in the light of Hughling Jackson's doctrines. Brain. 1936b;59:135–59 [1.2, 4.1, 7.5].
Foerster O, Altenburger H. Elektrobiologische vorgänge an der menschlichen hirnrinde. Dtsch Z Nervenheilkd. 1935;135:277–88 [1.2].
Foerster O, Penfield W. The structural basis of traumatic epilepsy and results of radical operation. Brain. 1930a;53:99–120 [1.2, 3.1].
Foerster O, Penfield W. Der narbenzug am und im gehirn bei traumatischer epilepsie in seiner bedeutung für das zustandekommen der anfälle und für die therapeutische bekämpfung derselben. Z Ges Neurol Psychiat. 1930b;125:475–572 [7.5].
Fox WL. Chapter 1. Neurological surgery before Walter E. Dandy: a brief introduction. In: Dandy of Johns Hopkins. Baltimore: Williams & Wilkins; 1984. p. 1–7 [1.1].
Freeman JM, Arroyo S, Vining EPG, Breiter SN, Barker PB, Pardo CA, Carson BS, Zuckerberg AL. Insular seizures: a study in Sutton's Law. Epilepsia. 1994;35 Suppl 8:49. (Abstr). [12.2.10].
French JD, Gernandt BE, Livingston RB. Regional differences in seizure susceptibility in monkey cortex. AMA Arch Neurol Psychiatry. 1956;75:260–74 [4.3.4.1].
Gardner WJ. Removal of cerebral hemisphere for glioma. Proceedings of 5th international congress on neurology, vol. 4. Lisbon, 1953. p. 307–13 [12.1.2].
Gardner WJ, Karnosh LJ, McClure CC, Gardner AK. Residual function following hemispherectomy for tumour and for infantile hemiplegia. Brain. 1955;78:487–502 [12.1.2].
Girvin JP. Basic aspects of chronic stimulation of excitable tissue. In: Cooper IS, editor. Chronic cerebellar stimulation. New York: Raven Press; 1978. p. 1–12 [4.2.1].
Girvin JP. Neurosurgical considerations and general methods for craniotomy under local anesthesia. Int Anesthesiol Clin. 1986a;24:89–114 [3.3.2, 3.5.5.1].
Girvin JP. Resection of intracranial lesions under local anesthesia. Int Anesthesiol Clin. 1986b;24:133–55 [3.3.2].
Girvin JP. Chapter 73. Complications of epilepsy surgery. In: Luders HO, editor. Epilepsy surgery. New York: Raven Press; 1991. p. 653–60 [13.2.6, 13.3.2].
Girvin JP. Chapter 11. Temporal lobectomy. In: Apuzzo MLJ, editor. Neurosurgical aspects of epilepsy. Park Ridge: American Association of Neurological Surgeons; 1992. pp. 157–70 [6.2.1].
Girvin JP, Baeesa SS. Functional hemispherectomy for the treatment of intractable seizures. Neurosciences. 2006;11:72–7 [12.2.1].
Girvin JP, McGlone J, McLachlan RS, Blume WT. Validity of the sodium amobarbital test for memory in selected patients [abstract]. Epilepsia. 1987;28:636 [4.6.5].
Gloor P. The temporal lobe and limbic system. Oxford: Oxford University Press; 1997. 865 pp. [6.2.7].
Goodall RJ. Cerebral hemispherectomy: present status and clinical indications. Neurology. 1957;7:151–62 [12.1.2].
Graham Brown T, Sherrington CS. On the instability of a cortical point. Proc Roy Soc. 1912;85B:250–77 [4.3.4].
Griffith HB. Cerebral hemispherectomy for infantile hemiplegia in the light of the late results. Ann R Coll Surg Engl. 1967;41:183–201 [12.1.4].
Grünbaum ASF, Sherrington C. Observations on physiology of the cerebral cortex of some of the higher apes. Proc R Soc London. 1901;69:206–9 [4.3.4].

Grunbaum ASF, Sherrington C. Observations on the physiology of the cerebral cortex of the anthropoid apes. Proc Roy Soc. 1903;72:152–5 [4.3.4].

Helmstaedter C, Kurthen M, Lux S, Reuber M, Elger CE. Chronic epilepsy and cognition: a longitudinal study in temporal lobe epilepsy. Ann Neurol. 2003;54:425–32 [6.7.4, 13.2.8].

Hermann BP, Stone JL. A historical review of the epilepsy surgery program at the University of Illinois medical center: the contributions of Bailey, Gibbs, and collaborators to the refinement of anterior temporal lobectomy. J Epilepsy. 1989;2:155–63 [1.2].

Hillier WF. Total left cerebral hemispherectomy for malignant glioma. Neurology. 1954;4:718–21 [12.1.2].

Hitzig E. Hughlings Jackson and the cortical motor centres in the light of physiological research. Brain. 1900;23:544–81 [1.1].

Holmes G. Disturbances of vision by cerebral lesions. Br J Ophthalmol. 1918;2:353–84, 449–68, 506–16. [4.6.4].

Holmes G. The cortical localization of vision. Br Med J. 1919;2:193–9 [4.6.4].

Holmes G. A contribution to the cortical representation of vision. Brain. 1931;54:470–9 [4.6.4].

Holmes G. The organization of the visual cortex in man. Proc R Soc London. 1945;132:348–61 [4.6.4].

Holmes G, Lister WT. Disturbances of vision from cerebral lesions, with special reference to the cortical representation of the macula. Brain. 1916;39:34–73 [4.6.4].

Hori T, Tabuchi S, Kurosaki M, Kondo S, Takenobu A, Watanabe T. Subtemporal amygdalohippocampectomy for treating medically intractable temporal lobe epilepsy. Neurosurgery. 1993;33:50–7 [6.4].

Horsley V. Brain-surgery. Br Med J. 1886;2:670–5 [1.2, 2.2.1, 4.1].

Horsley V. Ten consecutive cases of operation upon the brain and cranial cavity to illustrate the details and safety of the method employed. Br Med J. 1887;1:863–5 [1.2, 2.2.1, 4.1].

Horsley V, Schäfer EA. A record of experiments upon the functions of the cerebral cortex. Philos Trans R Soc London B. 1888;179:1–45 [7.5].

Invik RJ, Sharbrough FW, Laws ER. Effects of anterior temporal lobectomy kon cognitive function. J Clin Psychol. 1987;43:128–37 [6.7.4, 13.2.8].

Jackson JH, Colman WS. Case of epilepsy with tasting movements and 'dreamy state' with very small patch of softening in the left uncinate gyrus. Brain. 1898;21:580–90 [1.1].

King M, Stephanson JBP, Ziervogel M, Doyle D, Galbraith S. Hemigalencephaly—a case for hemispherectomy? Neuropediatrics. 1985;16:46–55 [12.2.2].

Krause F. Die operative behandlung der epilepsie. Med Klin Berlin. 1909;5:1418–22 [1.2].

Krause F. Die Sehbahnen in chirurgischer Beziehung und die faradische Reizung des Sehzentrums. Klin Wschr. 1924;3:1260–5 [1.2, 4.1, 4.6.4].

Krause F, Schum H. Die spezielle Chirugie der Gehirnkrankheiten. In: Kuttner H, editor. Neue Deutsche Chirugie, 3 Bände. II. Band. Die epileptischen Erkrankungen. Enke, Stuttgart 1931;49a:482–6 [1.2, 4.1, 4.6.4].

Krynauw RA. Infantile hemiplegia treated by removing one cerebral hemisphere. J Neurol Neurosurg Psychiatry. 1950;13:243–67 [12.1.3].

Kubu CS, Girvin JP, McLachlan RS, Pavol M, Harnadek MCS. Does the intracarotid amobarbital procedure predict global amnesia after temporal lobectomy? Epilepsia. 2000;41:1321–9 [4.6.5].

Laine E, Pruvot P, Osson D. Résultats éloignés de l'hémisphérectomie dans les d'hémiatrophie cérébrales infantile génératrice d'épilepsie. Neurochi Rugie. 1964;10:507–22 [12.1.4].

Lehman R, Andermann F, Olivier A, Tandon PN, Quesney LF, Rasmussen TB. Seizures with onset in the sensorimotor face area: clinical patterns and results of surgical treatment in 20 patients. Epilepsia. 1994;35:1117–24 [8.4.1].

Leyton ASF, Sherrington CS. Observations on the excitable cortex of the chimpanzee, orang-utan, and gorilla. Quart J Exp Physiol. 1917;11:135–222 [4.3.4, 7.5].

L'Hermitte J. L'ablation complète de l'hémisphère droit dans les cas de rumeur cérébrale localisée compliquée d'hémiplégie: la décérébration suprathalamique unilateréale chez l'homme. Encéphale. 1928;23:314–23 [12.1.2].

Libet B. Chapter 19. Electrical stimulation of cortex in human subjects and conscious sensory aspects. In: Iggo A, editor. Handbook of sensory physiology, vol. II, somatosensory system. Berlin-Heidleberg: Springer-Verlag; 1973. pp. 743–90 [4.2.2].

Libet B, Alberts WW, Wright EW, Levin G, Feinstein B. Sensory perception by direct stimulation of human cerebral cortex: stimulus parameters. Fed Proc. 1959;18:92 [4.2.2].

Libet B, Alberts WW, Wright EW, Levin G, Feinstein B. Cirect excitation of human somatosensory cortex. Electroenceph Clin Neurophysiol. 1961;13:498 [4.2.2].

Libet B, Alberts WW, Wright EW, Delattre LD, Levin G, Feinstein B. Production of threshold levels of conscious sensation by electrical stimulation of human somato-sensory cortex. J Neurophysiol. 1964;27:546–78 [4.2.2].

Liddell EGT, Phillips CG. Thresholds of cortical representation. Brain. 1950;73:125–40 [4.6.2].

Lilly JC. Injury and excitation by electric currents: the balanced pulse-pair waveform. In: Sheer DE, editor. Electrical stimulation of the brain. Austin: University of Texas Press; 1961. p. 60–4 [4.2.1].

Lilly JC, Austin GM, Chambers WM. Threshold movements produced by excitation of cerebral cortex and efferent fibers with some parametric regions of rectangular current pulses (cats and monkeys). J Neurophysiol. 1952;15:319–41 [4.2.1].

Lilly JC, Hughes JR, Alvord EC, Galkin TW. Brief, non-injurious electric wave form for stimulation of the brain. Science. 1955a;121:468–9 [4.2.1].

Lilly JC, Hughes JR, Galkin TW, Alvord EC. Production and avoidance of injury to brain tissue by electrical current and threshold values. EEG Clin Neurophysiol. 1955b;7:458–9 [4.2.1].

Lloyd JH, Deaver JB. A case of focal epilepsy successfully treated by trephining and excision of the motor centres. Am J Med Sci. 1888;96:477–87 [1.1].

Lüders H, Lesser RP, Hahn J, Dinner DS, Morris H, Resor S, Harrison M. Basal temporal language area demonstrated by electrical stimulation. Neurology. 1986;36:505–10 [6.7.1].

Luessenhop AJ. Interhemispheric commissurotomy: (the split brain operation) as an alternate to hemispherectomy for control of intractable seizures. Am Surg. 1970;36:265–8 [11.1.4].

Luessenhop AJ, dela Cruz TC, Fenichel GM. Surgical disconnection of the cerebral hemispheres for intractable seizures: results in infancy an childhood. JAMA. 1970;213:1630–6 [11.1.4].

MacIntyre WJ, Bidder TG, Rowland V. The production of brain lesions with electric currents. In: Quastler H, Morowitz HJ, editors. Proc Nat Biophys Conf (1st, 1957), Columbus, Ohio: Yale University Press, New Haven; 1959. p. 723–32 [4.2.1].

MacIntyre WJ, Bidder TG, Rowland V. Effect of electric currents on brain tissue: stimulation and electrolytic lesion production. In: Glasser O, editor. Medical physics, vol. III. Chicago: Yearbook; 1960. p. 102–5 [4.2.1, 4.2.3].

Mattingly JB, Husain M, Rorden C, Kennard C, Driver J. Motor role of unman inferior parietal lobe revealed in unilateral neglect patients. Nature. 1998;392:179–82 [9.1].

Maxwell RE, Gates JR, Gumnit RJ. Corpus callosotomy at the university of Minnesota. In: Engel J, editor. Surgical treatment of the epilepsies. New York: Raven Press; 1987. p. 659–66 [11.1.4, 11.2.1-2].

McCulloch W, Dusser de Barenne JG. Extinction: local stimulatory inactivation within the motor cortex. Am J Physiol. 1935;224:97–8 [4.3.4].

McFie J. The effects of hemispherectomy on intellectual functioning in cases of infantile hemiplegia. J Neurol Neurosurg Psychiatry. 1961;24:240–9 [12.1.4].

McKenzie KG. The present status of a patient who had the right cerebral hemisphere removed. JAMA. 1938;111:168–83 [12.1.3].

McKissock W. Infantile hemiplegia. Proc R Soc Med. 1953;46:431–4 [12.1.3-4].

McKissock W. The operative technique for cerebral hemispherectomy in the treatment of infantile hemiplegia. Zentralbl Neurochir. 1954;14:42–8 [12.1.3].

McNaughton FL. The innervation of the intracranial blood vessels and dural sinuses. ARNMD. 1937;18:178–200 [3.5.4, 3.5.5.3].

Meador KJ, Loring DW, Flanigin HF. History of epilepsy surgery. J Epilepsy. 1989;2:21–5 [1.2].

Meyers R. Recent advances in the neurosurgery of cerebral palsy. In: Illingworth RS, editor. Recent advances in cerebral palsy. London: Churchill; 1958. p. 330–86 [12.1.3].

Mihailović L, Delgado JMR. Electrical stimulation of monkey brain with various fragments and pulse durations. J Neurosurg. 1956;19:21–36 [4.2.2].

Milner B. Psychological defects produced by temporal lobe excision. Res Publ Assoc Res Nerv Ment Dis. 1958;36:244–57 [6.7.4].

Milner B, Branch C, Rasmussen T. Study of short-term memory after intracarotid injection of sodium amytal. Trans Am Neurol Assoc. 1962;87:224–6 [4.6.5].

Moosa ANV, Gupta A, Jehi L, Marashly A, Cosmo G, Lachhwani D, Wyllie E, Kotagal P, Bingaman W. Longitudinal seizure outcome and prognostic predictors after hemispherectomy in 170 children. Neurology. 2013;80:253–60 [12.2.1].

Morrell F. Multiple subpial transection for the surgical treatment of focal epilepsy. EEG Clin Neurophysiol. 1973;34:714 [abstract]. [8.2, 8.6.1].

Morrell F, Whisler WW, Bleck TP. Multiple subpial transection: a new approach to the surgical treatment of focal epilepsy. J Neurosurg. 1989;70:231–9 [8.2, 8.6.1].

Munk H. Über die Functionen der Grosshirnrinde. In: Hirschwald A, editor. Gesammelte Mittheilungen aus den Jahren 1877-80, mit Einleitung und Ammerkungen, Berlin. 1881 [7.5].

Nancrede NB. The operative treatment of Jacksonian and focal epilepsy. Ann Surg. 1896;24:122–30 [1.1].

Niemeyer P. The transventricular amygdala-hippocampectomy in temporal lobe epilepsy. In: Baldwin M, Bailery P, editors. The temporal lobe epilepsy. Springfield: Charles C Thomas; 1958. p. 461–82 [6.4].

Nieuwenhuys R, Voogd J, van Huijzen C. The human central nervous system: a synopsis and atlas. 3rd ed. New York: Springer; 1988. p. 37 [7.4].

Noetzel H. Diffusion von Blutfarbstoff in der inneren Randzone und äusseren Oberfläche des Zentralnervensystems bei subarachnoidaler Blutung. Arch Psychiatr Nervkrankh. 1940;111:129–38 [12.1.4].

Ojemann GA, Dodrill CB. Verbal memory deficits after left temporal lobectomy for epilepsy. Mechanism and intraoperative prediction. J Neurosurg. 1985;62:101–7 [6.7.4, 13.2.8].

Ojemann GA, Dodrill C. Intraoperative techniques for reducing language and memory deficits with left temporal lobectomy. Adv Epileptol. 1987;16:327–30 [6.7.4, 13.2.8].

Okonma SV, Blount JP, Gross RE. Planning extent of resection in epilepsy: limited versus large resections. Epilepsy Behav. 2011;20:233–40 [5.6].

O'Leary JL, Goldring S. Chapter 16. Role of neurological surgery in the treatment of epilepsy. In: Science and epilepsy: neuroscience gains in epilepsy research. New York: Raven Press; 1976. p. 227–50 [1.1, 1.2].

Olivier A. Cortical resections (commentary). In: Engel J, editor. Surgical treatment of epilepsy. New York: Raven Press; 1987. p. 405–16 [6.4].

Olivier A. Surgical techniques in temporal lobe epilepsy. Clin Neurosurg. 1997;44:211–41 [6.1, 6.4].

Olivier A. Transcortical selective amygdalohippocampectomy in temporal lobe epilepsy. Can J Neurol Sci. 2000;27 Suppl 1:S68–76 [discussion, pp. 92–6]. [6.4].

Olivier A. Epilepsy surgery at the MNI: from Archibald to the creation of the Shirley and Mark Rayport fellowship in surgery of epilepsy. Epilepsia. 2010;51 Suppl 1:97–100 [1.2, 6.1].

Oppenheimer DR, Griffith HB. Persistent intracranial bleeding as a complication of hemispherectomy. J Neurol Neurosurg Psychiatry. 1966;29:229–40 [12.1.4].

Pasquet A. Combined regional and general anesthesia for craniotomy and cortical exploration. Part II. Anesthetic considerations. Curr Res Anesth Analg. 1954;33:156–64 [3.1, 3.7.2, 3.8].

Patchell RA, Young AB, Tibbs PA. Benjamin Winslow Dudley and the surgical treatment of epilepsy. Neurology. 1987;37:290–1 [1.1].

Penfield W [1.2, 2.2.1, 2.3].

Penfield W. A contribution to the mechanism of intracranial pain. Proc Assoc Res Nerv Mental Dis. 1934;15:399–416 [3.5.4, 3.5.5.3].

Penfield W. The cerebral cortex in man. I. The cerebral cortex and consciousness. Arch Neurol Psychiatry. 1938;40:417–42 [8.1.2].

Penfield W. The epilepsies: with a note on radical therapy. N Engl J Med. 1939;221:209–18 [1.2, 2.2.1].

Penfield W. Bilateral frontal gyrectomy and postoperative intelligence. Chapter XXIII – symposium on gyrectomy, part 1. Res Publ Ass Nerv Ment Dis. 1947;27:519–34 [1.2, 2.2.1, 2.2.3.2, 7.5].

Penfield W. The supplementary motor area in the cerebral cortex of man. Arch Psych Zeit Neurol. 1950;185:670–4 [1.2, 7.5].

Penfield W. Combined regional and general anesthesia for craniotomy and cortical exploration. Part I. Neurosurgical considerations. Curr Res Anesth Analg. 1954a;33:145–55 [1.2, 3.2, 3.5.4, 3.5.4.2, 3.5.5.1, 3.5.5.3].

Penfield W. Temporal lobe epilepsy. Br J Surg. 1954b;41:337–43 [1.2, 6.2.5, 6.7.4].

Penfield W. Vestibular sensation and the cerebral cortex. Ann Otol. 1957;66:691–8 [6.6].

Penfield W. Pitfalls and success in surgical treatment of focal epilepsy. Br Med J. 1958;1:669–72 [4.5.1, 6.7.2, 13.2.1-2, 13.2.4].

Penfield W, Baldwin M. Temporal lobe seizures and the technique of subtotal temporal lobectomy. Ann Surg. 1952;136:625–34 [1.2, 2.2.1, 6.1].

Penfield W, Boldrey E. Somatic motor and sensory representation in the cerebral cortex of man as studied by electrical stimulation. Brain. 1937;60:389–443 [4.6.2].

Penfield W, Evans J. The frontal lobe in man: a clinical study of maximum removals. Brain. 1935;58:115–33 [1.2, 2.2.1, 7.6].

Penfield W, Flanigin H. Surgical therapy of temporal lobe seizures. Arch Neurol Psychiatry. 1950;64:491–500 [1.2, 5.6].

Penfield W, Jasper H. Epilepsy and the functional anatomy of the human brain. Boston: Little, Brown and Co; 1954. 896 pp. [1.1, 1.2, 4.2.2, 4.3.3, 4.3.5, 8.4.1, 10.1.2].

Penfield W, McNaughton F. Dural headache and innervation of the dura mater. Arch Neurol Psychiatry. 1940;44:43–75 [3.5.4, 3.5.5.3].

Penfield W, Paine K. The results of surgical therapy for focal epileptic seizures. In: Proceedings of the fifth international neurological congress, Lisbon, 1953 [1.2].

Penfield W, Paine K. Results of surgical therapy for focal epileptic seizures. Can Med Assoc J. 1955;73:515–31 [1.2, 5.6, 6.7.1].

Penfield W, Rasmussen T. A clinical study of localization of function. In: The cerebral cortex of man. New York: MacMillan; 1950. p. 184–6 [8.4.1].

Penfield W, Rasmussen T. The cerebral cortex of man. New York: Macmillan; 1952. p. 135–47, 165–6. [10.1.2].

Penfield W, Rasmussen T. The cerebral cortex of man: a clinical study of localization of function. New York: Hafner Publishing Company; 1968. 248 pp. [4.3.4, 4.6.4, 6.6, 7.5, 8.1.2, 8.4.1].

Penfield W, Roberts L. Speech and brain-mechanisms. Princeton: Princeton University Press; 1959. 286 pp. [3.1, 8.4.1].

Penfield W, Steelman H. The treatment of focal epilepsy by cortical excision. Ann Surg. 1947;126:740–62 [1.2, 2.2.5, 7.5].

Penfield W, Welch K. Instability of response to stimulation of the sensorimotor cortex of man. J Physiol. 1949;109:358–65 [1.2].

Penfield W, Welch K. The supplementary motor area of the cerebral cortex: a clinical and experimental study. AMA Arch Neurol Psychiatry. 1951;66:289–317 [1.2, 7.5].

Penfield W, Lende RA, Rasmussen T. Manipulation hemiplegia. An untoward complication in the surgery of focal epilepsy. J Neurosurg. 1961;28:760–76 [6.1, 6.7.2].

Perrin, R. Personal communication [3.6.3].

Pilcher WH, Rusyniak WG. Complications of epilepsy surgery. Neurosurg Clin N Am. 1993;4:311–25 [6.7.1, 7.5, 9.4.1, 11.2.6].

Polani PE. Encephalo-trigeminal angiomatosis (Sturge-Weber syndrome) treated by removal of the affected cerebral hemisphere. Proc R Soc Med. 1952;45:860–2 [12.1.3].

Rasmussen T. (Personal communication) [2.1.5*, 2.2.3.1, 5.6, 6.7.2, 7.1, 8.1.1, 8.4, 8.4.2, 9.1, 9.3.3*, 9.4.2, 13.2.7].
Rasmussen T. Surgical therapy of frontal lobe epilepsy. Epilepsia. 1963;4:181–98 [1.2, 5.6].
Rasmussen T. Postoperative superficial hemosiderosis of the brain, its diagnosis, treatment and prevention. Trans Am Neurol Assoc. 1973;98:133–7 [12.1.4, 12.2.10].
Rasmussen T. Cortical resection in the treatment of focal epilepsy. In: Purpura DP, Penry JK, Walter RD, editors. Advances in neurology, vol. 8. New York: Raven Press; 1975a. p. 139–54 [1.2, 8.4.1, 9.1].
Rasmussen T. Surgery for epilepsy arising in regions other than the temporal and frontal lobes. In: Purpura DP, Penry JK, Walter RD, editors. Advances in neurology, vol. 8. New York: Raven Press; 1975b. p. 206–26 [1.2, 8.4.1, 9.4.1, 12.1.4].
Rasmussen T. Surgical treatment of epilepsy. Can Med Assoc J. 1977;116:1369–70 [1.2].
Rasmussen T. Hemispherectomy for seizures revisited. Can J Neurol Sci. 1983a;10:71–8 [1.2, 12.1.4, 12.2.10].
Rasmussen T. Characteristics of a pure culture of frontal lobe epilepsy. Epilepsia. 1983b;24:482–93 [1.2, 7.1].
Rasmussen T. Surgical treatment of complex partial seizures: results, lessons and problems. Epilepsia. 1983c;24 Suppl 1:S65–76 [1.2].
Rasmussen T. Commentary: extratemporal cortical excisions and hemispherectomy. In: Engel J, editor. Surgical treatment of the epilepsies. New York: Raven Press; 1987. pp. 417–24 [1.2, 8.2, 12.2.10].
Rasmussen T, Andermann F. Hemispherectomy for seizures revisited. Can J Neurol Sci. 1983;10:71–8 [1.2, 12.1.4, 12.2.10].
Rasmussen T, Branch C. Temporal lobe epilepsy: indications for the results of surgical therapy. Postgrad Med. 1962;31:9–14 [1.2, 5.6].
Rasmussen T, Feindel W. Temporal lobectomy: review of 100 cases with major hippocampectomy. Can J Neurol Sci. 1991;18:601–2 [6.1].
Rasmussen T, Jasper H. Temporal lobe epilepsy: indications for operations and surgical technique. In: Baldwin M, Bailey P, editors. Temporal lobe epilepsy. Springfield: Charles C. Thomas; 1958. p. 440–60 [1.2, 5.6, 6.1].
Rasmussen T, Milner B. Clinical and surgical studies of the cerebral speech areas in man. In: Zulch KJ, Creutzfeldt O, Galbraith GC, editors. Cerebral localization: an Otfrid Foerster symposium. New York: Springer; 1975. p. 238–57 [4.2.2, 4.6.1.1-3, 4.6.5, 4.7*, 9.3.4*].
Ray BS, Wolff HG. Experimental studies on headache—pain-sensitive structures of the head and their significance in headache. Arch Surg. 1940;41:813–56 [3.5.5.3].
Roberts DW. Corpus callosotomy: surgical technique. In: Reeves AG, editor. Epilepsy and the corpus callosum. New York: Plenum Press; 1985. p. 259–67 [11.2.2].
Roberts DW, Siegel AM. Corpus callosotomy. In: Lüders HO, Comair YG, editors. Epilepsy surgery. 2nd ed. Philadelphia: Lippincott Williams & Wilkins; 2001. pp. 747–56 [11.2.2].
Rosenørn J, Diemer NH. Reduction of regional cerebral blood flow during brain retraction pressure in the rat. J Neurosurg. 1982;56:826–9 [13.2.3].
Rossi GFD. Considerations on the principles of surgical treatment of partial epilepsies. Brain Res. 1975;95:395–402 [5.6].
Rougier A, Saint-Hillaire J-M, Loiseau P, Bouvier G. Evaluation and surgical treatment of the epilepsies. Neurochirurgie. 1992;38:3–12 [6.4].
Rowland V, MacIntyre WJ, Bidder TG. The production of brain lesions with electric currents. II. Bidirectional currents. J Neurosurg. 1960;17:55–69 [4.2.1, 4.2.3].
Sachs E. The subpial resection of the cortex in the treatment of Jacksonian Epilepsy (Horsley operation) with observations on areas 4 and 6. Brain. 1935;58:492–503 [1.2, 2.2.1].
Salanova V, Andermann F, Rasmussen T, Olivier A, Quesney LF. Tumoural parietal lobe epilepsy: clinical manifestations and outcome in 34 patients treated between 1934 and 1988. Brain. 1995;118:1289–304 [9.1].
Schramm J. Hemispherectomy techniques. Neurosurg Clin N Am. 2002;13:113–34 [12.2.1].

Semmes J, Weinstein S, Ghent L, Teuber HL. Somatosensory changes after penetrating brain wounds in man. Cambridge, MA: Harvard University Press; 1960 [5.4].

Sherman EMS, Wiebe S, Fay-McClymont B, Tellez-Zenteno J, Metcalfe A, Hernandez-Ronquillo L, et al. Neuropsychological outcomes after epilepsy surgery: systematic review and pooled estimates. Epilepsia. 2011;52:857–69 [6.7.4, 13.2.8].

Smith A, Sugar O. Development of above normal language and intelligence 21 years after left hemispherectomy. Neurology. 1975;25:813–8 [12.1.4].

Smith S. The surgical treatment of epilepsy, with statistical tables, comprising all recorded cases of ligature of the carotid artery; and also of trephining the cranium by American surgeons. NY J Med. 1852;18:220–42 [1.1].

Spencer DD, Spencer SS, Mattson RH, Williamson PD, Novelly RA. Access to the posterior medial temporal lobe structures in the surgical treatment of temporal lobe epilepsy. Neurosurgery. 1984;15:667–71 [6.2.9].

Spencer SS, Gates JR, Reeves AR, Spencer DD, Maxwell RE, Roberts D. Corpus callosum section. In: Engel J, editor. Surgical treatment of the epilepsies. New York: Raven Press; 1987. p. 425–44 [11.1.4].

Steelman HF. Technique of cortical excision: an experimental study of postoperative cicatrization. Arch Neurol Psychiatry. 1949;62:479–92 [2.2.1].

Stensaas SS, Eddington DK, Dobelle WH. The topography and variability of the primary visual cortex in man. J Neurosurg. 1974;40:747–55 [4.5.2*, 10.2.1].

Sveinbjornsdottir KS, Duncan JS. Parietal and occipital lobe epilepsy: a review. Epilepsia. 1993;34:493–521 [9.1].

Tanriverdi T, Poulin N, Olivier O. Psychosocial status before and after temporal lobe epilepsy: a prospective clinical study. Neurosurgery. 2008;62:1071–9 [6.7.4].

Temkin O. The falling sickness. 2nd ed. Baltimore: The Johns Hopkins Press; 1971 [1.1].

Tinuper P, Andermann F, Villemure JG, Rasmussen TB, Quesney LF. Functional hemispherectomy for treatment of epilepsy associated with hemiplegia: rationale, indications, results, and comparison with callosotomy. Ann Neurol. 1988;24:27–34 [12.1.4].

Urban H. Zur Physiologie der Occipital region des Menschen. Z Ges Neurol Psychiat. 1937;158:257–61 [4.1, 4.6.4].

Van Wagenen WP, Herren RY. Surgical division of commissural pathways in the corpus callosum: relation to spread of an epileptic attack. Arch Neurol Psychiatry. 1940;44:740–59 [11.1.4, 11.2.1].

Villemure JG, Daniel RT. Peri-insular hemispherotomy. Childs Nerv Syst. 2006;22:967–81 [12.2.10].

Villemure JG, Daniel RT. Chapter 163. Hemispherectomy. In: Lozano AM, Gildenberg PL, Tasker R, editors. Textbook of stereotactic and functional neurosurgery. 2nd ed. Berlin/Heidelberg: Springer-Verlag; 2009. pp. 2741–60 [12.2.10].

Villemure J-G, Mascott CR. Hemispherotomy: the periinsular approach. Technical aspects. Epilepsia. 1993;34 Suppl 6:48. (abstract). [12.2.10].

Villemure JG, Mascott CR. Peri-insular hemispherotomy: surgical principles and anatomy. Neurosurgery. 1995;37:975–81 [12.2.10].

Villemure JG, Rasmussen T. Functional hemispherectomy: methodology. J Epilepsy. 1990;3(Suppl):177–82 [12.1.4, 12.2.10].

Villemure JG, Mascott CR, Anderman F, Rasmussen T. Is removal of the insular cortex in hemispherectomy necessary? Epilepsia. 1989;30:721 (Abstr). [12.2.10].

Villemure JG, Adams CBT, Hoffman HJ, Peacock WJ. Hemispherectomy. In: Engel J, editor. Surgical treatment of the epilepsies. 2nd ed. New York: Raven Press; 1993. p. 511–8 [12.2.1, 12.2.10].

Vogt C, Vogt O. Allgemeinere Ergebnisse unserer Hirnforschung. J Psychol Neurol. 1919;25: 273–462 [7.5].

Wada J. A new method for the determination of the side of cerebral speech dominance: a preliminary report on the intracarotid injection of sodium amytal in man. Med Biol. 1949;14:221–2 (Japanese). [4.6.1.3].

Wada JA. Epilepsy surgery revisited: conceptual reassessment of generalized seizure. Folia Psychiatr Neurol Jpn. 1982;36:233–5 [4.6.1.3, 4.6.5].
Wada J, Rasmussen T. Intracarotid injection of sodium Amytal for the lateralization of cerebral speech dominance: experimental and clinical observations. J Neurosurg. 1960;17:266–82 [4.6.1.3, 4.6.5].
Wada J, Rasmussen T. Intracarotid injection of sodium amytal for the lateralization of speech dominance: experimental clinical observations. Epilepsia. 1963;4:181–98 [4.6.1.3].
Walker AE. Electrocorticography in epilepsy. EEG Clin Neurophysiol. 1949a;2(Suppl):30–7 [4.3.5].
Walker AE. Post-traumatic epilepsy. Springfield: Charles Thomas; 1949b. 86 pp. [4.3.5].
Walker AE. Temporal lobectomy. J Neurosurg. 1967;26:642–9 [6.1, 6.2.4].
Walker AE, Johnson HC, Kollros JJ. Penicillin convulsions: the convulsive effect of Penicillin applied to the cerebral cortex of monkey and man. Surg Gynec Obstet. 1945;81:692–701 [4.3.4.1].
Ward AA. The epileptic neuron: chronic foci in animals and man. In: Jasper HH, Ward AA, Pope A, editors. Basic mechanisms of the epilepsies. Boston: Little, Brown & Co; 1969. p. 263–88 [5.3].
Wennberg R, Quesney F, Olivier A, Rasmussen T. Electrocorticography and outcome in frontal lobe epilepsy. EEG Clin Neurophysiol. 1998;106:357–68 [7.1].
Whisler WW. Multiple subpial transection. Tech Neurosurg. 1995;1:40–4 [8.6.1].
Wiebe S, Berg AT. Big epilepsy surgery for little people: what's the full story on hemispherectomy? Neurology. 2013;80:232–3 [12.2.1].
Wieser HG. Selective amygdalohippocampectomy: indications, investigative technique and results. In: Symon L, Brihaye J, Guidetti B, editors. Advances and technical standards in neurosurgery, vol. 13. Vienna: Springer; 1986. p. 39–133 [6.4].
Wieser HG. Selective amygdalo-hippocampectomy for temporal lobe epilepsy. Epilepsia. 1988;29 Suppl 2:100–13 [6.4].
Wieser HG. Selective amygdalo-hippocampectomy: indications and follow-up. Can J Neurol Sci. 1991;18:617–27 [6.4].
Wieser HG, ILAE. Mesial temporal lobe epilepsy with hippocampal sclerosis. Epilepsia. 2004;45:695–714 [5.7].
Wieser HJ, Yasargil MG. Die to "Selektive Amygdala-Hippokampektomie" als chirurgische Behandlungsmethode der mediobasal-limbischen Epilepsie. Neurochirurgia. 1982a;25:39–50 [6.4].
Wieser HG, Yasargil MG. Selective amygdalohippocampectomy as a surgical treatment of mesiobasal limbic epilepsy. Surg Neurol. 1982b;17:445–57 [6.4].
Williams DJ, Scott JW. The functional responses of the sympathetic nervous system of man following hemidecortication. J Neurol Neurosurg Psychiatry. 1939;2:313–22 [12.1.3].
Williamson PD, Boon PA, Thadani VM, Darcey TM, Spencer DD, Spencer SS, Novelly RA, Mattson RH. Parietal lobe epilepsy: diagnostic considerations and results of surgery. Ann Neurol. 1992;31:193–201 [9.1].
Wilson DH, Culver C, Waddington M, Gazzaniga M. Disconnection of the cerebral hemispheres: an alternative to hemispherectomy for the control of intractable seizures. Neurology. 1975;25:1149–53 [11.1.4].
Wilson DH, Reeves A, Gazzaniga M, Culver C. Cerebral commissurotomy for control of intractable seizures. Neurology. 1977;27:708–15 [11.1.4].
Wilson DH, Reeves A, Gazzaniga G. Division of the corpus callosum for uncontrollable epilepsy. Neurology. 1978;28:649–53 [11.1.4].
Wilson DH, Reeves AG, Gazzaniga G. "Cerebral" commissurotomy for intractable generalized epilepsy: series two. Neurology. 1982;32:687–97 [11.1.4, 11.2.2.].
Wilson PJE. Cerebral hemispherectomy for infantile hemiplegia. A report of 50 cases. Brain. 1970a;93:147–80 [12.1.4].
Wilson PJE. More 'second thoughts' on hemispherectomy in infantile hemiplegia. Dev Med Child Neurol. 1970b;12:799–800 [12.1.4].
Wolff HG. Headache and other head pain. Oxford: Oxford University Press; 1948 [3.5.5.3].

Wyler AR. Chapter 88. Multiple subpial transections. In: Lüders HO, editor. Epilepsy surgery. 2nd ed. New York: Raven Press; 2001. p. 807–11 [8.6.3].

Wyler AR, Hermann BP. Comparative results of temporal lobectomy under local or general anesthesia: seizure outcome. J Epilepsy. 1988;1:121–5 [3.1].

Wyler AR, Hermann BP, Somes G. Extent of medial temporal resection on outcome from anterior temporal lobectomy: a randomized prospective study. Neurosurgery. 1995a;37:982–91 [6.1].

Wyler AR, Wilkus RJ, Vossler DG. Multiple subpial transections for partial seizures in sensory-motor cortex. Neurosurgery. 1995b;37:1122–8 [8.6.3].

Yasargil MG, Teddy PJ, Roth P. Selective amygdalohippocampectomy: operative anatomy and surgical technique. In: Symon L, Brihaye J, Guidetti B, editors. Advances and technical standards in neurosurgery, vol. 12. Vienna: Springer; 1985. p. 93–123 [6.4].

Yasargil MG, Wieser HG, Valavanis A, von Ammon K, Roth P. Surgery and results of selective amygdala-hippocampectomy in one hundred patients with nonlesional limbic epilepsy. Neurosurg Clin N Am. 1993;4:243–61 [6.4].

Zollinger R. Removal of left cerebral hemisphere. Report of a case. Arch Neurol Psychiatry. 1935;34:48–63 [12.1.2].

Index

J.P. Girvin, *Operative Techniques in Epilepsy*,
DOI 10.1007/978-3-319-10921-3

MIX
Papier aus verantwortungsvollen Quellen
Paper from responsible sources
FSC® C105338

If you have any concerns about our products,
you can contact us on
ProductSafety@springernature.com

In case Publisher is established outside the EU,
the EU authorized representative is:
Springer Nature Customer Service Center GmbH
Europaplatz 3, 69115 Heidelberg, Germany

Printed by Libri Plureos GmbH
in Hamburg, Germany